BIOMEDICAL
PSYCHIATRIC
THERAPEUTICS

BIOMEDICAL PSYCHIATRIC THERAPEUTICS

Edited by

John L. Sullivan, M.D.

Professor of Psychiatry, Georgetown University, George Washington University and Duke University Schools of Medicine; Psychiatrist-in-Chief, Veterans Administration Medical Center, Washington, D.C.; Former Deputy Director of Medical Research for the Veterans Administration

Paula DeRemer Sullivan, Ph.D.

Clinical Psychologist, Suburban Psychiatric Associates, Bethesda, Maryland

With 27 contributing authors

Foreword by Morris A. Lipton, Ph.D., M.D.
Introduction by John M. Davis, M.D.

BUTTERWORTH PUBLISHERS
Boston • London
Sydney • Wellington • Durban • Toronto

Copyright © 1984 by Butterworth Publishers
All rights reserved.

No part of this publication may be reproduced, stored in a
retrieval system, or transmitted, in any form or by any means,
electronic, mechanical, photocopying, recording, or otherwise,
without the prior written permission of the publisher.

Every effort has been made to ensure that the drug dosage
schedules within this text are accurate and conform to standards
accepted at time of publication. However, as treatment
recommendations vary in light of continuing research and clinical
experience, the reader is advised to verify drug dosage schedules
herein with information found on product information sheets.
This is especially true in cases of new or infrequently used drugs.

Library of Congress Cataloging in Publication Data
Main entry under title:

Biomedical psychiatric therapeutics.

   Bibliography: p.
   Includes index.
   1. Psychopharmacology. 2. Mental illness—
Physiological aspects. I. Sullivan, John L. (John
Lawrence), 1943- . II. Sullivan, Paula DeRemer.
[DNLM: 1. Mental disorders—Therapy. WM 400 B6155]
RC483.B54 1984   616.89'18   83-26328
ISBN 0-409-95151-X

Butterworth Publishers
80 Montvale Avenue
Stoneham, MA 02180

10 9 8 7 6 5 4 3 2 1

Printed in the United States of America

To our families

CONTENTS

FOREWORD

Over the past 30 years, biological psychiatry has moved ahead of psychoanalysis as the dominant force in psychiatric training, research, and treatment. The brain is no longer a "black box" impervious to investigation except by its output as seen in the behavior of patients, especially in their transactions with therapists. It is now recognized as the complex organ of the mind which interacts constantly with the rest of the body, responding to changes in the internal milieu and, through its output, regulating most bodily functions. It also responds to the external milieu and is altered by it. With modern technology, it is a researchable organ which is attracting the attention and efforts of our best young people.

These remarkable changes started with two simultaneous developments. The first was the empirical discovery of drugs which in small doses could alter perception, mood, thinking, and behavior. Since drugs are chemicals which cannot influence metapsychological constructs but instead must act on chemical systems within the brain, the nature of the changes they produce in the brain has become the subject of intense investigation. At about the same time, the chemical theory of neurotransmission superseded electrical theories and it became evident that neuronal cells communicate with each other across synapses by means of very specific chemical neurotransmitters and receptors for them. Psychotropic drugs, it was soon found, influence the production, storage, and release of neurotransmitters in presynaptic neurons and their reception by postsynaptic neurons. Thus, a very profitable partnership between basic and clinical neurobiology was initiated and continues vigorously to this day. In recent years, the number of identified neurotransmitters, including the peptides, has increased to more than 20. The nature of receptors is being clarified. Endogenous ligands such as the endorphins are being discovered for several of the receptors. An intellectual fusion between neurobiology and molecular biology and genetics is also taking place.

The shift in perspective toward biological mechanisms has had profound consequences on psychiatric training and practice. Modern programs for the training of psychiatrists do not neglect the subjective, psychological, and social factors that influence health and illness, but to them are added training in basic and clinical neurobiology. The depth and breadth of information which the young psychiatrist must master is now substantially greater than was required in the past. A second consequence is that psychiatry has moved closer to the mainstream of medical thinking and practice. Greater rigor in diagnosis, greater specificity in the choice of treatment, and greater objectivity in the measurement of change are now demanded. Instruments have been developed for these purposes and are under constant refinement.

Drugs are the primary therapeutic agents in biological psychiatry. For many reasons, their use is far from simple, and that fact is made clear throughout this book. Drugs are not "magic bullets," absolutely specific for a given disease and devoid of side effects. Illnesses such as anxiety, depression, and schizophrenia are probably syndromes, each of which has several biological etiologies. The various members of a "labeled" class of drugs, such as, for example, the antidepressants, are not equally effective in all patients. Probably this is partly attributable to the etiological heterogeneity of the syndromes being treated. Certainly it is due to the genetic heterogeneity of human beings, which influences the rate at which drugs may be absorbed and metabolized. Thus, with a given dose, individual patients achieve different blood levels and have varying pharmacokinetic patterns, and these can be measured by appropriate laboratory tests. The chronic effects of drugs often differ from their acute effects. Drugs interact with each other, a matter of considerable importance to the patient receiving drugs for a medical illness along with psychotropic agents. Drugs sometimes have surprising effects. The tricyclic antidepressants and monoamine oxidase inhibitors so commonly identified as antidepressants are also effective in the treatment of panic attacks. Why this is so is not yet clearly understood.

The information explosion in biological psychiatry has been so great that a single individual can no longer write a text. Moreover, no student, scholar, or practitioner can possibly keep up with the wealth of material that appears daily in refereed journals, monographs, reviews, and specialty texts. Practitioners especially, who must make daily diagnostic and therapeutic decisions, lack the time to reflect at leisure while controversies are being resolved and must depend heavily upon the information and critical judgments offered to them by the authors of texts. The editors of this volume have chosen their authors wisely. Not only are they experienced clinicians and clinical researchers, they are also teachers who present their material lucidly. The result is an up-to-date, "state-of-the-art" text with a bonus from Dr. Wyatt, one of our most distinguished investigators in biological psychiatry, who attempts to predict the future. This is always chancy, but Dr. Wyatt is undoubtedly correct in believing that the syndrome of schizophrenia will be broken down into subgroups that can then be understood and treated more effectively. He anticipates that the new technologies of positron emission tomography, nuclear magnetic resonance, and electrophysiological mapping of the cortex will yield new insights. His forecasts will probably prove correct, but part of the adventure of research is its unpredictability. Newer discoveries about the roles of the peptides and neurotransmitters, about genetic markers and genetic engineering, may surprise us as much a generation from now as did the psychotropic drugs when they emerged in the 1950s.

Every text is a compromise between the requirements of the publishers, the wishes of the authors, and the value system of the editor. What topics shall be chosen and what will be omitted? To what extent should the basic science substrates of the clinical information be expounded? How shall areas of controversy be discussed? This book is an excellent compromise in a format which can readily be revised in later editions. Not the least of its virtues are bibliographies which offer both original articles and up-to-date reviews for those who wish greater depth on pertinent topics.

A potential concern in a book such as this has been alluded to by Leon Eisenberg, who warned: "Biological psychiatry threatens to become so myopic in its clinical vision that it threatens to substitute mindless psychiatry for the brainless psychiatry of the past. It is disregarding its social and psychological context" (Eisenberg, L. The subjective in medicine. Perspect Biol Med 27:24, 1983). Comprehensive medical care involves human transactions for which drugs will never be a total substitute, and any text which focuses on the biomedical aspects of psychiatry risks neglecting that fact. Fortunately, no one knows this better than the editors and authors of this book. In addressing major psychosocial considerations relevant to biomedically oriented treatment, they underscore the importance of a balanced therapeutic perspective in the comprehensive care of the patient.

Morris A. Lipton, Ph.D., M.D.

PREFACE

The last several decades have witnessed psychiatry's evolution as a scientifically based and practical medical specialty, with attendant differentiation along subspecialty lines in order to accommodate the burgeoning depth and diversity of the discipline. One of the most rapidly evolving of these subspecialty areas, biomedical psychiatry, deals with the biological basis of mental illness, biological diagnostic and treatment techniques, and special problems associated with the biomedical treatment of psychiatric patients with concurrent nonpsychiatric medical illness.

Most of the significant developments in biomedical psychiatry have impacted on the management of psychiatric patients in a variety of clinical settings. Therefore, we have attempted to develop a book that can serve as a general reference text on biomedical psychiatric therapeutics for students, house staff, and practitioners engaged in the care of psychiatric patients or patients with a psychiatric component to their illness.

The text is divided into three parts: (1) general treatment approaches, (2) special topics, and (3) future directions. The first part primarily addresses basic principles of biomedical psychiatric therapeutics, and the second part discusses special areas of major clinical importance where biomedical psychiatry interfaces with other medical specialties or psychiatric subspecialties. Although a number of other special areas such as the chemical dependencies, pediatric psychopharmacology, and consultation-liaison psychiatry, to name just a few, could also have been selected for this part, we have limited ourselves to several areas that have seen substantive changes in recent years or that are fundamentally important to the clinical practice of biomedical psychiatric therapeutics. The third part discusses advances in biological exploration of psychiatric disorders that are expected to have a significant impact on biomedical psychiatric therapeutics in the near future.

In preparing this text, we have been constantly mindful of what is, perhaps, the most significant advance for American psychiatry in recent years: the realization of the increasingly scientific, and integrated, nature of the discipline. This achievement is reflected in the virtual disappearance of a philosophic orientation for psychiatry based upon theory and dogma alone, without due regard for observation and experience, as well as erosion of a strict dichotomous approach to the biological and psychosocial aspects of the discipline. Consonant with this evolutionary advance, we are hopeful that our readers appreciate our focus on an important area of psychiatry that, under appropriate circumstances, can contribute meaningfully to the comprehensive care of the patient.

The editors and contributors of this volume are indebted to the support, encouragement, and inspiration of a number of our colleagues, residents, and students in the preparation of the manuscript, including Ms. Pearl Anderson; Herbert Baganz, M.D.; Sam Barondes, M.D.; Hollis Boren, M.D.; Keith Brodie, M.D.; William Bunney, M.D.; Ewald Busse, M.D.; Mr. William Carey; Bernard Carroll, M.D., Ph.D.; James Collins, M.D.; Don Custis, M.D.; Ms. Annie Dunn; Jack Ewalt, M.D.; James Finkelstein, M.D.; Earl X. Freed, Ph.D.; Robert Friedel, M.D.; Mr. Al Gavazzi; Richard Greene, M.D., Ph.D.; George Higgins, M.D.; Jeff Houpt, M.D.; Lewis Judd, M.D.; Douglass Kay, M.D.; Kenneth Keller, Ph.D.; Alex Kelly, M.D.; John Kurtzke, M.D.; C. Raymond Lake, M.D., Ph.D.; Robert Lindeman, M.D.; Markku Linnoila, M.D., Ph.D.; John Lipkin, M.D.; Arnold Mandell, M.D.; Victor McKusick, M.D.; Dennis Murphy, M.D.; Barbara Palmeri, M.D.; Douglas Price, M.D.; Charles Rackley, M.D.; Louis Rittelmeyer, M.D.; Allan Schwartzberg, M.D.; David Segal, Ph.D.; Ms. Cynthia Smith; Vincent Tomasino, M.D.; Philip Tumulty, M.D.; Jerry Wiener, M.D.; William Wilson, M.D.; and James Wyngaarden, M.D.

Finally, we thank Butterworth Publishers and our editors Mr. Arthur Evans, Ms. Nancy Megley, Ms. Karen Myer, Ms. Elizabeth O'Neill, and Ms. Patricia Sheehan for their patience and support in this venture.

J. L. S.
P. D. S.

CONTRIBUTING AUTHORS

Jesse O. Cavenar, Jr., M.D.
Professor of Psychiatry, Duke
University School of Medicine;
Psychiatrist-in-Chief, VA Medical
Center, Durham, North Carolina

Mary G. Cavenar, R.N., M.S.N.
Johnston Scholar, University of
North Carolina, Chapel Hill,
North Carolina

C. Edward Coffey, M.D.
Assistant Professor of Psychiatry
and Medicine (Neurology), Duke
University School of Medicine;
Chief, Neuropsychiatric Imaging
Program, Duke University Medical
Center, Durham, North Carolina

Joseph Cools, M.D.
Clinical Associate in Psychiatry,
Duke University School of
Medicine; Chief, Inpatient
Psychiatry Division, Duke
University Medical Center,
Durham, North Carolina

Tim Covington, Pharm.D.
Associate Professor of Clinical
Pharmacy, West Virginia
University School of Medicine;
Coordinator of Clinical Pharmacy,
West Virginia University
Medical Center, Morgantown,
West Virginia

Jonathan Davidson, M.D.
Associate Professor of Psychiatry,
Duke University School of
Medicine; Attending Psychiatrist,
VA Medical Center, Durham,
North Carolina

John M. Davis, M.D.
Gilman Professor of Psychiatry,
University of Illinois College of
Medicine; Director of Research,
Illinois State Psychiatric Institute,
Chicago, Illinois

Lynn E. DeLisi, M.D.
Staff Psychiatrist, Laboratory of
Psychology and Psychopathology,
National Institute of Mental
Health, Bethesda, Maryland

William E. Fann, M.D.
Professor of Psychiatry and
Associate Professor of
Pharmacology, Baylor College of
Medicine; Psychiatrist-in-Chief,
VA Medical Center, Houston,
Texas

D. Ted George, M.D.
Clinical Associate, Laboratory of
Clinical Science, National Institute
of Mental Health, Bethesda,
Maryland

Richard L. Goldberg, M.D.
Assistant Professor of Psychiatry,
Georgetown University School of
Medicine; Director of Residency
Training, Department of
Psychiatry, Georgetown University
Medical Center, Washington, D.C.

David M. Goldstein, M.D.
Assistant Professor of Psychiatry,
Georgetown University School of
Medicine; Chief, Adult Outpatient
Division, Department of
Psychiatry, Georgetown University
Medical Center, Washington, D.C.

Martha M. Letterie, M.D.
Instructor in Psychiatry,
Georgetown University School
of Medicine; Attending
Psychiatrist, VA Medical Center,
Washington, D.C.

Morris A. Lipton, Ph.D., M. D.
Sarah Graham Kenan Professor of
Psychiatry, University of North
Carolina School of Medicine;
Director, Biological Sciences
Research Center of the Child
Development Research Institute,
Chapel Hill, North Carolina

Steve Mahorney, M.D.
Associate in Psychiatry, Duke
University School of Medicine;
Attending Psychiatrist,
VA Medical Center, Durham,
North Carolina

Allan A. Maltbie, M.D.
Associate Professor of Psychiatry,
Duke University School of
Medicine; Chief, Consultation-
Liaison Division, Duke University
Medical Center, Durham, North
Carolina

E. Wayne Massey, M.D.
Associate Professor of Medicine
(Neurology), Duke University
School of Medicine; Attending
Neurologist, Duke University
Medical Center, Durham, North
Carolina

Wesley M. Pitts, M.D.
Assistant Professor of Psychiatry,
Baylor College of Medicine;
Attending Psychiatrist, VA
Medical Center, Houston, Texas

Manuel Rodriguez-Garcia, M.D.
Assistant Professor of Psychiatry,
Baylor College of Medicine;
Attending Psychiatrist, VA
Medical Center, Houston, Texas

Donald R. Ross, M.D.
Attending Psychiatrist, Sheppard
and Enoch Pratt Hospital,
Baltimore, Maryland

John L. Sullivan, M.D.
Professor of Psychiatry,
Georgetown University, George
Washington University and Duke
University Schools of Medicine;
Psychiatrist-in-Chief, VA Medical
Center, Washington, D.C.; Former
Deputy Director of Medical
Research for the Veterans
Administration

Paula DeRemer Sullivan, Ph.D.
Clinical Psychologist, Suburban
Psychiatric Associates, Bethesda,
Maryland

Ronald J. Taska, M.D.
Assistant Professor of Psychiatry,
Duke University School of
Medicine; Associate Director of
Residency Training, Department of
Psychiatry, Duke University
Medical Center, Durham, North
Carolina

Daniel R. Weinberger, M.D.
Chief, Clinical Neuropsychiatry
and Neurobehavior Section, Adult
Psychiatry Branch, National
Institute of Mental Health,
Washington, D.C.

Richard D. Weiner, M.D., Ph.D.
Associate Professor of Psychiatry,
Duke University School of
Medicine; Attending Psychiatrist,
VA Medical Center, Durham,
North Carolina

Jeanine C. Wheless, B.A.
Special Assistant, Department of
Psychiatry, Baylor College of
Medicine, Houston, Texas

Thomas N. Wise, M.D.
Professor of Psychiatry,
Georgetown University School of
Medicine; Associate Professor of
Psychiatry, The Johns Hopkins
University School of Medicine;
Psychiatrist-in-Chief, The Fairfax
Hospital, Falls Church, Virginia

Richard Jed Wyatt, M.D.
Chief, Adult Psychiatry Branch,
National Institute of Mental
Health, Washington, D.C.

William W. K. Zung, M.D.
Professor of Psychiatry, Duke
University School of Medicine; VA
Medical Center, Durham, North
Carolina

BIOMEDICAL PSYCHIATRIC THERAPEUTICS

Introduction

John M. Davis

This is a textbook on physical treatments in psychiatry, principally psychotropic drugs and electroconvulsive treatment (ECT). Although psychiatry has lagged behind general medicine in the development of pharmacotherapies, this lag represents only a modest number of years when considered in the context of the history of medicine from antiquity to the present. In the past 50 years, general medicine has seen the development of a substantial number of safe and efficacious drug treatments for a variety of disorders. Physical treatments in psychiatry had their beginning before World War II with the development of ECT and the serendipitous discovery that amphetamine has a beneficial effect on children with what at that time was called hyperactive behavior. The antimanic effect of lithium was discovered in 1949, but chemotherapy and psychiatry really became one with the discovery of the antipsychotic properties of chlorpromazine and reserpine in 1952. Their use became widespread throughout the world in the late 1950s and early 1960s.

The discovery of effective treatments has substantially altered the fate of mental patients. In real life, it is rare that any treatment completely prevents illness or produces a permanent cure in every patient all the time, although this does occur on occasion. For example, smallpox as a disease has been completely eliminated from the world. More typically, drugs suppress a disorder, but continuous administration is necessary to prevent recurrences. Even though the miracle antibiotics may produce a dramatic cure in a patient with an infectious disease, they do not prevent recurrences in patients who have suitable predisposing factors.

It is relevant, therefore, to ask: What is the increment in therapeutics achieved through the use of drugs in psychiatry? Such a question is semiquantitative. For any new treatment, one can ask: How well do patients do, now that we have this new treatment, in comparison to how they would have done with the older treatment? For comparison, let us take the first two antibiotics discovered: penicillin and streptomycin. At the time streptomycin was discovered, the standard treatment for tuberculosis was a prolonged period of bed rest in a sanatorium. In a controlled trial done by the British Medical Research Council, patients were randomly assigned to regimens of streptomycin plus bed rest or bed rest alone. Two out of three patients recovered with streptomycin, and one out of three recovered with standard treatment. At the time penicillin was discovered, sulfur was the standard treatment for

1

pneumococcal pneumonia, and approximately 11% of patients were dying. With penicillin, the death rate was reduced to 6%. For both of these antibiotics, then, the increment to medical practice was either to double the number of patients who made a reasonable recovery (tuberculosis) or to cut by 50% the number of patients who died (pneumococcal pneumonia).

How well do the psychiatric drugs perform in comparison? To quantify this, we use the percentage of patients who do relatively well with the new treatment in comparison with the percentage who do well with the standard treatment. The National Institute of Mental Health (NIMH) double-blind study of antipsychotics found that about 30% of patients showed a reasonable recovery with placebo, but this recovery rate could be increased to about 70% with the use of antipsychotic drugs, more than doubling the efficacy. It is, of course, important to remember that there is a qualitative distinction in that continuous administration of drugs in psychiatry is generally required to prevent relapses. It is relevant to note that about 35 double-blind studies on the maintenance use of antipsychotic drugs to prevent relapse found that in four to six months about 53% of patients relapsed on placebo. This can be reduced to 20% by maintenance antipsychotic drugs. Again, drugs produce a doubling of the number of patients doing relatively well. Similarly, in 30 double-blind studies on imipramine for depression, approximately 65% of patients recovered with imipramine in three or four weeks and only 32% recovered with placebo. Seven studies on maintenance tricyclics to prevent recurrence showed that, in approximately four to six months, half the patients relapsed on placebo but one-fourth relapsed when treated with maintenance antidepressants. Similarly, in seven double-blind studies of lithium for unipolar and bipolar recurrent affective disease, 4 out of 5 patients relapsed in six months or a year, whereas only 1 out of 3 relapsed when treated with maintenance medication. In terms of producing an increment in the number of patients who do well with our present chemotherapy in comparison with the numbers who would have done as well without these new innovations, we have nothing to be ashamed of in psychiatry.

With the development of such effective pharmacotherapies, the need arises for adequate textbooks in which the medical student, the house officer, and the practitioner can learn about drug treatment of mental illness and related topics. This book admirably fulfills these needs and serves as a means of updating the practicing psychiatrist. In addition, many primary care physicians, internists, and other practitioners who see a great variety of patients with major psychiatric problems in fact do a fair amount of psychiatric chemotherapy. This text is ideal for introducing the general physician to psychotropic drugs. In addition to primary learning, the text provides an excellent review for psychiatrists preparing for board examinations and is comprehensive enough to serve as a general reference text for the practicing psychiatrist.

The authors have a gift for concise, declarative statements, and the text is very readable. It is a clearly written, medium-length book that can be read in the time it would take to read a much shorter but less skillfully written book. This textbook covers the basic chemotherapy of anxiety, the affective disorders, and schizophrenia. It also has a chapter on ECT. Although the effectiveness of modern pharmacotherapy is such that ECT is not now used as much as it once was, at present there is clearly a role for ECT in psychiatry. With the increasing age of our population, the care of a wide variety of dementias and deliriums becomes an increasingly important problem, and this topic is well covered. In recent years, it has become apparent that some patients who have chronic pain are in fact suffering from depressions, and this text reviews the new information on chronic pain.

With any innovation of treatment, there is always a price to pay in side effects. These are covered here in the various chapters on the specific treatments. Drug–drug interactions are a consequence of having many drugs in medicine but, like side effects, the physician must learn to cope with these, and this topic is reviewed in a separate chapter. Unfortunately, both prescription and nonprescription drugs can lead to psychiatric complications, and the psychiatrist deals with many patients who are suffering from mental disorders either as a consequence of drugs their physician administers or consequent to self-administration of nonprescription medications, as well as the abuse of drugs. With any technological advances, there are new problems to solve, and it is important that physicians be trained in how to handle these new problems.

The discovery of effective drug treatments has other consequences for the practice of psychiatry. Biological psychiatrists are studying the mechanisms by which drugs produce their beneficial effects. My work, for example, has focused on looking at the common denominators of the biologic mechanisms of actions of the drugs that can either benefit a given psychiatric disorder or produce a psychiatric disorder as a complication. For example, reserpine when used to treat hypertension can cause depression, and we now know that it lowers brain norepinephrine levels. Virtually all drugs used to treat depression can potentiate norepinephrine. This line of reasoning led to the catecholamine hypothesis of depression. A similar line of reasoning has implicated serotonin and acetylcholine in depression. This general paradigm led to the development of the so-called dopamine theory of schizophrenia.

In addition to adding to our general knowledge of biologic factors, the medical model has sharpened diagnostic distinctions and led to the development of laboratory tests for mental illness. Knowledge about the clinical pharmacology of drugs may allow us to use drugs more effectively. Plasma-level monitoring may be helpful with dose adjustment, in understanding the various mechanisms, and in evaluating the seriousness of overdose. This text covers the use of laboratory results in psychiatry. Psychiatry has developed the technology to measure the effectiveness of psychotropic drugs (quantitative rating scales with known reliability, double-blind design, random assignment, and so on). The development of this technology has enhanced the development of psychiatry as a scientific specialty.

This book also covers future directions in biologic psychiatry. In using the drugs, physicians must also deal with patients psychologically, and this text covers psychodynamic and psychoanalytic considerations relevant to the medically oriented psychiatric treatments. This is an important textbook in fulfilling a training need so practitioners and students can gain a better understanding of the various medically oriented therapies and be able to use these treatments with greater understanding and, hence, a greater degree of efficacy and safety.

PART I

General Treatment Approaches

CHAPTER 1

Chemotherapy of Anxiety

John L. Sullivan,
Paula D. Sullivan,
Steve Mahorney,
and
Richard L. Goldberg

The nature and meaning of anxiety have provided an issue for speculation, observation, and experimentation since the earliest periods of civilization. Normal anxiety is often considered to be a warning signal that serves to protect psychobiologic functioning. However, for reasons that are poorly understood, anxiety can reach dimensions that threaten the integrity of psychobiologic functioning and thus constitute a pathologic condition. For example, adaptive as well as creative behaviors appear to be more successful if there is an optimal element of anxiety, but pathologic anxiety can incapacitate such behaviors to the extent that they become ineffective. Anxiety stems from anticipation of impending danger in which the source and character of the danger cannot be clearly defined, whereas fear is an emotional reaction to a specific and known danger (1). Both of these emotional reactions are responses to organismic stress. Thus, anxiety can be viewed as an adaptive mechanism that has survival value if it falls within a normative range.

Anxiety itself reflects a complex emotional response to a variety of human circumstances. It is generally regarded as an unpleasant feeling that is similar in certain respects to fear. At pathologic levels, anxiety reflects an emotional response to danger that is disproportionate to the objective degree of the threat, and the psychophysiologic manifestations of anxiety may resemble extreme fear and panic. Because anxiety is a phenomenon which is often difficult to evaluate and quantify, exact figures about its prevalence and magnitude within any given social group are difficult to obtain. In large measure, we must rely on subjective reports of anxiety, since there are few widely accepted and objectively verifiable composite measures for the phenomenon. A number of self-rating and observer-rating tests that measure specific, subjective impressions, and behavioral variables have been designed to quantify some of the more commonly agreed upon manifestations of anxiety.

A distinction that has gained some popularity in recent years is the differentiation between state anxiety and trait anxiety. State anxiety concerns an emotion felt at a given time in response to a specific circumstance or set of circumstances, whereas trait anxiety refers to a personal characteristic of an individual, including a baseline of anxiety and susceptibility to anxiety in response to stress. According to this concept, state anxiety can be superimposed on trait anxiety, and the results of treatment may vary in these two types. Although this concept of anxiety has theoretical implications, the evaluation of potentially therapeutic agents that are effective in alleviating anxiety (anxiolytics) relies in large measure on the determination of generally excessive anxiety at the time of treatment.

The central role of anxiety in subjective and objective human behaviors states has been appreciated for millenia by philosophers, but Sigmund Freud was the first to attempt to explain anxiety in scientific terms. Freud conceived that anxiety was fundamentally composed of inherited biologic factors that were influenced significantly by developmental and social factors, and that perturbations in any or all of these systems could result in pathologic anxiety, as manifested in a variety of psychopathologic states. Unfortunately, much of Freud's work remained in the theoretical realm during his lifetime because of the relative technical inadequacies of psychobiologic inquiry that prevailed during his lifetime.

The notion that anxiety can be conceptualized as a functional state subject to maladaptive influence suggests that abnormal anxiety may result in symptomatic disease states in much the same way that adrenal tumor or cardiogenic shock may result in hypertension or hypotension, respectively. Most of the knowledge that we have acquired about the phenomenon of pathologic anxiety has emphasized the consequences of excessive amounts of anxiety. Therefore, the development of medicinals to treat pathologic anxiety has focused on pharmacologic compounds that serve as effective antianxiety agents.

BENZODIAZEPINES

Benzodiazepines are considered to be the most effective class of medicinals for the treatment of anxiety, except perhaps, for separation anxiety associated with panic attacks and the phobic-anxiety syndrome, which are discussed later (1). Since the introduction of benzodiazepines for clinical use, there has been a marked increase in the prescription of anxiolytics. For the past decade, the benzodiazepines, particularly diazepam and chlordiazepoxide, have been among the most frequently administered prescription drugs in the United States, as well as in many other countries throughout the world. It is interesting that the majority of prescriptions for these anxiolytics is written by non-psychiatrists and that fewer than half of the prescriptions are dispensed to patients with a formal psychiatric diagnosis.

An important neurochemical mechanism associated with the anxiolytic properties of benzodiazepines appears to be facilitation of chemical transmission in the central nervous system's gamma aminobutyric acid (GABA -ergic) neuronal system. Starting in 1977, a number of research groups independently demonstrated the existence of very specific central nervous system binding sites for benzodiazepines on brain membranes. Research indicates that this benzodiazepine receptor is, in fact, the GABA receptor—a supramolecular structure with two recognition sites (2). GABA binds to one site and benzodiazepines bind to the second site. GABA, the neurotransmitter of about 30 percent of the neurons in the brain, has long been recognized as the most important inhibitory neurotransmitter in the brain; it is known to act on all areas of the central nervous system to inhibit neuronal firing. Anxiety is probably associated with hyperexcitability of certain neural pathways—that is, an excessive neural firing rate. When a benzodiazepine is administered, the drug binds to its site on the GABA receptor, enhancing the binding of GABA and potentiating its effect.

Other studies have also identified several compounds, the purines inosine and hypoxanthine and nicotinamide, that competitively inhibit the binding of (^{3}H) diazepam and that may function as naturally occurring antianxiety substances, or endogenous benzodiazepines. These findings correlate with animal studies that have shown potential anxiolytic properties for a new class of purinelike agents, the thiazolopyridazines (1,2).

Dosage Ranges

Dosage ranges (mg/day) for the most frequently used benzodiazepines in clinical practice are given in Table 1.1. Although no significant tolerance usually develops to their anxiolytic properties, tolerance often develops to sedating and other central nervous system effects of the benzodiazepines. Therefore, physicians should counsel their patients to approach important decisions and complex motor functions with particular caution when benzodiazepine treatment is initiated and when there is an upward adjustment in dosage. When benzodiazepine treatment is initiated, side effects can often be minimized with a divided dose schedule in which two-thirds of the dose is given one or two hours before bedtime and the remainder is given once or twice during the day. With this type of a regimen, the initial sedative-hypnotic properties of the benzodiazepines can also be maximized. Although there is no pharmacokinetic rationale to support continuation of such a regimen for a prolonged period of time, some individuals appear to derive more psychological benefit from this multiple-dose regimen as compared to a once-a-day regimen (3). However, potentially troublesome side effects can result from accumulation of the parent compound and active metabolites when these drugs are prescribed several times a day for an extended period of time. These side effects include sedation, confusion, and motor incoordination.

Table 1.1 Pharmacology of the Benzodiazepine Anxiolytics

Duration of Action (Half-life in hr)	Drug	Adult Daily Dose (mg)	Dose to Peak Serum Concentration Time (hr)
Short (5 to 10)	oxazepam (Serax)	15 to 120	2.5
Intermediate (10 to 20)	lorazepam (Ativan)	1 to 10	2.5
	halazepam (Paxipam)[a]	40 to 160	2
	alprazolam (Xanax)	0.5 to 4	1.5
Long (2 to 200)	chlordiazepoxide (Librium)[a]	10 to 100	8
	diazepam (Valium)[a]	4 to 40	1
	clorazepate (Tranxene)[a]	7.5 to 60	1
	prazepam (Centrax)[a]	20 to 60	8

[a]Has active metabolites.

Side Effects

Some concern has been expressed that use of benzodiazepines in the symptomatic management of anxiety may preclude effective psychotherapeutic treatment in some patients; however, no systematic evidence currently exists to identify such a subset of anxious patients. As appropriate treatment with anxiolytic medication can facilitate the learning process by reducing high levels of anxiety, chemotherapeutic and psychotherapeutic treatments of anxiety are often synergistic.

Perhaps the most controversial issue with respect to the use of benzodiazepines is the issue of drug dependence, particularly since withdrawal symptoms may follow abrupt discontinuation of benzodiazepine medication. However, if the patient has not taken any drug with which the benzodiazepine is cross tolerant (e.g., barbiturates, alcohol) before the use of usual therapeutic doses of the benzodiazepine and has taken this dosage for less than twenty weeks, there appears to be little risk of a withdrawal reaction (4). Length of administration appears to be the critical factor for withdrawal risk when benzodiazepine medication alone is taken within the therapeutic range and may account for some of the reported cases of withdrawal (5). Although long-term (greater than four months) usage of benzodiazepines has not been thoroughly assessed by systematic clinical studies, this strategy appears to be useful in some chronically anxious patients (6). The risk of withdrawal reactions in patients treated for eight months or more is much greater as compared to patients treated continuously for less than eight months. However, withdrawal reactions can be readily managed by gradually tapering medication when benzodiazepine treatment is discontinued (7).

An important consideration with respect to the use of benzodiazepines in the geriatric population is the altered metabolism of these drugs as a consequence of the aging process. These alterations result in increased sensitivity to the effects of the benzodiazepines as well as qualitative changes in the behavioral effects that can produce adverse consequences such as toxic confusional states or increased irritability. These adverse effects can be particularly troublesome when benzodiazepines are used by older individuals with concurrent serious illnesses such as myocardial ischemia or acute myocardial infarction. Oxazepam, which has no significant active metabolite and a relatively short half-life of four to twenty-four hours, appears to be less troublesome in regard to these potential problems in the geriatric population, as compared to the other benzodiazepines. Therefore, oxazepam, normally in a total daily dose of about 45 mg, appears to be particularly useful for the treatment of anxiety in older individuals; younger adults usually require 60 to 120 mg per day (8).

Of particular interest, behavioral side effects of the benzodiazepines include a paradoxical aggressiveness. Essentially, patients with poorly controlled hostile impulses have been observed to develop aggressive behaviors as a side effect following benzodiazepine treatment. A group setting appears to be a prominent variable due to the fact that poorly controlled hostile and angry impulses with psychological and social determinants may be released following benzodiazepine treatment. This paradoxical effect appears to involve metabolic and pharmacologic factors as well; for example, oxazepam appears less likely to produce hostile or aggressive behaviors than other benzodiazepines. Some evidence also indicates that the aggressive effects of the benzodiazepines may occur more often at doses lower than the dose range associated with anxiolytic properties of the compound. Thus, increasing the dose of the benzodiazepine may attenuate this paradoxical effect (1).

Neurological side effects of the benzodiazepines include vertigo, nystagmus, ataxia, dysarthria, and paresthesias (9). Headaches have been reported as a possible side effect, although it is often difficult to distinguish headaches associated with the anxiety syndrome as opposed to anxiolytic medication administration. Although benzodiazepines have fewer autonomic side effects than the neuroleptics and tricyclic antidepressants, they have been reported to cause hypotension, palpitations, dry mouth, dysuria, constipation, and disturbances in sexual potency.

Hematological side effects are quite rare but include agranulocytosis, leucopenia, aplastic anemia, leucocytosis, and eosinophilia. Dermatologic side effects that have been reported include urticaria, photoallergic eruptions, erythema nodosum, erythema multiforme, and purpura.

Benzodiazepines have also been reported to cause gastrointestinal disturbances, increased appetite, and weight gain (unassociated with anxiolytic efficacy), and rarely, cholestatic jaundice and hepatocellular jaundice.

Side effects associated with the female reproductive system include suppression of ovulation, galactorrhea, and amenorrhea. Large doses of benzodiazepines administered during pregnancy or before delivery may result in hypotonia, apnea, lethargy, and feeding difficulties in the neonate.

Experimental and clinical reports indicate that benzodiazepines are relatively safe in overdose. A fatal overdose from benzodiazepine medication has never been conclusively documented, although there are numerous reports of deaths following a multiple-drug overdose in which one of the medications is a benzodiazepine (1). As the relevance of a benzodiazepine in multiple-drug overdose resulting in death is still controversial, benzodiazepines cannot be considered to be suicide proof.

NON-BENZODIAZEPINE ANXIOLYTICS

The sedative antihistaminic hydroxyzine (Vistaril, Atarax), at oral dosage levels between 30 and 200 mg daily, and neuroleptics (in low doses) have some anxiolytic action. Although these agents are not usually as effective in alleviating anxiety as the benzodiazepines, they have less potential for psychological and physical dependence and are also relatively safe in overdose (10). Therefore, these compounds may be effective for the treatment of anxiety in some individuals with a propensity for benzodiazepine abuse or who respond poorly to the benzodiazepines.

Antidepressants have a special use in the treatment of phobic anxiety and spontaneous panic attacks although amitriptyline's anticholinergic side effects render it somewhat less suitable than the other compounds (11). Some evidence suggests that the anxiolytic properties of the tricyclic antidepressants are associated, at least in part, with monoamine oxidase (MAO) inhibition. This action may play a role in the effectiveness of imipramine and the tricyclics in the treatment of panic attacks and phobic-anxious patients (12,13,14). Imipramine dosage requirements are highly variable, and these patients commonly respond to as little as 10 mg orally, administered once a day in the morning or evening. Patients who respond positively to tricyclics, even for several weeks or months, may experience a breakthrough phenomenon with the reoccurrence of panic. When this occurs, it may be necessary to increase the dosage of medication. Patients should be cautioned about this phenomenon at treatment onset in order to prevent demoralization (15). MAO inhibitor antidepressants like phenelzine also have anxiolytic effects and appear to be particularly useful in the medical management of severe phobic anxiety in the same dosage range as when these compounds are used for their antidepressant effect (16,17) (see Chapter 2).

Clonidine, a centrally acting α_2-adrenergic agonist which is currently used as an antihypertensive agent, may also be effective in the chemotherapeutic management of panic disorders (18). Two side effects from clonidine administration, hypotension and sedation, tend to limit its therapeutic efficacy (19). Also, more systematic research with clonidine needs to be done before its proper role in the treatment of panic disorder can be fully assessed.

As there is an unusually high incidence of prolapsed mitral valves in patients with panic disorders (20,21) it has been proposed that a hyperdynamic central β-adrenergic state may be functioning in both disorders (22). When these conditions occur together judicious use of either imipramine or phenelzine has been reported to be effective in treating the panic disorder (22,23), perhaps as a consequence of α_2-adrenergic autoreceptor desensitization and subsequent dampening of central β-adrenergic discharge. Neither imipramine nor phenelzine exert significant physiological effects upon the prolapsed mitral valve.

MAO inhibitors have also been used as a treatment for anxious depression or mixed anxiety-depression with somatic symptoms. However, the triazolobenzodiazepine alprazolam (Xanax), which is associated with fewer and less severe side effects compared to the MAO inhibitors, is also effective in the treatment of these conditions (24), as discussed in Chapter 2. There are, as yet, no studies published which compare the relative efficacy of alprazolam and MAO inhibitors in anxious-depressive conditions.

Neuroleptics may have a special role for treating anxiety in borderline and severe obsessive-compulsive individuals, although the supporting evidence for this is rather sparse (8). Neuroleptics with anxiolytic properties include fluphenazine (4 mg/day), prochlorperazine (20 mg/day), molindone (10 mg/day), and chlorpromazine (100 mg/day). Neuroleptics can also be useful in the management of anxious, agitated geriatric patients with dementia.

However, when the neuroleptics are used for their anxiolytic effects, the dose should be initiated and maintained at the lowest therapeutic level. Unfortunately, even in low doses, neuroleptics can produce disturbing side effects such as drowsiness, ataxia, dry mouth, and blurred vision. Extrapyramidal side effects are usually mild akathisia or inner restlessness, which can exacerbate the anxiety syndrome. The possibility also exists that long-term use of neuroleptics for management of anxiety could result in tardive dyskinesia.

Another agent that has been shown to have some anxiolytic properties, presumably as a consequence of its anticatecholaminergic effects, is the β-blocking agent DL-propranolol (Inderal) in oral dosages of 30 to 120 mg per day given in three to four divided doses. The β-adrenoreceptor blockade following propranolol administration diminishes sympathetic manifestations of anxiety such as atrial tachyarrhythmias, tremor, and hyperventilation. Although the relative efficacy and indications for propranolol are still uncertain, this compound may be used effectively for its adjunctive effects on anxiety associated with other medical disorders for which β-adrenergic blockade is helpful (e.g., hypertension, certain forms of cardiac arrhythmia, and thyrotoxicosis) (25).

Prominent adverse effects of propranolol include sinus bradycardia, first-degree atrioventricular block, and complete heart block with cardiac arrest. Patients with preexisting first-degree or second-degree heart block are particularly at risk for complete heart block. Propranolol may also precipitate or aggravate congestive heart failure, obstructive pulmonary disease, asthma, mental depression, claudication, cold extremities, Raynaud's phenomenon, and diabetes mellitus. In regard to the latter effect, it is important to note that propranolol-induced β-blockade often masks the important signs and symptoms of hypoglycemia. Other effects of propranolol include insomnia, nightmares, perceptual disturbances, mood alterations, fatigue, headache, dizziness, muscle cramps, fever, conjunctival dryness, purpura, skin rashes, and gastrointestinal disturbances.

The two other major classes of compounds with anxiolytic properties, the propanediols (e.g., meprobamate) and the barbiturates, are less effective than the benzodiazepines. These two classes of compounds also have a significant potential for toxicity and substance abuse, and they are infrequently prescribed for the treatment of anxiety. Anther chemical group, the azaspirodecanediones (e.g., buspirone), has been reported to be more anxioselective than the benzodiazepines in clinical trials. In addition, this group appears to lack sedative, muscle-relaxing, and anticonvulsive effects; cross tolerance with alcohol or barbiturates; and major drug-abuse potential. However, the place of this new group of antianxiety drugs in clinical practice remains to be determined.

TREATMENT OF ALCOHOL WITHDRAWAL

Since anxiety is often a prominent manifestation of alcohol withdrawal and since anxiolytics can substitute at least in part, pharmacologically, for alcohol in the treatment of alcohol withdrawal, benzodiazepines are currently in wide use for the treatment of alcohol withdrawal. They are at least as effective and usually less toxic than the antihistamines, neuroleptics, barbiturates, and paraldehyde. Although most benzodiazepine derivatives including diazepam, chlordiazepoxide, oxazepam, flurazepam, lorazepam, and chlorazepate have been used in the medical treatment of alcohol withdrawal (26), no clear evidence indicates that any one benzodiazepine is superior over another for this condition. Although benzodiazepine treatment alleviates much of the clinical symptomatology associated with withdrawal, continuous seizures and hallucinations appear to be relatively refractory to the effects of these medications (27).

Ethanol has no role in the proper medical management of alcohol withdrawal because its administration perpetuates the numerous metabolic dysfunctions associated with alcohol abuse, and in addition, the rapid biotransformation of ethyl alcohol requires frequent dosages in order to maintain blood alcohol concentrations. Also, treatment of the alcoholic with alcohol may perpetuate the patient's primary drug dependence.

Chlordiazepoxide is the prototype benzodiazepine for alcohol withdrawal because it has been the most frequently studied benzodiazepine derivative for this condition. It is more effective than placebo in decreasing anxiety, restlessness, tremor, seizure frequency, and the development of delirium tremens. However, as with the other benzodiazepines, it does not have significant anti-hallucinatory activity. Although both chlordiazepoxide and diazepam are effective, both of these compounds have some potential complicating factors when they are used for treating alcohol withdrawal. For example, both have relatively long half-lives (approximately twelve hours for chlordiazepoxide and thirty-five hours for diazepam). Therefore, drug accumulation can occur with chronic administration.

The half-lives of these compounds vary threefold to fourfold among individuals, and bioavailability after intramuscular (IM) injection is relatively poor (28). Also, the high degree of protein binding makes chlordiazepoxide and diazepam metabolism susceptible to genetic variation in albumin binding as well as to changes in albumin concentration and displacement. Since the hepatic metabolism of chlordiazepoxide and diazepam is slowed down with liver disease and advancing age and since both drugs have active metabolites with excretion rates often slower than the parent compound, proper estimation of clinical effect can be troublesome in the treatment of alcohol withdrawal complicated by hepatic disease and/or advancing age.

However, oxazepam (Serax) and lorazepam (Ativan) may be differentially advantageous in the medical management of alcohol withdrawal because neither has active metabolites and the metabolic disposition of both of these compounds is not altered to a significant degree by hepatic disease or aging (27). However, more carefully controlled studies are needed in regard to this issue.

Routine dosage schedules with benzodiazepines for the management of alcohol withdrawal are not advisable because of the variability in metabolism of these drugs as well as the variability in duration and severity of the withdrawal syndrome. On the first day of treatment, 100 to 400 mg of chlordiazepoxide or equivalent dosage of another benzodiazepine is usually administered, but up to 1,600 mg of chlordiazepoxide or its equivalent may be required. Dosage can then be decreased by about 15 to 20 percent per day. If the withdrawal syndrome is particularly severe, a benzodiazepine can be administered cautiously by the intravenous (IV) route, with appropriate dosage adjustments.

When hallucinations are a prominent component of the withdrawal syndrome, the butyrophenone haloperidol (Haldol) may be effective either alone or in combination with a benzodiazepine. As haloperidol appears to have fewer cardiovascular, seizure-inducing, hepatotoxic, and sedative side effects than other neuroleptics (8), it is currently the neuroleptic of choice in the treatment of alcohol withdrawal. The occurrence of significant dystonic reactions is unusual given the relatively small doses (2 to 5 mg per day) of haloperidol that are usually required to treat alcohol withdrawal.

When severe tremors are present, the β-blocking agent propranolol may be useful (29,30). However, alcoholics have an increased incidence of myocardial depression, hypoglycemia, and bronchospasm, all of which are relative contraindications to the use of propranolol. Also, the nightmares that can occur with propranolol administration may complicate the withdrawal syndrome, and in addition, propranolol does not have antiseizure activity. Therefore, propranolol appears to be most useful as an adjunct to benzodiazepine treatment in selected patients with severe tremors.

USE OF ANXIOLYTICS IN PATIENTS WITH MEDICAL ILLNESS

Gastrointestinal Disorders

A number of reports indicate that diazepam and other benzodiazepines are useful in the treatment of the so-called functional gastrointestinal disorders such as irritable colon and intestinal spasms, since anxiety has been associated with altered colonic motility. Deutsch (31), for example, reported anxiety reduction in a double-blind study of patients treated for functional gastrointestinal disorders, where improvement in emotional status was significantly better with a diazepam-propantheline combination when compared to a placebo-propantheline combination. Voegtlin also (32) reported that diazepam was an effective adjunct in the management of functional gastrointestinal disorders with associated anxiety. The chlordiazepoxide-clidinium combination (Librax) has been reported to be especially useful in the management of functional gastrointestinal disorders (33), and some researchers believe that the effects of Librax are related to the anticholinergic properties of clidinium, which result in decreased gastrointestinal secretions and motility, as well as the anxiolytic properties of chlordiazepoxide. Kasich (34) concluded that clorazepate was superior to placebo and comparable to diazepam in the management of functional gastrointestinal disorders with associated anxiety. Kasich (35) also showed that lorazepam was comparable to diazepam in the adjunctive management of gastrointestinal disease with associated anxiety.

Since many clinicians believe that emotional stress is a contributory factor in the development of peptic ulcer disease, it is interesting to note that the administration of a number of antianxiety drugs has been associated with reduced basal gastric acid secretion. Roberts and Oldrey (36) conducted a study with dyspeptic patients that indicated that IV diazepam significantly suppressed gastric acid secretion after the effect of pentagastrin administration had worn off. However, they also noted that diazepam had no effect on nocturnal basal gastric acid secretion. These findings and related data indicate that benzodiazepines may act by inhibition of centrally mediated secretory stimulation during wakefulness. For example, a study by Stacher and associates indicated that lowered basal gastric acid secretion as well as insulin-stimulated gastric acid secretion after bromazepam administration was due to the central effect of the drug (37,38).

Of practical concern, several reports indicate that cimetidine administration reduces plasma clearance of diazepam, chlordiazepoxide, and alprazolam and increases the elimination half-life of these benzodiazepines. This pharmacokinetic effect can manifest itself clinically as excessive sedation. Animal studies indicate that cimetidine reduces metabolic degradation of these compounds by inhibiting hepatic microsmal activity. The benzodiazepines oxazepam and lorazepam, which are metabolically degraded by glucuronidation, are apparently spared this type of drug interaction (39).

Although adjunctive treatment with benzodiazepines for gastrointestinal disorders associated with anxiety has been associated with improvement in the patient's clinical status, it is still unclear as to what extent anxiety functions in precipitating and sustaining various gastrointestinal illnesses. Clearly, more controlled studies are needed in this area. For example, carefully controlled studies indicate that anxiolytics hasten recovery from functional gastrointestinal disorders and peptic ulcer disease or that adjunctive therapy with anxiolytics is effective in prophylaxis for these conditions.

Migraine

Psychotropic agents, including the anxiolytics, have also been used in the treatment of migraine. In a double-blind study of eighty patients suffering from migraine, Okasha and colleagues (40) showed that doxepin in a dosage of 10 mg three times a day gave the best response and that amitriptyline in a dosage of 10 mg three times a day was the next most effective. Diazepam in a dosage of 2 mg three times daily was also superior to placebo. However, few reports in the literature demonstrate superior efficacy of psychotropics alone in the treatment of migraine. As a single treatment, ergot derivatives still appear to be the most effective treatment for acute attacks (41). In addition, once established, most migraine attacks seem to be helped with an analgesic regimen combined with judicious use of an appropriate psychotropic medication.

The benzodiazepines may also be useful in conjunction with methysergide for migraine prophylaxis by reducing anxiety and emotional stress; small doses of tricyclic antidepressants also appear to be effective (31). However, this area of medical therapy also requires more carefully controlled clinical trials.

Respiratory Disorders

The anxiolytics have also been used in the adjunctive management of asthma and related respiratory disorders. For example, hydroxyzine has been used in this regard. Blerman and associates (42) reported that ephedrine had no effect on postexercise asthma, that hydroxyzine had a weak therapeutic effect, and that theophylline had a strong therapeutic effect. However, the additive effect of the three compounds together was superior to theophylline alone. Alanko and colleagues (43) compared an ephedrine-theophylline-hydroxyzine combination with salbutamol in fifteen asthmatic patients. Criteria for improvement included measurements of peak expiratory flow, number of isoproterenol inhalations per day, and severity of respiratory symptomatology. The results of the study indicated that the combination therapy was better than salbutamol. Similar conclusions were obtained by Chodosh and Doraiswami (44) when they added hydroxyzine to a theophylline-ephedrine regimen; the addition of hydroxyzine resulted in a greater improvement in most pulmonary function tests compared to the theophylline-ephedrine regimen.

However, although antianxiety medication may be helpful in the prophylactic management of asthma, particularly when there is a concomitant emotional factor (41), the respiratory depressant effects of the benzodiazepines may limit their particular usefulness in acute asthmatic attacks. For example, the benzodiazepines have been shown to produce respiratory depression in individuals with and without respiratory disorders. It is interesting that diazepam sensitivity has also been implicated in acute asthmatic attacks (45). In fact, when benzodiazepines were administered to some patients with acute asthma or chronic obstructive pulmonary disease, blood gases deteriorated out of proportion to the degree of bronchospasm or obstruction. The use of anxiolytics has also been shown to suppress restlessness as a symptomatic presentation of progressive respiratory failure.

The utility of benzodiazepines in stable chronic respiratory disease is also controversial and requires more controlled clinical studies. Kroneberg and associates (46) administered diazepam orally to stable patients with severe chronic obstructive pulmonary disease and hypercapnia. They could not detect any significant change in the forced expiratory volume or arterial blood gases when the patients took 10 mg four times a day for the first week, and these individuals continued to take 5 to 15 mg per day for up to two years without adverse effect. Zsigmond and colleagues (47) showed that diazepam in a dose of 0.15 mg/kg could be administered safely intravenously in patients with stable severe pulmonary obstructive disease. However, contradictory findings were observed by Catchlove and Kafer (48) when they studied patients recovering from an acute exacerbation of obstructive pulmonary disease.

The antihistaminic and bronchodilating properties of hydroxyzine indicate that judicious use of this drug represents the current antianxiety management of choice in the adjunctive management of respiratory illness complicated by anxiety (41). However, the specific value of hydroxyzine during acute episodes of respiratory decompensation needs to be determined particularly carefully. The agitation, mental confusion, and restlessness that frequently accompany progressive respiratory decompensation (hypercapnia and/or hypoxemia) do not currently constitute an indication for the use of hydroxyzine because administration of this compound suppresses symptomatic manifestation of the respiratory decompensation. More controlled studies are also needed on the prophylactic value of chronic hydroxyzine administration in the management of asthma and asthmatic patients with chronic pulmonary disease complicated by anxiety.

Cardiac Disorders

Antianxiety medication is also often prescribed in the medical management of patients with angina pectoris or myocardial infarction. Although there is an intuitive belief that anxiolytics may be effective in alleviating the emotional stresses that presumably can precipitate an anginal attack, there is currently no compelling evidence that anxiolytics reduce the frequency of anginal attacks. Therefore, they are currently used, for the most part, for alleviating the anxiety and emotional tension that are precipitated by the acute anginal attacks. Additional controlled studies are needed to evaluate the specific prophylactic value of anxiolytics in patients with angina pectoris.

Melsom and colleagues (49) conducted a controlled study of thirty-eight hospitalized post-myocardial-infarction patients in which half of the patients received diazepam. They concluded that the patients who received anxiolytic medication were less tense and fearful and required lower dosages of analgesic medication. On the basis of these conclusions, the authors suggested that prophylactic use of benzodiazepine medication in appropriate post-myocardial-infarction patients may decrease stress reactions and, thus, the frequency of serious arrhythmias and progressive myocardial damage. Dunbar et al. (50) have indicated also that the benzodiazepines may be useful in the adjunctive management of cardiac arrhythmias; Gedeon and Varkonyi (51) obtained similar results. In addition, IV diazepam does not seem to have significant adverse hemodynamic effects in patients with cardiac dysfunction (52). In their double-blind randomized study of fifty-eight patients in a coronary care unit, Hackett and Cassem (53) concluded that patients who received chlordiazepoxide required less analgesic medication and remained in the coronary care unit for shorter periods of time. However, additional clinical investigations are required to address the issue as to whether the benzodiazepines decrease the morbidity and mortality associated with serious cardiac arrhythmias and myocardial infarction.

Hypertension

Greenblatt and colleagues (54) have discussed the controversial use of anxiolytic medication in hypertensive patients, and they, as well as others (33), concluded that there is no indication for substituting anxiolytic medication for specific antihypertensive medication on the premise that anxiety reduction will alleviate hypertension. Oral administration of benzodiazepines has not been demonstrated to exert sustained therapeutic effects, although decreases in systolic and diastolic blood pressures have been demonstrated following IV administration of diazepam. However, even with IV administration, rapid tolerance significantly limits the therapeutic utility of diazepam for the specific treatment of hypertension.

Insomnia

Diazepam and, to a somewhat lesser degree, other benzodiazepine anxiolytics have sedative-hypnotic properties (24). Therefore, these compounds, particularly diazepam, can be effective for the symptomatic management of insomnia associated with anxiety.

There are also several benzodiazepines with short elimination half-lives which have been developed principally as hypnotics: flurazepam (Dalmane), 15–30 mg orally at bedtime; temazepam (Restoril), 15–30 mg orally at bedtime; and triazolam (Halcion), the shortest-acting benzodiazepine derivative available in the U.S., with recommended dosage of 0.25 to 0.5 mg orally at bedtime (0.125 mg in older patients).

At present, none of the available benzodiazepine hypnotics are clearly more efficacious than the others. Although triazolam has no long-acting metabolites that could accumulate to produce psychomotor impairment—in contrast with flurazepam, whose metabolite desalkylflurazepam has a half-life up to 150 hours—there are potential problems associated with its ultra-brief half-life, which causes a rapid fall in blood levels (55). Triazolam's pharmacokinetic profile may be related to reports of rebound insomnia, a significant worsening of sleep beyond the original insomnia after discontinuing the drug, as well as early morning insomnia and daytime anxiety, consequent to a mini-withdrawal effect. The molecular mechanisms underlying these clinical effects may also involve a lag in production of endogenous benzodiazepine-like compounds or some other disruption of GABA-ergic neurochemical transmission in the central nervous system (56). Although both triazolam and flurazepam have a slightly more rapid onset of action as compared to temazepam, the choice of which benzodiazepine hypnotic to use should be based on a careful assessment of the individual patient.

SUMMARY

The development of medicinals to treat pathologic anxiety constitutes a major contribution to twentieth century psychiatry. Although there are still important questions to be answered regarding the most effective utilization of anxiolytics in clinical practice, general guidelines have been developed to significantly reduce abuse and potential toxicity of these compounds. Furthermore, advances in our understanding of the neurochemical mechanism of action of antianxiety agents and the metabolic basis of anxiety promise to productively increase our understanding of the interrelationships between brain function and behavior.

Although the various benzodiazepines are currently considered to be most effective for treating pathologic anxiety in a variety of settings, specific uses have been proposed for heterocyclic antidepressants, monoamine oxidase inhibitors, β-blockers, antihistamines, and, perhaps, neuroleptics, and clonidine, to increase the specificity and sensitivity of our therapeutic arma-mentarium. In addition, work with other classes of compounds which demon-strate anxiolytic properties such as the thiazolopyridazines and azaspirodecanediones, continues to refine our ability to provide effective and safe chemotherapy for the anxiety disorders.

REFERENCES

1. Sullivan, J.L.; Taska, R.J.; and Davidson, J. Antianxiety medications. In *Critical Problems in Psychiatry*, Cavenar, J.O. and Brodie, H.K.H., eds. Philadelphia: J.B. Lippincott Company, 1982, pp. 25–48.
2. Snyder, S.H. Opiate and benzodiazepine receptors. *Psychosomatics* 22:986–989, 1981.
3. Hollister, L.E. Valium: A discussion of current issues. *Psychosomatics* 28:44–58, 1977.
4. Ayd, F.J. Benzodiazepines: dependence and withdrawal. *JAMA* 242:1401–1402, 1979.
5. Prescribing of minor tranquilizers. *FDA Drug Bulletin* 10:2–3, 1980.
6. Rickels, K.; Case, G.; Downing, R.W.; and Winokur, A. Long-term diazepam ther-apy and clinical outcome. *JAMA* 250:767–771, 1983.
7. Tyer, P.; Owen, R.; and Dawling, S. Gradual withdrawal of diazepam after long-term therapy. *Lancet* 1:1402–1406, 1983.
8. Rickels, K. Use of antianxiety agents in anxious outpatients. *Psychopharmacology* 58:1–17, 1978.
9. Edwards, J.G. Unwanted effects of psychotropic drugs IV—Drugs for anxiety. *The Practitioner* 219:117–212, 1977.
10. Hollister, L.E. *Clinical Use of Psychotherapeutic Drugs*. Springfield, Ill.: Charles C Thomas, 1973.
11. Baldessarini, R.J. *Chemotherapy in Psychiatry*. Cambridge: Harvard University Press, 1977.
12. Sullivan, J.L.; Dackis, C.; and Stanfield, C. In vivo inhibition of platelet MAO activ-ity by tricyclic antidepressants. *Am. J. Psychiatry* 134:188–190, 1977.
13. Sullivan, J.L.; Zung, W.W.K.; Stanfield, C.N.; and Cavenar, J.O. Clinical correlates of tricyclic antidepressant-mediated inhibition of platelet monamine oxidase. *Biol. Psychiatry* 13:399–407, 1978.
14. Davidson, J.; Linnoila, M.; Raft, D.; and Turnbull, C.D. MAO inhibition and con-trol of anxiety following amitriptyline therapy. *Acta Psychiatr. Scand.* 63:147–152, 1981.
15. Muskin, P.R.; and Fyer, A.J. Treatment of panic disorder. *J. Clin. Psychopharmacol.* 1: 81–90, 1981.
16. [Medical News]. New studies confirm MAO inhibitors' efficacy in treating severe anxiety. *JAMA* 245:1799–1801, 1981.
17. Raft, D.; Davidson, J.; Wasik, J.; and Mattox, A. Relationship between response to phenelzine and MAO inhibition in a clinical trial of phenelzine, amitriptyline and placebo. *Neuropsychobiology* 7:122–126, 1981.
18. Hoehn-Saric, R.; Merchant, A.F.; and Keyser, M.L. Effects of clonidine on anxiety disorders. *Arch. Gen. Psychiatry* 38:1278–1282, 1981.

19. Liebowitz, M.R.; Fyer, A.S.; and McGrath, P. Clonidine treatment of panic disorders. *Psychopharmacol. Bull.* 17:122–123, 1981.
20. Praiser, S.F.; Pinta, E.R.; and Jones, B.A. Mitral valve prolapse syndrome and anxiety neurosis/panic disorder. *Am. J. Psychiatry* 135:246–247, 1978.
21. Praiser, S.F.; Jones, B.A.; Pinta, E.R.; Young, E.A.; and Fontena, M.E. Panic attacks: diagnostic evaluations of 17 patients. *Am. J. Psychiatry* 136:105–106, 1978.
22. Gorman, J.M.; and Fyer, A.S.; Glich, J.; King, D.; and Klein, D.S.F. Effect of imipramine on prolapsed mitral valves of patient with panic disorder. *Am. J. Psychiatry* 138:977–978, 1981.
23. Evan, D.G.; and Kolina, K. Effect of phenelzine on the prolapsed mitral valve in patient with agorophobia and panic attacks. *J. Clin. Psychopharmacol.* 3:36–38, 1983.
24. Feighner, J.P.; Aden, G.C.; Fabre, L.F.; Rickels, K.; and Smith, W.T. Comparison of alprazolam, imipramine, and placebo in the treatment of depression. *JAMA* 249: 3057–3064, 1983.
25. Tinklenberg, J.R. Antianxiety medications and the treatment of anxiety. In *Psychopharmacology*, Barchas, J.D., Berger, P.A., Ciaranello, R.D., and Elliott, G.R., eds. New York: Oxford University Press, 1977, pp. 226–242.
26. Sellers, E.M., and Kalant, Harold. Alcohol intoxication and withdrawal. *N. Engl. J. Med.* 294:757–762, 1976.
27. Sellers, E.M. Antianxiety drugs in alcohol withdrawal. *Curr. Psychiatr. Ther.* 18: 157–163, 1978.
28. Greenblatt, D.J.; Shader, R.I.; MacLeod, S.M.; Sellers, E.M.; Franke, K.; and Giles, H.G. Absorption of oral and intramuscular chlordiazepoxide. *Eur. J. Clin. Pharmacol.* 13(4):267–274, 1978.
29. Sellers, E.M.; Degani, N.C.; and Zilm, D.H. Letter: Propranolol-decreased noradrenaline excretion and alcohol withdrawal. *Lancet* 1(7950):94–95, 1976.
30. Sellers, E.M.; Zilm, D.H.; and Degani, N.C. Comparative efficacy of propranolol and chlordiazepoxide in alcohol withdrawal. *J. Stud. Alcohol* 38(11):2096–2108, 1977.
31. Deutsch, E.M. Relief of anxiety and related emotions in patients with gastrointestinal disorders. A double-blind controlled study. *Am. J. Dig. Dis.* 16:1091–1094, 1971.
32. Voegtlin, W.L. Management of functional gastrointestinal disorders with diazepam. *Appl. Ther.* 6:801–805, 1964.
33. Krogh, C.; McLean, W.M.; and LaPierre, Y.D. Minor tranquilizers in somatic disorders. *Can. Med. Assoc. J.* 118(9):1097, 1100–1108, 1978.
34. Kasich, A.M. Chloraxepate dipotassium in the treatment of anxiety associated with chronic gastrointestinal disease. *Curr. Ther. Res.* 15:83–91, 1973.
35. Kasich, A.M. Lorazepam in the management of anxiety associated with chronic gastrointestinal disease: A double-blind study. *Curr. Ther. Res.* 19(3):292–306, 1976.
36. Roberts, D.M., and Oldrey, T.B. The effect of diazepam on pentagastrin-stimulated and nocturnal (sleeping) gastric secretion in man. *Am. J. Gastroenterol.* 63(5): 396–399, 1975.
37. Stacher, G., and Starker, D. Inhibitory effect of bromazepam on insulin-stimulated gastric acid secretion in man. *Am. J. Dig. Dis.* 20(2):156–161, 1975.
38. Stacher, G.; Bauer, P.; and Brunner, H. Gastric acid secretion, serum-gastrin levels and psychomotor function, under the influence of placebo, insulin-hypoglycemia and/or bromazepam. *Int. J. Clin. Pharmacol. Biopharm.* 13(1):1–10, 1976.
39. Ruffalo, R.L., and Thompson, J.F. Effect of cimetidine on the clearance of benzodiazepines. *N. Engl. J. Med.* 303(B):753–754, 1980.

40. Okasha, A.; Ghaleb, H.A.; and Sadek, A. A double blind trial for the clinical management of psychogenic headache. *Br. J. Psychiatry* 122:181–183, 1973.
41. Parkes, J.D. Diseases of the central nervous system. Relief of pain: Headache, facial neuralgia, migraine, and phantom limb. *Br. Med. J.* 4(5988):90–92, 1975.
42. Blerman, C.W.; Pierson, W.E.; and Shapiro, G.G. Treatment of asthma. *Pediatrics* 56(suppl.):919–925, 1975.
43. Alanko, K.; Lahdensuo, A.; and Mattila, M.J. Bronchodilator effect of oral salbutamol and an ephedrine + theophylline + hydroxyzine combination in asthmatic out-patients. *Scand. J. Respir. Dis.* 55(6):340–350, 1974.
44. Chodosh, S., and Doraiswami, S. An evaluation of theophylline/ephedrine with and without hydroxyzine in asthma. *Curr. Ther. Res.* 18(6):773–784, 1975.
45. Blumberg, M.Z., and Young, S. Diazepam-associated asthma. *Pediatrics* 54(6): 811–812, 1974.
46. Kroneberg, R.S.; Cosio, M.G.; and Stevenson, J.E. Letter: The use of oral diazepam in patients with obstructive lung disease and hypercapnia. *Ann. Intern. Med.* 83(1): 83–84, 1975.
47. Zsigmond, E.K.; Shirely, J.G.; and Flynn, K. Diazepam and meperidine on arterial blood gases in patients with chronic obstructive pulmonary disease. *J. Clin. Pharmacol.* 15(5–6):464–469, 1975.
48. Catchlove, R.F., and Kafer, E.R. The effects of diazepam on respiration in patients with obstructive pulmonary disease. *Anesthesiology* 34:14–18, 1971.
49. Melsom, M.; Andreassen, P.; and Melsom, H. Diazepam in acute myocardial infarction. Clinical effects and effects on catecholamines, free fatty acids, and cortisol. *Br. Heart J.* 38(8):804–810, 1976.
50. Dunbar, R.W.; Boettner, R.B.; and Haley, J.V. The effect of diazepam on the antiarrhythmic response to lidocaine. *Anesth. Analg.* 50:685–692, 1971.
51. Gedeon, A., and Varkonyi, S. Symptomatic treatment of myocardial infarction and acute psychosyndrome with Seduxen injections. *Ther. Hung.* 21:41–42, 1973.
52. Cote, P.; Gueret, P.; and Bourassa, M.G. Effect of diazepam on coronary circulation and myocardial metabolism in subjects with normal coronary arteries and patients with coronary arteriosclerosis. *Union Med. Can.* 104(1):46–56, 1975.
53. Hackett, T.P., and Cassem, N.H. Reduction of anxiety in the coronary care unit. A controlled double-blind comparison of chlordiazepoxide and amobarbital. *Curr. Ther. Res.* 14:649–656, 1972.
54. Greenblatt, D.J.; Shader, R.I.; and Lofgren, S. Rational psychopharmacology for patients with medical diseases. *Ann. Rev. Med.* 27:407–420, 1976.
55. Donaldson, S.R. Triazolam (Halcion): New entry in the sleeper sweepstakes. *Massachusetts General Hospital Newsletter — Biological Therapies in Psychiatry* 6: 33, 1983.
56. Kales, A., Soldatos, C.R., Bixler, E.O., and Kales, J.D. Early morning insomnia with rapidly eliminated benzodiazepines. *Science* 220: 95–97, 1983.

CHAPTER 2

Chemotherapy of Affective Disorders

John L. Sullivan,
Ronald J. Taska,
Thomas N. Wise,
and
David M. Goldstein

No widely accepted pharmacological treatment existed for affective disorders prior to the 1950s, although these illnesses are among the most common major psychiatric disorders. Sympathomimetic drugs, like amphetamines, had been tried for depressions characterized by psychomotor retardation, and barbiturates had been tried for agitated depressions, with little success. In 1951, isoniazid and its isopropyl derivative, iproniazid, were developed for the treatment of tuberculosis. It was soon found that both compounds, especially iproniazid, had mood-elevating effects in patients with tuberculosis. As a result, iproniazid was studied in depressed patients and was discovered to have antidepressant properties. Iproniazid was also discovered to be a potent and irreversible inhibitor of the amine-catabolizing enzyme, monoamine oxidase (MAO). Other MAO inhibitors subsequently were discovered to have antidepressant activity and were introduced into psychiatric practice.

HETEROCYCLIC ANTIDEPRESSANTS

During the late 1950s, the second major class of antidepressant drugs, the heterocyclic antidepressants (HCAs), was introduced into psychiatric practice. The prototypic compound of this class is the phenothiazine analog imipramine. Although the standard HCAs (tricyclic antidepressants, or TCAs) are the most widely used antidepressant agents, their efficacy is somewhat limited. Improvement rates following treatment with a standard HCA have been in the 66 to 75 percent range, while placebo response rates are often in the 20 to 40 percent range (1,2,3,4). However, advances in pharmacokinetics and delineation of subtypes of depressive illness indicate that these reported improvement rates for the HCAs are on the low side. While the expectation for improvement following treatment with an HCA is generally better in cases of endogenous or major depression, excellent results have been obtained in some apparently "pure" cases of reactive depression (5).

Mechanisms of Action

Since the work of Axelrod and his colleagues in the 1960s (6), researchers have known that imipramine and other typical HCAs block the inactivation of norepinephrine by reuptake or transport at adrenergic nerve terminals in central neuronal systems and also in the sympathetic and peripheral neuronal systems. These agents also have weak effects against the uptake of dopamine and variable effects against the uptake of serotonin.

The demethylated antidepressants (secondary amines) such as desipramine, nortriptyline, and protriptyline are very potent against norepinephrine uptake but relatively weak against serotonin reuptake inactivation. Desipramine is the demethylated metabolite of the tertiary amine HCA imipramine, and nortriptyline is the demethylated metabolite of the tertiary amine HCA amitriptyline. The secondary amine HCAs are normally less sedating than the tertiary amine compounds.

Evidence concerning the blockade of serotonin reuptake inactivation indicates limited potency of most HCAs although some of the newer experimental agents, such as clomipramine and fluoxetine, are quite potent in this regard. However, while facilitation of central serotonergic neurotransmission may produce sedation or antianxiety effects, the relationship of this pharmacologic action to true antidepressant activity remains unclear (7).

If potentiation of the action of norepinephrine is an important effect of many HCAs, it is likely to be mediated through postsynaptic (α_1 and β) neuronal receptors for norepinephrine. Thus, although the in vitro and in vivo potency against norepinephrine uptake correlates only weakly with clinical potency (not efficacy) of the HCAs, there is a significant inverse correlation of clinical potency with α_1-blocking potency (7). Clinical potency also correlates significantly with the ratio of potencies of blocking norepinephrine uptake to blocking α_1 receptors, although the effects on uptake and $\dot{\alpha}_1$ receptors are not significantly intercorrelated.

Evidence is also increasing that presynaptic (α_2) noradrenergic receptors may become less sensitive after repeated treatment with HCAs (7). This change presumably leads to increased neuronal release of norepinephrine since α_2 autoreceptors are believed to decrease the synthesis and release of norepinephrine as their sensitivity (or density) increases. This action is particularly interesting because changes in neuronal activity and metabolism following several weeks of antidepressant treatment are more likely to provide clues to the actions of antidepressants associated with their clinical efficacy.

It has also been observed that repeated administration of several chemical classes of antidepressants (including HCAs, MAO inhibitors, and some of the new, atypical antidepressants) as well as electroconvulsive therapy (ECT) results in diminished sensitivity of postsynaptic β-adrenergic receptors in the brain (8,9,10). Although the functional significance of this apparently short-lived and reversible downregulation of norepinephrine sensitivity is uncertain, such a change is more likely to reflect restoration of homeostasis in central neural transmission rather than a true loss of noradrenergic neurotransmission (7).

With respect to the dopamine systems, some investigators have reported neurophysiologic (11) and behavioral (12) changes consistent with decreased sensitivity of presynaptic dopamine autoreceptors, associated with repeated (long-term) HCA treatment as well as with ECT (13). This decreased sensitivity of the presynaptic autoreceptor would presumably result in increased functional activity of dopamine at postsynaptic dopamine receptors, an effect that may contribute to the mood-elevating and/or behavior-activating effects of the antidepressants.

Some interesting findings are also emerging in regard to the serotonin systems. For example, decreased platelet binding of tritiated imipramine has been reported in some depressed patients (14), and considerable evidence indicates that these binding sites are functionally, and probably structurally, associated with membrane uptake (transport) sites for serotonin. However, there is still some uncertainty as to whether this finding is an artifact of antidepressant drug exposure. Some researchers also have reported decreases in binding site strength and/or density for both types 1 and 2 serotonin receptors following long-term HCA treatment. However, these results contradict the results of neurophysiological and behavioral studies that demonstrate increased sensitivity to serotonin in the brain after repeated treatment (weeks) with antidepressant chemicals of both the typical and atypical classes (7).

Although it is virtually certain that no single biochemical or neurophysiological hypothesis accounts for the actions of all antidepressants, it appears that the combination of blockade of norepinephrine reuptake inactivation, low potency against postsynaptic α_1-adrenergic blockade, desensitization of α_2-adrenergic autoreceptors, and a tendency to down regulation of β-adrenergic receptors may characterize a number of effective HCAs. However, the role of brain amine neurotransmitter deficiency in the pathogenesis of depressive disorders is still uncertain, and a major limitation to understanding how antidepressants work is the likelihood that depressions are biologically heterogeneous. HCAs may also work by lengthening circadian rhythms, thereby readjusting the physiological patterns of body temperature, cortisol, and REM sleep which are shortened in major depressions. (See Chapter 5 for phenylethylamine theory of affective disorders and REM latency studies.)

The typical HCAs are metabolized by hydroxylation, and the water soluble hydroxylated metabolites are rapidly excreted. Barbiturates (15,16) and cigarette smoking stimulate the enzymatic rate of hydroxylation, thus increasing the rate of urinary excretion and decreasing the plasma levels of the HCAs. Phenothiazines, methylphenidate, and amphetamine conversely inhibit the enzymatic rate of hydroxylation, thus decreasing the rate of urinary excretion and increasing the plasma levels of the HCAs. Elderly patients, likewise, have slower enzymatic rates of hydroxylation and hence develop higher plasma levels than nonelderly adults (17). Thus, elderly patients should be treated with one-half to two-thirds of the HCA dose that nonelderly adults receive.

Dosages and Therapeutic Blood Level Monitoring

Dosage ranges for HCAs are given in Table 2.1. Most of the commonly used HCAs can usually be initiated at a dose of 50 mg/day in nonelderly adults, and the dose is then increased about 50 mg every other day until a total dose of 150 to 200 mg is reached. Patients are usually maintained on this dose for two to three weeks in order to receive an adequate therapeutic trial. The dose of nortriptyline is not usually increased above 150 mg per day. The dose of imipramine, desipramine, amitriptyline, or doxepin can be increased to as much as 300 mg per day if the patient does not respond to the lower doses. The half-lives of the HCAs are such that most of the daily dosage of these drugs can be given at night. Such a bedtime regimen often increases medication compliance

Table 2.1   Dosages of Antidepressant Drugs

Generic Name	Daily Dosage (mg)[a]
Heterocyclics	
Standard heterocyclics	
Imipramine HCl	100 to 300
Amitriptyline HCl	100 to 300
Protriptyline HCl	15 to 60
Desipramine HCl	100 to 300
Nortriptyline HCl	75 to 150
Doxepin HCl	100 to 400
New heterocyclics	
Trimipramine maleate	75 to 300
Amoxapine HCl	200 to 600
Maprotiline HCl	100 to 300
MAO inhibitors	
Phenelzine sulfate	15 to 90
Tranylcypromine sulfate	20 to 40
Isocarboxazid	10 to 60
Atypical antidepressants	
Trazodone HCl	150 to 600
Alprazolam[b]	6 to 12

[a]Lower doses may be required for adolescent and geriatric patients.
[b]Antidepressant dose is not yet precisely established.

by decreasing the number of times during the day that the medication needs to be taken. Doxepin has been reported to be less potent in vivo than most of the other HCAs (18) and, hence, may need to be used at slightly higher doses to produce equivalent antidepressant activity.

In the interest of providing optimal treatment regimens for individuals receiving antidepressant medication, a large body of literature has evolved that addresses the use of chemical assays of blood drug levels of the HCAs (Table 2.2). Unfortunately, we still know comparatively little about the clinical value of therapeutic monitoring of antidepressant drug blood levels. For example, the metabolic variance between individuals receiving presumably adequate doses of an HCA appears to be so great that it is difficult to define optimal blood levels for groups of patients (7). However, there is some evidence that the demethylated (secondary amine) HCAs, specifically nortriptyline and perhaps desipramine, may have a biphasic or curvilinear (inverted-U) relationship between blood level and clinical response (19,20,21). For endogenously depressed patients treated with nortriptyline, improvement is most likely when plasma levels are roughly between 50 and 150 ng/ml, while higher or lower doses of the drug have been reported to be associated with relatively poor clinical outcome. There is some evidence, although not incontrovertible, that for methylated (tertiary amine) HCAs, specifically imipramine and perhaps amitriptyline, there is a more linear, positive correlation. Endogenously depressed, nondelusional patients have been reported most likely to improve when blood levels of the parent drug plus its major demethylated metabolite total roughly 200 ng/ml or above. However, the risk of toxicity is significant with levels above 500 ng/ml, at least with respect to the standard HCAs (22).

Although commercial laboratories are making assays for blood concentrations of antidepressant drugs readily available, their value remains unclear for the routine management of depressive patients. However, these blood-drug assays may be helpful in the evaluation of patients who demonstrate a poor

Table 2.2 Heterocyclic Antidepressant Blood (Plasma) Levels

Drug	Half-life (hr)	Levels (ng/ml)
Secondary amines		
Desipramine	33	100 to 300 (?)
Nortriptyline	52	50 to 150
Protriptyline	126	100 to 200
Amoxapine	30	?
Maprotiline	48	200 to 500
Tertiary amines		
Imipramine	16	150 to 300
Amitriptyline	30	100 to 250
Doxepin	34	100 to 200

response to conventionally adequate doses of medication administered for several weeks where questions of noncompliance or atypical pharmacokinetics arise, patients who become toxic with antidepressant medication treatment, and elderly or cardiac patients or patients who have concurrent major medical illnesses who thus may be at significant risk for toxicity. Some evidence indicates that antidepressant drug levels may also be useful in confirming an overdose in the absence of accurate historical information and in anticipating major adverse effects when HCA plasma levels are greater than 1,000 ng/ml (23).

Several additional cautions are also necessary when evaluating HCA blood levels. Specifically, valid assays require appropriate techniques of blood drawing, as per the specific instructions of the laboratory. For example, blood should be drawn for assay approximately twelve hours after the last dose of the HCA. Also, not every laboratory that offers the assays has demonstrated consistent reliability. The reliability of laboratories can be assessed, to a certain degree, by sending occasional split samples to different laboratories or to the same laboratory if internal consistency is in question. (See Chapter 5 for additional discussion of HCA blood levels.)

Other Clinical Laboratory Tests and Treatment Response Potentiators

Various other laboratory tests may also be useful as biological markers of depression or as predictors of response to biomedical treatments for depression. These laboratory tests include the dextroamphetamine challenge test, urinary 3-methoxy-4-hydroxyphenylglycol, cerebrospinal fluid 5-hydroxyindoleacetic acid, the dexamethasone suppression test, the thyroid-releasing hormone (TRH) stimulation test, and the sleep electroencephalogram (EEG) test (polysomnography).

In the dextroamphetamine challenge test (24,25), the depressed patient is interviewed and then given 30 mg of dextroamphetamine orally. If during subsequent interviews (about two hours after the administration of the oral dextroamphetamine), the patient shows improvement of the depressed mood, then he or she is said to have a positive dextroamphetamine challenge test. If the patient shows no improvement in mood, this is interpreted as a negative dextroamphetamine challenge test. Several groups of investigators (24,25) have shown that a positive dextroamphetamine challenge test is correlated with a therapeutic response to imipramine or desipramine. The remaining tests are discussed in Chapter 5.

Despite judicious selection of HCA therapy on the basis of clinical signs and symptoms and the use of appropriate clinical laboratory measures, including blood level measurements, some patients do not respond effectively to HCA treatment alone. In a number of these cases, particularly in patients with a major depression who respond poorly to imipramine or amitriptyline, the addition of 25 to 50 mg of triiodothyronine daily may be significantly beneficial (26). Lower doses or a gradual increase in daily dosage may be advisable in patients with cardiovascular disease. The relationship of this apparent synergism between a HCA and thyroid hormone to thyroid function or a positive TRH stimulation test has not been clearly established.

There is also evidence that, in a number of individuals with HCA-resistant depression, the antidepressant effect of the HCA may be potentiated by lithium (see following section on lithium for dosage). The first report of this possible synergism was the double-blind, placebo-controlled trial of Lingjaerde and associates in which various HCAs were combined with lithium (27). More recently, other investigators have demonstrated marked improvement occurring within several days to a week after adding lithium to the treatment regimen of patients with depression refractory to a variety of HCAs (28,29). The prophylactic value of this combination of a HCA and lithium as compared to the HCA alone in such patients has not yet been sufficiently evaluated. Interestingly, the atypical antidepressant bupropion is also effective in a significant number of patients with (typical) HCA-resistant depression.

The use of a HCA in combination with a neuroleptic has benefited some patients with psychotic (delusional) depression. The side effects from this combination of medications, particularly the anticholinergic effects, have also limited the value of this form of treatment (30). Electroconvulsive therapy is still the most effective treatment for psychotic depression (30a), as discussed in Chapter 4.

Side Effects

The HCAs, except for maprotiline and some of the atypical agents, have significant anticholinergic side effects including dry mouth, blurred vision, exacerbation of acute narrow-angle glaucoma, urinary retention, constipation, palpitations, and tachycardia. As reviewed by Taska (31), the incidence of these side effects shows little correlation with HCA plasma levels. The urinary retention side effect can often be alleviated by treatment with bethanecol chloride, a peripherally acting cholinergic agonist that does not cross the blood-brain barrier (32). Bethanecol can be administered orally in 5 to 10 mg doses on an hourly basis until satisfactory response occurs or until a maximum of 50 mg has been given.

The anticholinergic activity of the more traditional HCAs, as assayed by competition with the potent muscarinic antagonist ^{3}H-quinuclidinyl benzilate (^{3}H-QNB) or stimulation of cyclic guanosine monophosphate (GMP) synthesis by neural tissues, correlates to a certain degree with anticholinergic side effects. These studies indicate that amitriptyline is most potent in this regard, followed in descending order of potency by protriptyline, doxepin, imipramine, desipramine, and nortriptyline (7).

Cardiac side effects are also potentially troublesome for individuals receiving HCAs because they are often cardiotoxic following overdose. However, some studies have demonstrated that, in healthy adult patients, traditional HCAs in standard doses are usually free of clinically significant adverse cardiovascular effects, except for postural (orthostatic) hypotension (33,34) (see

Chapter 3 for treatment considerations). Glassman (35) reported that 14 percent of his patients on imipramine had either falls or ataxia, presumably as a consequence of orthostatic hypotension. For another 7 percent, treatment was stopped or modified because of severe dizziness. Although with time, most patients develop some tolerance to the anticholinergic side effects of the HCAs, at least one study showed that orthostatic hypotension remained unchanged during four weeks of treatment with imipramine (35). The use of HCAs in patients with cardiovascular disease, except for cardiac conduction abnormalities and congestive heart failure, is primarily limited by the occurrence of significant postural hypotension.

It is interesting that Veith et al. (36), in their investigation of the cardiovascular effects of therapeutic doses of HCAs in patients with well-defined, significant heart disease, found that the HCAs are often safe in many patients with overt heart disease. Depressed patients with atrial or ventricular arrhythmias often showed improvement with HCA treatment and, although orthostatic hypotension was noted in a number of patients, the magnitude was less pronounced in comparison to earlier studies, perhaps due to a lower starting dose and gradual increments in dosage. Depressed heart patients with preexisting bundle-branch block or congestive heart failure appear to be at greatest risk for cardiovascular side effects of HCAs and may, perhaps, best be treated with alprazolam, bupropion, or other atypical agents not yet available in the United States when antidepressant medication is required. (See later section on atypical antidepressants.)

Of potential clinical significance is the fact that a number of drugs commonly used to treat hypertension can cause or aggravate depression, including reserpine, clonidine, methyldopa, propranolol, and guanethidine. At times, antidepressant medication may be necessary to terminate these drug-induced depressions, in addition to changing the antihypertensive medication regimen. (Also see following section on MAO inhibitors.)

When depression occurs in patients with chronic renal failure, treatment regimens with HCAs must take into account the possible effects of compromised excretion. For example, although the mean steady-state serum levels of nortriptyline have been demonstrated to be similar in depressed patients with chronic renal failure and depressed patients with normal renal function, much wider fluctuations in serum levels occurred in the patients with renal failure (37). Standard dialysis techniques had only minimal effects on the serum levels of nortriptyline and its active 10-hydroxymetabolite. When HCAs are used to treat depression in patients with renal failure, one of the compounds with demonstrated value in monitoring serum levels should probably be used in order to obtain sufficient precision in adjusting the dosage.

Neuropsychiatric side effects of the HCAs include a reduction of seizure threshold (38), as compared to the MAO inhibitors that may have anticonvulsant actions (39). HCAs can interact with sedative medications and ethanol, as well as precipitate an anticholinergic psychosis characterized by delirium, confusion, and disorientation. The risk of such an anticholinergic psychosis is increased if other drugs with anticholinergic properties such as antipsychotic or antiparkinsonian drugs are used simultaneously with an HCA. An anticholinergic psychosis can usually be treated with one or two milligrams of IM or IV physostigmine, but IV physostigmine should be used with caution since it can produce grand mal seizures. Physostigmine has a short duration of action: only about thirty minutes. Another potential psychotic complication of HCA therapy is precipitation of a manic episode or shortening of the cycle length in susceptible bipolar patients (40).

There has been considerable controversy concerning whether a schizophrenic who develops depressive symptoms should be treated with antidepressant medication because antidepressants have been reported to worsen schizophrenic symptoms (41). Although this issue is still not completely resolved, the impression is that adequate treatment of the schizophrenic illness, including judicious use of neuroleptic medication, often resolves the depressive component of the illness (see Chapter 3).

HCAs have also been associated with sexual dysfunction, including slowness in achieving erection, delayed ejaculation, nonejaculation, and retrograde ejaculation (42). Motoric complications of the HCAs include precipitation or worsening of tardive dyskinesia, presumably related to effects on catecholaminergic and cholinergic neuronal systems (43). The incidence of this complication appears to be low and may be associated principally with long-term prophylactic use of the HCAs. Lithium added to the HCA regimen may be of value in treating tardive dyskinesia in depressed patients who require chronic use of a HCA (44).

Maintenance and Prophylaxis

If a patient responds to an HCA, then he or she should be maintained on this medication for about a year in order to prevent a relapse. A patient who has multiple episodes of depression should perhaps be maintained on the HCA for an even more extended period of time, although systematic data regarding this issue are relatively sparse. Studies have demonstrated that maintenance on HCAs significantly reduces the probability of relapse during the year after the patient has recovered from a depressive episode (45,46,47). Quitkin et al. (48) estimated that HCA maintenance lowers the probability of relapse during the first year after recovery by 20 to 50 percent. Seager and Bird (49) reported that 69 percent of placebo-treated patients relapsed, whereas only 17 percent of HCA-treated patients relapsed during the first six months after remission. Since nausea, vomiting, malaise, myalgias, dizziness, and coryza have been reported in some patients after the abrupt discontinuation of HCAs (50), it may be advisable to taper HCA medication slowly rather than to discontinue the drug abruptly when treatment is terminated.

Toxicity and Overdosage

Toxicity of the HCAs contributes a potentially serious problem because over-doses can be fatal. Lethal overdoses are usually in the range of two grams and over of imipramine or amitriptyline and equivalent doses of the other com-pounds (51), although smaller doses can be fatal in children. Hence, if the pa-tient has any suicidal risk, prescriptions for HCAs should take this into account since as ingestion of a ten-to-fourteen-day supply of the standard HCAs carries a high risk of fatal outcome. In fact, HCAs are rapidly overtaking barbiturates as the medication most frequently involved in serious overdose. Recent studies show that patients taking HCAs constitute up to 30 percent of persons hospi-talized for drug overdose (52).

The initial reaction to HCA overdosage is characterized primarily by an anticholinergic syndrome, including delirium, hyperreflexia, and supra-ventricular tachycardia. Recovery usually occurs within twenty-four hours if the overdose is not serious. A more serious form of overdosage is marked by convulsions, metabolic and respiratory acidosis, and both atrioventricular and intraventricular cardiac conduction defects. The most serious forms of over-dosage can progress to respiratory arrest, bradyarrhythmias, hypotension, ventricular arrhythmias, and cardiac arrest.

Clinical indications of serious HCA overdosage include some combination of the following: seizures, anticholinergic symptoms, and conduction defect, particularly QRS prolongation (greater than 0.10 milliseconds) on the electro-cardiogram (ECG). Although the occurrence of cardiac arrhythmias up to one week following HCA overdosage has been considered a potentially significant risk, new data indicate that patients may not be at risk for this complication if their level of consciousness and ECG have returned to normal and remain sta-bilized for twenty-four hours after discontinuation of any specific therapy for overdosage and if no other toxic signs and symptoms appear (53,54). This clin-ical judgment should be made on the basis of a twenty-four-hour period of inpatient cardiac monitoring, except in very mild cases, as well as observation, and may not apply in cases with preexisting cardiac disease.

The life-threatening complications of the HCA overdose are usually hy-potension and dysrhythmia. Therefore, the use of physostigmine, a reversible cholinesterase inhibitor that carries the risk of life-threatening bradyar-rhythmias, is usually contraindicated in cases of serious HCA overdose. Vaso-pressor agents, save for dobutamine, are also contraindicated because of the poor response and potential enhancement of ectopic dysrhythmic activity. However, HCA-induced hypotension and dysrhythmias are often responsive to intravenous infusion of fluid and alkalinization of arterial pH to 7.50–7.55. The success of alkalinization therapy may be at least partially the result of in-creased HCA protein binding (55). The value of alkalinization in HCA overdose also appears to have a precedent in the efficacy of such therapy in cases of quinidine overdose. The most effective second line of treatment for patients who remain hypotensive after both volume expansion and alkalinization ap-pears to be calcium and, if necessary, dobutamine (56,57), although there are no systematic data in this area. There is also some evidence that polyresin (not charcoal) hemoperfusion is effective in treating serious cases of HCA overdosage, perhaps by keeping the plasma level of the drug and its metabolites below a critical level (58,59,60).

If seizures, arrhythmias, or conduction defects persist, the most effective treatment appears to be phenytoin, 1 gram intravenously, given at a rate of no more than 50 mg/min (56). Diazepam may be helpful, when necessary, to achieve seizure control. Electrical pacing can be used in cases of refractory, life-threatening heart block. Cardiac conduction defects should not be treated with quinidine, procainamide, or disopyramide because these antiarrhythmic drugs share important pharmacologic properties with the HCAs that may result in an additive toxic effect (61).

New Imipramine-like Heterocyclics

Finally, the addition of amoxapine, trimipramine, and maprotiline raises the complement of imipramine-like or typical HCAs to nine (Table 2.1). Although the initial suggestion that these newer HCAs had a more rapid onset of action compared to the standard HCAs has not held up with more extensive clinical use, it does appear that maprotiline has a lower incidence of anticholinergic side effects and orthostatic hypotension. Clomipramine (3-chloroimipramine), a potent antagonist of serotonin uptake as well as norepinephrine uptake, is undergoing advanced clinical trials in the United States, and there is a preliminary suggestion that this compound may be useful in certain obsessive-compulsive conditions.

MONOAMINE OXIDASE INHIBITORS

The MAO inhibitors appear to effect their antidepressant action, in part, by blocking the metabolic degradation of brain norepinephrine and/or serotonin by MAO. More recently, this antidepressant action has been related to enhanced transmission in critical noradrenergic systems, with subsequent downregulation of presynaptic and postsynaptic noradrenergic receptors. Iproniazid, the first MAO inhibitor useful in treating depression, has been removed from the market because of its reported association with hepatotoxicity (2).

Dosage and Monitoring of Therapeutic Response

In addition, there has been a traditional reluctance to use other MAO inhibitors because of reports of marked toxicity and dangerous interactions with other agents, as well as unfavorable results in placebo-controlled clinical trials (2). However, there has been a more recent renaissance of interest in the MAO inhibitors following the demonstration of outcome results in the treatment of depression similar to those of the standard HCAs with doses of phenelzine (Nardil) high enough to inhibit blood platelet MAO activity by more than 85 percent (39,62). The correlation between inhibition of platelet MAO (mainly type B in humans) and significant clinical efficacy has resulted in the currently accepted clinical practice of often using relatively high doses of phenelzine (45 to 90 mg/day). Preliminary data suggest that this approach may also be feasible with another hydrazine MAO inhibitor, isocarboxazid (Marplan) but probably not with the nonhydrazine MAO inhibitor tranylcypromine (Parnate), which produces strong MAO inhibition at clinically ineffective doses (7).

Inhibition of platelet MAO is probably not a useful test for the experimental propargylamine MAO inhibitor clorgyline either, because this compound is selective against type A MAO. Type A MAO is present in brain, skin, and human gut but is not in human platelets. Although some evidence indicates that another experimental propargylamine compound, depenyl, which is selective as a type B MAO inhibitor, may be safer than other MAO inhibitors with respect to toxicity, it appears to be less effective than the other MAO inhibitors as an antidepressant (63). It is interesting that the prototype propargylamine MAO inhibitor pargyline (Eutonyl) is currently used primarily as an antihypertensive rather than as an antidepressant (64), although it has been advocated for the concurrent treatment of depression and mild to moderate hypertension. However, this use of pargyline has not been carefully evaluated in prospective, controlled clinical trials. The potential blood-pressure-lowering effect of pargyline and other MAO inhibitors appears to be related, at least in part, to the neuronal accumulation and release of the weak adrenergic false neurotransmitter octopamine.

A number of drugs of the hydrazine class, including phenelzine, undergo metabolism via acetylation. Rates of acetylation have strong genetic determinants and show substantial interindividual variation (65,66,67). Thus, on the basis of studies that have categorized patients by their rates of acetylation of isoniazid or one of the sulfa compounds, it has been suggested that the clinical effects of phenelzine treatment may be different in so-called fast as compared to slow acetylators. Side effects of phenelzine, for example, have been reported to be more common among slow acetylators (68), and Johnstone and March (69,70) have reported that slow acetylators may also show greater clinical responsiveness to phenelzine. However, since other investigators (67) have found no relationship between acetylator status and clinical response to phenelzine, this approach has not provided a useful clinical laboratory test.

Even considering the relatively recent advances that have been made regarding the MAO inhibitors, they are still not widely prescribed because of the need for prudent dietary restrictions as a safeguard against potential hypertensive crises; they are prescribed mostly for patients who are unresponsive or develop intolerable side effects to the HCAs. MAO inhibitors are also useful in patients who give a history of previous response to an MAO inhibitor and perhaps also in patients with rejection-sensitive (hysteroid) dysphoria, a mixed anxiety-depression state or phobic anxiety (see Chapter 1). The standard daily dosage range is 15 to 90 mg for phenelzine and 20 to 40 mg for tranylcypromine (Table 2.1).

Side Effects and Toxicity

With regard to side effects, MAO inhibitors have no significant anticholinergic activity (71), and hence, in contrast to the HCAs, they do not have troublesome anticholinergic side effects. However, hypertensive reactions can result if a patient treated with MAO inhibitor eats food rich in tyramine, dopamine, or tyrosine or is medicated with sympathomimetic compounds (see Chapter 9). Foods that need to be regulated during treatment with MAO inhibitors include aged cheese, yogurt, chianti wine, foreign beer, coffee, liver, snails, pickled herring, cream, chocolate, broad beans, citrus fruits, raisins, soy sauce, yeast products, bananas, avocados, and canned figs. Some medications that are relatively contraindicated when patients are treated with MAO inhibitors include L-dopa, epinephrine, norepinephrine, methylphenidate, dextroamphetamine, ephedrine, phenylephrine, and antihistamines.

Because combined HCA and MAO inhibitor therapy may also produce a central adrenergic syndrome characterized by hypertension, hyperpyrexia, and grand mal seizures, a drug-free period of two weeks is recommended before switching from an MAO inhibitor to an HCA or vice versa. Ananth and Luchins (72) contend, however, that it is less dangerous to start the two drugs concomitantly or to start the HCA first than to add an HCA once an MAO inhibitor has been started (see Chapter 9).

MAO inhibitors irreversibly destroy MAO, and the process of producing new MAO takes about two weeks. Therefore, as noted with the HCAs, patients should be advised to wait two weeks before taking an incompatible drug or eating tyramine-containing foods after they have discontinued an MAO inhibitor.

If a hypertensive reaction to an MAO inhibitor does occur (more likely after the second or third week than the first), then the patient should receive immediate attention. Treatment approaches may include the following:

- Administration of a vasodilator drug:

    An α-adrenergic blocking agent such as phentolamine, initially 5 mg IV slowly with subsequent treatment adjusted to response, or phenoxybenzamine, with 100 mg in 250 ml of a 5 percent dextrose solution infused over 90 to 120 minutes;

    Diazoxide, in a dosage of 300 mg IV slowly, may be preferable in some cases. The decrease in blood pressure usually lasts two to eight hours, and treatment can be repeated as indicated;

    Sodium nitroprusside, freshly prepared, 50 to 100 mg in 500 ml of 5 percent dextrose in water, may be advisable in severer cases. Continuous blood pressure monitoring is needed to titrate the therapeutic effect.

- Concomitant administration of a diuretic is advisable since the vasodilator may cause fluid retention. Furosemide, 40 mg IV slowly, is an effective adjunct because it both counteracts fluid retention and reduces blood pressure.

- In cases of MAO inhibitor overdosage, dialysis and hemoperfusion with exchange resin column may be useful (65,72,73,74).

- The treatment of malignant hyperpyrexia includes antipyretic drugs, topical cooling agents, and in the presence of serious convulsive episodes, curarization.

- Patients should be observed closely for several hours to several days after recovery from the acute event, until cardiovascular and other physiological parameters have clearly stabilized.

Because MAO inhibitors can also potentially exert a blood-pressure-lowering action, adding them to antihypertensive drug regimens may result in an additive effect (as with the HCAs). A small downward adjustment in the antihypertensive drug dosage is usually all that is required to counteract this potential drug-drug interaction, although some patients may not require another antihypertensive agent in addition to the MAO inhibitor.

Some patients who receive hydrazine MAO inhibitors develop a generalized edema. This effect usually subsides within a week or two although, uncommonly, it may persist longer. Dosage reduction does not appear to hasten the reduction of this side effect, which should not be confused with weight gain from increased caloric intake that is more common. Since inappropriate antidiuretic hormone secretion (SIADH) and hyponatremia have been reported as a syndrome associated with antidepressant medications, electrolytes should be evaluated when edema or other signs and symptoms of electrolyte imbalance are present. Peripheral neuropathy which is pyridoxine-reversible (25 mg/day) has also been associated with MAO inhibitors.

ATYPICAL ANTIDEPRESSANTS

Of the antidepressant agents that have been introduced, a number of which are currently experimental, most are pharmacologically similar to the imipraminelike HCAs. However, a few, such as iprindole, mianserin, trazodone, bupropion, and alprazolam, are considered to be atypical antidepressants in that they are neither MAO inhibitors nor do they exert significant blocking action on the neuronal reuptake inactivation of the monoamine neurotransmitters. However, it appears that most, if not all, antidepressant treatments, including the "second generation" atypical antidepressants, produce alterations in synaptic receptor sensitivity after long-term administration. Postsynaptic β-adrenergic sensitivity is reduced, while postsynaptic serotonergic and α-adrenergic stimulation are enhanced. Trazodone (Desyrel) has been approved for clinical use in the United States as an antidepressant agent. The tri-azolobenzodiazepine alprazolam (Xanax), which has been used previously as an antianxiety agent, has also been demonstrated to be an effective antidepressant, at slightly higher doses, for moderately depressed patients and patients with anxious depression or mixed anxiety-depression accompanied by somatic symptoms (75).

The purported major advantage of these atypical agents is their lack of certain undesirable side effects associated with the typical HCAs—most specifically, adverse anticholinergic and cardiovascular effects (including orthostatic hypotension). Nevertheless, trazodone has been reported to enhance myocardial irritability, and precipitate or aggravate cardiac arrhythmias (76). It appears that these compounds also are probably not as lethal in overdose when compared to the typical HCAs. For example, animal toxicity data show that trazodone is relatively safe, and no fatal overdoses that are attributable to trazodone ingestion in humans are reported in the literature (77). However, the possibility of a contribution to death from overdose involving ethanol or other medicinals must always be considered.

An important issue that is not completely resolved is how effective these atypical agents are in severely depressed or melancholic patients, since they have been most carefully evaluated in clinical trials involving outpatients with anxiety, somatic symptoms, and mild to moderate depression (7). Also, there is some concern that the supposed antidepressant effects of the atypical compounds may be largely anxiolytic or sedative actions. Yet evidence in regard to iprindole suggests that it may be even less anxiolytic than imipramine (78) and alprazolam's effect on depressive symptoms cannot be explained by its anxiolytic and sedative actions alone (75).

LITHIUM

In the late 1940s, John Cade discovered that lithium caused sedation in guinea pigs and reasoned that it might calm manic patients. He subsequently administered the drug to ten manic patients and reported substantial improvement in all of them (79). Since Cade's original report, a number of controlled investigations (80,81,82,83) have shown that lithium is effective in treating mania in over 80 percent of the patients studied.

Indications for Lithium Therapy

Lithium is currently the drug of choice in the treatment of mania (84). However, since seven to fourteen days may be required for lithium to exert a substantial clinical effect, a neuroleptic drug, in addition to lithium therapy, may be required initially in the treatment of moderate to severe, acute mania (see Chapter 3 for neuroleptic dosage). In some patients, continued use of the neuroleptic together with the lithium may be advantageous.

Cade (79) originally reported that lithium was not effective in the acute treatment of depression, and subsequent studies (85,86,87,88,89) have likewise reported that lithium does not have antidepressant activity. However, a number of other investigators (83,90,91,92,93,94) have found that lithium does have an antidepressant effect, especially in bipolar patients. Lithium has also been shown to potentiate the antidepressant effects of the HCAs, as previously discussed.

The prophylactic use of lithium was first reported in 1963 by Hartigan (87) and indicated that maintenance treatment with lithium carbonate prevented manic as well as depressive relapses in bipolar patients. Since then, a number of well-controlled studies (84,95,96,97,98) have clearly demonstrated the prophylactic effectiveness of lithium in preventing the recurrence of manic and depressive episodes in bipolar patients. A number of investigators (84,95,96) have also reported that lithium is prophylactically effective in preventing recurrent depressions in some unipolar patients, although some controversy exists as to whether these patients display variants of bipolar manic-depressive illness, manifested as recurrent, clinically significant depression with mild, spontaneous, subclinical euphoria or hyperactivity and mild insomnia (bipolar type II disorder) (99).

Substantial debate also has occurred concerning the effectiveness of lithium in treating schizophrenia. A number of investigators (100,101,102,103, 104) have reported that lithium is ineffective and may even be harmful in treating schizophrenia. Recently, in contrast, Alexander et al. (105) have reported a controlled study that showed that schizophrenic patients are responsive to lithium. In addition, Hirschowitz et al. (106) have reported that lithium is effective in treating so-called good-prognosis schizophrenia. Moreover, several investigators (107,108,109,110) have reported that lithium may be effective in treating schizoaffective patients, especially when the lithium is used as an adjunct to neuroleptic therapy. However, these reports must necessarily be tempered with support for the view that schizoaffective disorders cannot be distinguished meaningfully from bipolar manic-depressive illness (7) and that a number of so-called schizophrenics may be suffering from an affective illness.

Lithium therapy may also be effective in some cases of chronic alcoholism (111), impulsive aggressiveness (112), premenstrual tension (113), and cluster headaches (114,115), as well as in the prophylactic treatment of corticotropin-induced psychosis (116).

Dosages and Therapeutic Blood Level Monitoring

Lithium has no metabolites and is excreted almost entirely by the kidney in unchanged form with a half-life of about twenty-four hours. Lithium excretion is influenced by sodium intake and sodium excretion so that patients on low sodium diets will retain lithium. Patients who use sodium-depleting diuretics, who perspire heavily in hot weather, who have sodium-depleting diarrhea, and who have high fevers will also retain lithium. Although patients can be treated simultaneously with lithium and thiazide diuretics, careful observation and about a 30 percent reduction in the lithium dosage is usually required (117). Other conditions may require sodium replacement therapy as well as a reduction in the lithium dosage.

Prior to starting lithium therapy, kidney function should be evaluated. Since lithium is excreted primarily by the kidneys, patients with impaired renal function may be particularly susceptible to lithium toxicity. Baseline thyroid functions are also useful prior to starting treatment since lithium can produce thyroid side effects. If cardiovascular or renal disease is present, lithium treatment may require close monitoring.

In the United States, standard lithium carbonate is available in 300 mg capsules and tablets. Two slow-release lithium carbonate preparations are available—namely, Lithobid (300 mg) and Eskalith CG (450 mg). Lithium citrate, a liquid, contains 8 mEq/5 cc, the equivalent of 300 mg of lithium carbonate.

The recommended starting dosage for acute manic attacks in adults under 50 years of age is 600 mg three times a day (1,800 mg/day). Once remission occurs, 900 to 1,500 mg/day in divided doses is often required, and treatment programs must be carefully individualized within a range of about 600 to 3,600 mg/day.

Blood samples for serum lithium determinations should always be drawn as closely as possible to twelve hours after the last dose. Following initiation of treatment or change in dosage, approximately four to five days are required to reach steady-state serum levels. Consequently, unless toxicity is a concern, measuring serum levels more often than every five days is redundant and misleading. When the clinical condition of the patient and the blood level are stable, levels can be routinely monitored at longer intervals but usually should not exceed every three months. However, levels should also be checked whenever clinical conditions so indicate (118).

Although efforts to correlate serum levels absolutely with clinical response have been unsuccessful, therapeutic ranges have been developed. Most reports place the minimum effective level for the treatment of acute mania at 0.8 mEq/L and the maximum at 1.5 mEq/L. Because of interindividual differences in response and sensitivity, it is best to start at lower levels and increase the dosage, if necessary and tolerated. Recommended levels for the acute treatment of depression are similar, although they are based on less substantial data. For maintenance therapy, lower serum concentrations are usually required—between 0.6 and 1.2 m Eq/L. Some patients, including the elderly, can do well on even lower maintenance levels.

Side Effects and Toxicity

Severe toxic effects occur most often at serum levels above 1.5 mEq/L. With levels above 3 mEq/L, treatment with hemodialysis may be required to prevent serious complications. Serum lithium levels above 3.5 mEq/L may be frankly life threatening (118,119).

We should emphasize that close monitoring of side effects, not serum lithium levels, is the ultimate criterion for lithium toxicity. Cases of severe toxicity have been reported with serum lithium levels below 1.6 mEq/L (120), and elderly patients (121) and patients with preexisting brain damage (122) may be particularly susceptible to toxicity at therapeutic serum levels. If a patient develops signs and symptoms of lithium toxicity, then the lithium should be discontinued or decreased, regardless of the serum lithium level. Signs and symptoms of lithium toxicity or overdosage include weakness, ataxia, drowsiness, dysarthria, blurred vision, tinnitus, nausea, vomiting, hyperactive deep tendon reflexes, nystagmus, confusion, seizures, and coma.

Many patients will develop polydipsia and polyuria during their first few days of lithium therapy. This may resolve during the first week of treatment, although 5 to 10 percent of patients develop or sustain significant polyuria (daily output of urine in excess of four liters) and polydipsia after prolonged lithium therapy. This side effect may be manageable if the daily intake of salt and protein is reduced and a single daily dose treatment regimen is instituted. The addition of a thiazide diuretic to the lithium regimen can also be useful in treating this nephrogenic (vasopressin-resistant) diabetes insipidus-like syndrome. Concurrent administration of a thiazide diuretic has a paradoxical antidiuretic effect. Because this treatment is associated with lithium retention, it is usually necessary to lower the daily lithium dose. In some cases, lithium therapy may need to be discontinued and a trial course of carbamazepine instituted, as discussed below.

The possibility that lithium can produce structural renal damage is a controversial area. In 1977, Hestbach et al. (123) reported that fourteen patients on chronic lithium therapy had a significant reduction in creatinine clearance associated with nonspecific chronic renal lesions, including tubular atrophy, interstitial fibrosis, and glomerulosclerosis. Scully et al. (124) have reported a case of renal failure secondary to chronic interstitial nephritis that was possibly related to lithium therapy. Gerner et al. (125) did extensive testing of renal function in forty-three patients who had been taking lithium from 1 to 120 months. Their only abnormal finding was that the urine-concentrating ability of these patients was mildly to moderately impaired. Depaulo et al. (126) studied renal function in ninety-nine lithium-treated patients and reported a relationship between chronic lithium therapy and declining glomerular filtration rate. However, although lithium may cause some renal damage resulting in concentrating defects and concomitant polyuria, the consensus is that serious renal damage in patients treated with therapeutic serum levels of lithium is uncommon (124). It is interesting that lithium treatment can also result in pretibial and pedal edema, apparently unrelated to serious renal damage.

Lithium treatment, in some patients, can produce nausea, vomiting, and diarrhea. To control gastric distress, lithium is usually prescribed in small divided doses during the day and can also be prescribed with meals. Leukocytosis with white blood cell counts in the range of 10,000 to 14,000 has also been associated with lithium administration (119).

An increased incidence of cardiac abnormalities in the offspring of mothers treated with lithium during pregnancy and lithium-induced teratogenicity in animals have also been reported (127). Thus, lithium therapy should be avoided, if possible, during pregnancy, especially during the first trimester. Lithium should also be avoided, if possible, during nursing since it is excreted in breast milk (127).

Despite the frequency and diversity of lithium-associated changes in thyroid function, clinical manifestations are relatively uncommon (118). Clinical hypothyroidism and/or goiter have been estimated to occur in 5 percent of patients treated with lithium, and lithium-associated hyperthyroidism is much less common. Several studies reported the incidence of thyroid dysfunction in lithium-treated patients to be significantly higher in women (128,129). Lithium may also cause a biochemical hyperparathyroidism, with increased serum calcium concentrations, decreased serum phosphate concentrations, and decreased urinary calcium excretion (130,131,132,133,134,135).

Neurological side effects associated with lithium treatment include a hand tremor that can often be alleviated by the addition of 15 to 60 mg per day of propranolol to the lithium regimen. Lithium can also produce cogwheel rigidity (136,137,138,139), which is not responsive to anticholinergic medication.

Some evidence indicates that concomitant treatment with a neuroleptic and lithium may be associated, in some cases, with serious neurotoxicity. Cohen and Cohen (140) reported a series of four patients who developed serious, irreversible neurological complications while they were being treated with lithium and haloperidol. A careful review of these cases, however, raises the question of whether or not these patients were suffering from an encephalitis or some other illness not associated with drug toxicity. Baastrup et al. (141) retrospectively reviewed the records of 425 patients who had been treated with lithium plus haloperidol and found no cases of the type of neurotoxicity described by Cohen and Cohen. In 1979, Spring (142,143) described six cases of toxicity associated with combined neuroleptic and lithium therapy, five with thioridazine, and one with fluphenazine. Spring and Frankel (144) later reported a case of toxicity associated with combined lithium and haloperidol therapy and characterized by hyperpyrexia, severe rigidity, mutism, and the development of irreversible tardive dyskinesia. Although the incidence, dosages, length of treatment, types of neuroleptics, and other critical features of this presumably drug-drug interaction are unclear, caution is warranted when a neuroleptic and lithium are used concurrently until the issue of potential neurotoxicity is clarified.

Biological Markers

With regard to biological tests associated with lithium response, Sullivan et al. (145) have reported a positive association between platelet MAO activity and response to lithium therapy in manic patients. Subsequent studies by Nurnberger et al. (146) and Sullivan et al. (147) have indicated that platelet MAO activity is also associated with responsiveness to lithium in individuals with depression. Studies with multiple biological variables indicate that platelet MAO activity, augmentation of the average evoked response, and plasma dopamine-β-hydroxylase activity are positively correlated with lithium response in depressed patients, such that these three factors account for 44 percent of the variance in the response to lithium treatment (146). Although these observations suggest potentially useful clinical applications, more work is needed, including clarification of whether at least some of these markers are diagnostic measures of bipolar illness or affective disorder rather than lithium response per se. Other laboratory tests which may be useful in predicting lithium response are discussed in Chapter 5.

CARBAMAZEPINE

Carbamazepine, an anticonvulsant that has also been used effectively in other clinical conditions, has emerged as a potentially useful pharmacologic agent in the treatment of lithium refractory bipolar affective disorders (148,149,150, 151). Okuma and associates have shown an acute antimanic effect for carbamazepine equal to chlorpromazine, as did Ballenger and Post, who worked with a smaller patient sample. The latter investigators also indicated that many of their carbamazepine responders were unresponsive to lithium. Carbamazepine also appears to have antidepressant properties, although the data are not as extensive as the studies on acute mania.

Evidence has also been presented in regard to prophylatic benefits for carbamazepine in the treatment of cycling manic depressives. Ballenger and Post reported on four patients whose cycling was interrupted, and Okuma performed a double-blind study in which sixty percent of the patients had a prophylactic response that was at least moderately effective (150). Both groups indicated that lithium nonresponders responded to carbamazepine (148, 149,150).

Carbamazepine is also an antidiuretic agent that is used as a primary treatment for diabetes insipidus. The antidiuretic effect of carbamazepine is attributed to the induction of increased renal sensitivity to antidiuretic hormone (ADH), although central ADH release has been implicated as well. In manic-depressive, and, perhaps, schizoaffective illness associated with resistant, lithium-induced nephrogenic diabetes insipidus, carbamazepine may serve the dual therapeutic purpose of psychotropic agent as well as antidiuretic agent (152).

Carbamazepine is rapidly absorbed after oral administration, reaching peak levels in two to six hours, although there is considerable individual variability in metabolism. The therapeutic range for epilepsy is 4 to 12 μg/ml, and preliminary work suggests a therapeutic range of 6 to 12 μg/ml for manic-depressive disease (148,150). The full maintenance dose of carbamazepine (100 or 200 mg tablets) is usually in the range of 7 to 15 mg/kg/day for adults, divided into two or four doses. However, in order to avoid toxic side effects, the full maintenance dose should be gradually achieved over a three-week interval.

In summary, carbamazepine may be a useful alternative in the treatment of some lithium-refractory patients, including possibly those who are not able to tolerate lithium side effects. Carbamazepine has been used in combination with phenothiazines, butyrophenones, and tricyclic antidepressants without serious adverse effects (150). However, use with MAO inhibitors is not recommended (150,153), and reports regarding the safety of carbamazepine in combination with lithium are conflicting (154,155,156).

Side effects associated with carbamazepine use are similar to those found with other anticonvulsants and include, most commonly, dizziness, ataxia, slurred speech, clumsiness, diplopia, and drowsiness. These side effects are usually manageable by dosage adjustment. Cardiovascular, genitourinary, metabolic, and hepatic adverse effects appear to be quite infrequent. The most serious side effects are hematologic, with bone marrow suppression, aplastic anemia, and thrombocytopenia (148,150,153), although such adverse reactions appear to be rare. Nevertheless, physicians should be alert to signs or symptoms of fever, sore throat, petechiae, or hemorrhage in patients receiving carbamazepine, and a complete blood count should be obtained weekly for the first month of treatment, every other week for the second month, and then monthly for a period of time to observe for possible suppression of hematologic indexes.

NEW TREATMENTS FOR MANIC-DEPRESSIVE DISEASE

Two agents which may be useful as possible innovative treatments for bipolar patients in whom lithium, lithium plus a neuroleptic, or carbamazepine therapy is either ineffective or toxic are the antihypertensive clonidine (17 μg/kg/day orally in three divided doses) and the anticonvulsant benzodiazepine clonazepam (2 to 16 mg/day in divided doses) (157). Potentiation of lithium by tryptophan (6 to 9 grams/day in divided doses) is another possibly useful strategy for selected patients (158). However, the studies with these compounds are still preliminary, and more work needs to be done in order to carefully evaluate the possible role of these agents in the treatment of manic-depressive disease. For example, clonidine may raise the seizure threshold, which can complicate electroconvulsive therapy.

REFERENCES

1. Hollister, L.E. Tricyclic antidepressants. *N. Engl. J. Med.* 299:1106–1109, 1168–1172, 1978.
2. Baldessarini, R.J. *Chemotherapy in Psychiatry*. Cambridge: Harvard University Press, 1977.
3. Baldessarini, R.J. Drugs and the treatment of psychiatric disorders. In *The Pharmacological Basis of Therapeutics*, 6th ed., Gilman, A.G., Goodman, L.S., and Gilman, A., eds. New York: Macmillan, 1980, pp. 391–447.

4. Rogers, S.C., and Clay, P.M. A statistical review of controlled studies of imipramine and placebo in the treatment of depressive illnesses. *Br. J. Psychiat.* 127: 599–603, 1975.

5. Shepherd, M.; Lader, M.; and Rodnight, R. *Clinical Psychopharmacology.* London: The English Universities Press Ltd., 1968, p. 145.

6. Axelrod, J.; Whitby, L.G.; and Hertting, G. Effect of psychotropic drugs on the uptake of H^3-norepinephrine by tissues. *Science* 133:383–384, 1961.

7. Baldessarini, R.J. *Biomedical Aspects of Depression and Its Treatment.* Washington, D.C.: American Psychiatric Press, Inc., 1983.

8. Vetulani, J.; Stawarz, R.J.; and Dingell, J.V.; A possible common mechanism of action of antidepressant treatments. *Naunyn-Schmiedeberg's Arch. Pharmacol.* 293: 109–114, 1976.

9. Peroutka, S.J., and Snyder, S.H. Long-term antidepressant treatment decreases spiroperidol-labeled serotonin receptor binding. *Science* 210:88–90, 1980.

10. Crews, F.T.; Paul, S.M.; and Goodwin, F.K. Acceleration of β-receptor desensitization in combined administration of antidepressants and phenoxybenzamine. *Nature* 290:787–789, 1981.

11. Chiodo, L., and Antelman, S.M. Repeated tricyclics induce a progressive dopamine autoreceptor subsensitivity independent of daily drug treatment. *Nature* 287:451–454, 1980.

12. Serra, G.; Argiolas, A.; and Klimek, V. Chronic treatment with antidepressants prevents the inhibitory effect of small doses of apomorphine on dopamine synthesis and motor activity. *Life Sciences* 25:415–424, 1979.

13. Chiodo, L., and Antelman, S.M. Electroconvulsive shock: Progressive dopamine autoreceptor subsensitivity independent of repeated treatment. *Science* 210: 799–801, 1980.

14. Paul, S.M.; Rehavi, M.; and Skolnick, P. Depressed patients have decreased binding of tritiated imipramine to platelet serotonin 'transporter'. *Arch. Gen. Psychiat.* 38:1315–1317, 1981.

15. Burrows, G.D., and Davis, B. Antidepressants and barbiturates. *Br. Med. J.* 3:331–334, 1971.

16. Glassman, A.H., and Perel, J.M. The clinical pharmacology of imipramine. *Arch. Gen. Psychiat.* 28:649–653, 1973.

17. Nies, A.; Robinson, D.S.; Friedman, M.J.; Green, R.; Cooper, T.B.; Ravaris, C.L.; and Ives, J.O. Relationship between age and tricyclic antidepressant plasma levels. *Am. J. Psychiat.* 134:790–793, 1977.

18. Hollister, L.E. Doxepin hydrochloride. *Ann. Intern. Med.* 81:360–363, 1974.

19. Cooper, T.B.; Simpson, G.M.; and Lee, T.H. Thymoleptic and neuroleptic drug plasma levels in psychiatry: Current status. *Int. Rev. Neurobiol.* 19:269–309, 1976.

20. Baldessarini, R.J. Status of psychotropic drug blood level assays and other biochemical measurements in clinical practice. *Am. J. Psychiat.* 136:1177–1180, 1979.

21. Risch, S.C.; Janowsky, D.S.; and Huey, L.Y. Plasma levels of tricyclic antidepressants and clinical efficacy. In *Antidepressants: Neurochemical, Behavioral, and Clinical Perspectives*, Enna, S.J., Malick, J.B., and Richelson, E., eds. New York: Raven Press, 1981, pp. 183–217.

22. Laboratory tests for patients taking psychotropic drugs. *Massachusetts General Hospital Newsletter-Biological Therapies in Psychiatry* 6:5–7, 1983.

23. Rudorfer, M.V. Tricyclic antidepressant plasma levels in overdose. *JAMA* 245:703–704, 1981.

24. Fawcett, J., and Siomopoulos, V. Dextroamphetamine response as a possible predictor of improvement with tricyclic therapy in depression. *Arch. Gen. Psychiat.* 25:247–255, 1971.
25. Van Kammen, D.P., and Murphy, D.L. Prediction of imipramine antidepressant response by a one-day *d*-amphetamine trial. *Am. J. Psychiat.* 135:1179–1184, 1978.
26. Goodwin, F.K.; Prange, A.J.; Post, R.M.; Muscettola, G.; and Lipton, M.A. Potentiation of antidepressant effects by L-triiodothyronine in tricyclic nonresponders. *Am. J. Psychiat.* 139:34–38, 1982.
27. Lingjaerde, O.; Edlund, A.H.; and Gormsen, C.A. The effect of lithium carbonate in combination with tricyclic antidepressants in endogenous depression. *Acta Psychiatr. Scand.* 50:233–242, 1974.
28. De Montigny, C.; Grunberg, F.; Mayer, A.; and Deschenes, J.P. Lithium induces rapid relief of depression in tricyclic antidepressant drug non-responders. *Br. J. Psychiat.* 138:252–256, 1981.
29. Heninger, G.R.; and Charney, D.S. Lithium potentiation of antidepressant treatment. Presented at the annual meeting of the American Psychiatric Association, May 1982 (New Research Abstracts 66).
30. Linnoila, M.; George, L.; Guthrie, S. Interaction between antidepressants and perphenazine in psychiatric patients. *Am. J. Psychiat.* 139:1329–1331, 1982.
30a. Perry, P.J.; Morgan, D.E.; Smith, R.E.; and Tsuang, M.T. Treatment of unipolar depression accompanied by delusions: ECT versus tricyclic antidepressant-antipsychotic combinations. *J. Affective Disorders.* 4:195-200, 1982.
31. Taska, R.J. Clinical laboratory aids in the treatment of depression: Tricyclic antidepressant plasma levels and urinary MHPG. *Current Concepts in Psychiatry* 3:12–20, 1977.
32. Everett, H.C. The use of bethanechol chloride with tricyclic antidepressants. *Am. J. Psychiat.* 132:1202–1204, 1975.
33. Davidson, J., and Wenger, T. Using antidepressants in patients with cardiovascular disease. *Drug Therapy* 6:169–178, 1982.
34. Glassman, A.H., and Bigger, J.T. Cardiovascular effects of therapeutic doses of tricyclic antidepressants. *Arch. Gen. Psychiat.* 38:815–820, 1981.
35. Glassman, A.H. Clinical characteristics of imipramine-induced orthostatic hypotension. *Lancet* 1:468–472, 1979.
36. Veith, R.C.; Raskind, M.A.; Caldwell, J.H.; Barnes, R.F.; Gumbrecht, G.; and Ritchie, J.L. Cardiovascular effects of tricyclic antidepressants in depressed patients with chronic heart disease. *N. Engl. J. Med.* 305:954–959, 1982.
37. Dowling, S.; Lynn, K.; and Rosser, R. Nortriptyline metabolism in chronic renal failure: metabolite elimination. *Clin. Pharm. Ther.* 32:322–329, 1982.
38. Itil, T.M., and Myers, J.P. Epileptic and anti-epileptic properties of psychotropic drugs. In *International Encyclopedia of Pharmacology and Therapeutics*, 19 vols., Mercier, J., ed. 2:599–622, 1973.
39. Robinson, D.S.; Nies, A.; and Ravaris, C.L. Clinical pharmacology of phenelzine. *Arch. Gen. Psychiat.* 35:629–635, 1978.
40. van Scheyen, J.D., and Van Kammen, D.P. Clomipramine-induced mania in unipolar depression. *Arch. Gen. Psychiat.* 36:560, 1979.
41. Prusoff, B.A.; Williams, D.H.; Weissman, M.W.; and Astrachan, B.M. Treatment of secondary depression in schizophrenia. *Arch. Gen. Psychiat.* 36:569–575, 1979.
42. Comfort, A. Effects of psychotropic drugs on ejaculation. *Am. J. Psychiat.* 136:124–125, 1979.

43. Baldessarini, R.J., and Tarsy, D. Tardive dyskinesia. In *Psychopharmacology: A Generation of Progress*, Lipton, M.A., DiMascio, A., and Killam, R.F., eds. New York: Raven Press, 1978, pp. 993–1004.
44. Rosenbaum, A.H.; Maruta, T.; and Duane, D.D. Tardive dyskinesia in depressed patients: successful therapy with antidepressants and lithium. *Psychosomatics* 21:715–719, 1980.
45. Klerman, G.L. Long-term treatment of affective disorders. In *Psychopharmacology: A Generation of Progress*, Lipton, M.A., DiMascio, A., and Killam, K.F., eds. New York: Raven Press, 1978, pp. 1303–1312.
46. Davis, J.M. Overview: Maintenance therapy in psychiatry: II. Affective disorders. *Am. J. Psychiat.* 133:1–3, 1976.
47. Cooper, A.; Ghose, K.; Montgomery, S.; Ramarao, V.A.; Bailey, J.; and Jorgensen, A. Continuation therapy with amitriptyline in depression. *Br. J. Psychiat.* 133:28–33, 1978.
48. Quitkin, F.; Rifkin, A.; and Klein, D.F. Prophylaxis of affective disorders: current status of knowledge. *Arch. Gen. Psychiat.* 33:337–341, 1976.
49. Seager, C.P., and Bird, R.L. Imipramine with electrical treatment in depression—A controlled trial. *J. Ment. Sci.* 108:704–707, 1962.
50. Kramer, J.C.; Klein, D.F.; and Fink, M. Withdrawal symptoms following discontinuation of imipramine therapy. *Am. J. Psychiat.* 118:549–550, 1961.
51. Biggs, J.T.; Spiker, D.C.; Petit, J.M.; and Ziegler, V.E. Tricyclic antidepressant overdose: Incidence of symptoms. *JAMA* 238:135–138, 1977.
52. Greenland, P., and Howe, T.A. Cardiac monitoring in tricyclic antidepressant overdose. *Heart and Lung* 10:856–859, 1981.
53. Pentel, P., and Sious, L. Incidence of late arrhythmias following tricyclic antidepressant overdose. *Clinical Toxicology* 18:543–548, 1981.
54. Fasoli, R.A., and Glauser, F.L. Cardiac arrhythmias and ECG abnormalities in tricyclic antidepressant overdose. *Clinical Toxicology* 18:155–163, 1981.
55. Hoffman, J.R., and McElroy, C.R. Bicarbonate therapy for dysrhythmia and hypotension in tricyclic antidepressant overdose. *Western J. Med.* 134:60–64, 1981.
56. Uhl, J.A. Phenytoin: The drug of choice in tricyclic antidepressant overdose? *Ann. Emerg. Med.* 10:270–274, 1981.
57. Ahmad, S. Cardiovascular complications of tricyclic antidepressant overdose. *Ann. Emerg. Med.* 9:281, 1980.
58. Pedersen, R.S. Haemoperfusion in tricyclic antidepressant poisoning (letter). *Lancet* 1:154–155, 1980.
59. Heath, A.; Wickstrom, I.; and Ahlmen, J. Haemoperfusion in tricyclic antidepressant poisoning (letter). *Lancet* 1:155, 1980.
60. Trafford, A.; Sharpstone, P.; and O'Neal, H. Haemoperfusion in tricyclic antidepressant poisoning (letter). *Lancet* 1:155, 1980.
61. Calesnick, B. Tricyclic antidepressant toxicity. *Am. Fam. Physician* 21:104–106, 1980.
62. Murphy, D.L.; Brand, E.; and Goldman, T. Platelet and plasma amine oxidase inhibition and urinary amine excretion changes during phenelzine treatment. *J. Nerv. Ment. Dis.* 164:129–134, 1977.
63. Mendis, N.; Pare, C.M.B.; and Sandler, M. Is the failure of (−)deprenyl, a selective monoamine oxidase B inhibitor, to alleviate depression related to freedom from the cheese effect? *Psychopharmacology* 73:87–90, 1981.
64. Levy, B.F. Treatment of hypertension with pargyline hydrochloride. *Curr. Ther. Res.* 8:343–346, 1966.

65. Evans, D.A.P.; Manley, K.A.; and McKusick, V. Genetic control of isoniazid metabolism in man. *Br. Med. J.* 2:485–491, 1960.

66. Evans, D.A.P., and White, T.A. Human acetylation polymorphism. *J. Lab. Clin. Med.* 63:391–403, 1964.

67. Maas, J.W., and Landis, D.H. In vivo studies of metabolism of norepinephrine in the central nervous system. *J. Pharmacol. Exper. Ther.* 163:147–162, 1968.

68. Evans, D.A.P.; Davison, K.; Pratt, R.I.C. The influence of acetylator phenotype on the effects of treating depression with phenelzine. *Clin. Pharmac. Ther.* 6:430–435, 1965.

69. Johnstone, E.C., and Marsh, W. Acetylator status and response to phenelzine in depressed patients. *Lancet* 1:567–570, 1973.

70. Johnstone, E.C. The relationship between acetylator status and inhibition of monoamine oxidase, excretion of free drug and antidepressant response in depressed patients on phenelzine. *Psychopharmacology* 46:289–294, 1976.

71. Snyder, S.H., and Yamamura, H.I. Antidepressants and the muscarinic acetylcholine receptor. *Arch. Gen. Psychiat.* 34:235–239, 1977.

72. Ananth, J., and Luchins, D. A review of combined tricyclic and MAOI therapy. *Comprehen. Psychiat.* 18:221–230, 1977.

73. Sheehan, D.V.; Claycomb, J.B.; and Kouretas, N. Monoamine oxidase inhibitors: Prescription and patient management. *Int'l. J. Psychiatry in Med.* 10:99–121, 1980.

74. Arena, J.M. T.M. poisoning—treatment and prevention. *JAMA* 232:1272–1275, 1975.

75. Feighner, J.P.; Aden, G.C.; Fabre, L.F.; Rickels, K.; and Smith, W.T. Comparison of alprazolam, imipramine, and placebo in the treatment of depression. *JAMA* 249:3057–3064, 1983.

76. Gelenberg, A.J., ed. Overdoses with trazodone (Desyrel). Massachusetts General Hospital Newsletter-Biological Therapies in Psychiatry 6:35–36, 1983.

77. Golden, R.N., and Gualtieri, C.T. A clinician's guide to the new antidepressants. *Medical Times* 111:101–107, 1983.

78. Rickels, K.; Chung, H.R.; and Csanalosi, I. Iprindole and imipramine in nonpsychotic depressed out-patients. *Br. J. Psychiat.* 123:329–339, 1973.

79. Cade, J.F.J. Lithium salts in the treatment of psychotic excitement. *Med. J. Australia* 36:349–352, 1949.

80. Schou, M.; Juel-Nielsen, N.; Stromgen, E.; and Vodby, H. The treatment of manic psychoses by the administration of lithium salts. *J. Neurol. Neurosurg. Psychiat.* 1:250–260, 1954.

81. Maggs, R. Treatment of manic illness with lithium carbonate. *Br. J. Psychiat.* 109:56–65, 1963.

82. Bunney, W.R., Jr.; Manson, J.W.; Roatch, J.F.; and Hamburg, D.A. A psychoendocrine study of severe psychotic depressive crises. *Am. J. Psychiat.* 122:72, 1965.

83. Goodwin, F.K.; Murphy, D.L.; and Bunney, W.E., Jr. Lithium carbonate treatment in depression and mania: A longitudinal double-blind study. *Arch. Gen. Psychiat.* 21:486–496, 1969.

84. Prien, R.F.; Klett, C.J.; and Caffey, F.M. Lithium carbonate and imipramine in prevention of affective disorders. *Arch. Gen. Psychiat.* 29:420–425, 1973.

85. Stokes, P.E.; Stoll, P.M.; Shamorian, C.A.; and Patton, M.J. Efficacy of lithium as acute treatment of manic-depressive illness. *Lancet* 1:1319–1325, 1971.

86. Gershon, S., and Yuwiler, A. Lithium ion: A specific pharmacological approach to the treatment of mania. *J. Neuropsychiat.* 1:229–251, 1960.

87. Hartigan, G.P. The use of lithium salts in affective disorders. *Br. J. Psychiat.* 109:810–814, 1963.

88. Gershon, S. Lithium prophylaxis in recurrent affective disorders. *Compr. Psychiat.* 15:365–373, 1974.

89. Fieve, R.R.; Platman, S.R.; and Plutchick, R.R. The use of lithium in affective disorders. I. Acute endogenous depression. *Am. J. Psychiat.* 125:487–491, 1968.

90. Goodwin, F.K.; Murphy, D.L.; and Dunner, D.L. Lithium response in unipolar vs. bipolar depression. *Am. J. Psychiat.* 129:44–47, 1972.

91. Mendels, J.; Secunda, S.K.; and Dyson, W.L. A controlled study of the antidepressant effects of lithium. *Arch. Gen. Psychiat.* 26:154–157, 1972.

92. Johnson, F. Antidepressant effects of lithium. *Compr. Psychiat.* 15:43–47, 1975.

93. Noyes, R.; Dempsey, G.M.; and Blum, A. Lithium treatment of depression. *Compr. Psychiat.* 15:187–190, 1974.

94. Mendels, J. Lithium in the treatment of depression. *Am. J. Psychiat.* 133:373–377, 1976.

95. Baastrup, P.C., and Schou, M. Lithium as a prophylactic agent: Its effect against recurrent depression and manic depressive psychosis. *Arch. Gen. Psychiat.* 16:167–172, 1967.

96. Coppen, A.; Noguera, R.; and Bailey, J. Prophylactic lithium in affective disorders. *Lancet* 2:275–279, 1971.

97. Hullin, R.P.; MacDonald, R.; and Allsopp, M.N.E. Prophylactic lithium in recurrent affective disorders. *Lancet* 1:1044–1046, 1972.

98. Stallone, F.; Shelley, E.; Mendlewicz, J.; and Fieve, R.R. The use of lithium in affective disorders. III. A double-blind study of prophylaxis in bipolar illness. *Am. J. Psychiat.* 130:1006–1010, 1973.

99. Fieve, R.R.; Kumbaraci, T.; and Dunner, D.L. Lithium prophylaxis of depression in bipolar I, bipolar II, and unipolar patients. *Am. J. Psychiat.* 133:925–929, 1976.

100. Hollister, L.E. Mental disorder—Antipsychotic and antimanic drugs. *N. Engl. J. Med.* 286:984–987, 1972.

101. Bailey, E.; Bond, P.A.; and Brooks, B.A. The medicinal chemistry of lithium. *Prog. Med. Chem.* 11:193–272, 1975.

102. Hekimian, L.J.; Gershon, S.; Hardesty, A.S. Drug efficacy and diagnostic specificity in manic depressive illness and schizophrenia. *Dis. Nerv. Syst.* 30:747–751, 1969.

103. Shopsin, B.; Kim, S.S.; and Gershon, S. A controlled study of lithium vs. chlorpromazine in acute schizophrenics. *Br. J. Psychiat.* 119:435–440, 1971.

104. Johnson, G. Differential response to lithium carbonate in manic depressive and schizoaffective disorders. *Dis. Nerv. Syst.* 31:613–615, 1970.

105. Alexander, P.E.; VanKammen, D.P.; and Bunney, W.E., Jr. Antipsychotic effects of lithium in schizophrenia. *Am. J. Psychiat.* 136:283–287, 1979.

106. Hirschowitz, J.; Casper, R.; Garver, D.L.; and Chang, S. Lithium response in good prognosis schizophrenia. *Am. J. Psychiat.* 137:916–920, 1980.

107. Taylor, M.A., and Abrams, R. The phenomenology of mania: A new look at some old patients. *Arch. Gen. Psychiat.* 29:550–552, 1973.

108. Dinsmore, P.R, and Ryback, R. Lithium in schizoaffective disorders. *Dis. Nerv. Syst.* 33:771–776, 1972.

109. Gleisinger, B. Evaluation of lithium treatment in treatment of psychotic excitement. *Med. J. Australia* 41:277–283, 1954.

110. Biederman, J.; Lerner, Y.; and Belmaker, R.H. Combination of lithium carbonate and haloperidol in schizoaffective disorder. *Arch. Gen. Psychiat.* 36:327–333, 1979.

111. Merry, J.; Reynolds, C.M.; Bailey, J.; and Coppen, A. Prophylactic treatment of alcoholism by lithium carbonate. A controlled study. *Lancet* 2:486–488, 1976.

112. Schou, M. The range of clinical uses of lithium. In *Lithium in Medical Practice,* Johnson, F.N., and Johnson, S., eds. Baltimore: University Park Press, 1978, pp. 21–39.

113. Sletten, I.W., and Gershon, S. The premenstrual syndrome: A discussion of pathophysiology and treatment with lithium ion. *Compr. Psychiat.* 7:197–206, 1966.

114. Ekbon, K. Lithium in the treatment of chronic cluster headache. *Headache* 17:39, 1977.

115. Kudrow, L. Lithium prophylaxis for chronic cluster headache. *Headache* 17:15, 1977.

116. Falk, W.E.; Mahnke, M.W.; and Poskanzer, D.C. Lithium prophylaxis or corticotropin-induced psychosis. *JAMA* 241:1011–1012, 1979.

117. Himmelhoch, J.M.; Forrest, J.; Neil, J.F.; and Detre, T.P. Thiazide-lithium synergy in refractory mood swings. *Am. J. Psychiat.* 134:149–152, 1977.

118. Jefferson, J.W.; Greist, J.H.; and Ackeman, D.L., *Lithium Encyclopedia for Clinical Practice.* Washington, D.C.: American Psychiatric Press, 1983.

119. Baldessarini, R.J., and Lipinsky, J.F. Lithium salts 1970–1975. *Ann. Int. Med.* 83:527–533, 1975.

120. Strayhorn, J.M., and Nash, J.L. Severe neurotoxicity despite "therapeutic" serum levels. *Dis. Nerv. Syst.* 38:107–111, 1977.

121. Van Der Velde, C. Toxicity of lithium carbonate in elderly patients. *Am. J. Psychiat.* 127:115–117, 1971.

122. Shopsin, B.; Johnson, G.; and Gershon, S. Neurotoxicity with lithium: Differential drug responsiveness. *Int. Pharmacopsychiat.* 5:170–182, 1970.

123. Hestbach, J.; Hanse, H.; Amdisen, A.; and Olsen, S. Chronic renal lesions following long-term treatment with lithium. *Kidney International* 12:205–213, 1977.

124. Scully, R.F.; Galdabini, J.J.; and McNeely, B.U. Case records of the Massachusetts General Hospital. *N. Engl. J. Med.* 304:1025–1032, 1981.

125. Gerner, R.H.; Psarras, J.; and Kirschenbaum, M.A. Results of clinical renal function tests in lithium patients. *Am. J. Psychiat.* 137:834–837, 1980.

126. Depaulo, J.R., Jr.; Correa, E.I.; and Sapir, D.G. Renal glomerular function and long-term lithium therapy. *Am. J. Psychiat.* 138:324–327, 1981.

127. Goldberg, H.L., and DiMascio, A. Psychotropic drugs in pregnancy. In *Psychopharmacology: A Generation of Progress,* Lipton, M.A., DiMascio, A., and Killam, K.F., eds. New York: Raven Press, 1978, pp. 1047–1055.

128. Gershon, S., and Shopsin, B. *Lithium: Its Role in Psychiatric Research and Treatment.* New York: Plenum Press, 1973.

129. Cho, J.T.; Bome, S.; Dunner, D.L.; Colt, E.; and Fieve, R.R. The effect of lithium treatment on thyroid function in patients with primary affective disorder. *Am. J. Psychiat.* 136:115–116, 1979.

130. Tupin, J.P.; Schlagenhauf, G.K.; and Creson, D.L. Lithium effects on electrolyte excretion. *Am. J. Psychiat.* 125:536–542, 1968.

131. Gerner, R.H.; Post, R.M.; and Spiegel, A.M. Effects of parathyroid hormone and lithium treatment on calcium and mood in depressed patients. *Biol. Psychiat.* 23:145–151, 1977.

132. Mellerup, E.T.; Lauritsen, B.; and Dan, H. Lithium effects on diurnal rhythms of calcium, magnesium, and phosphate metabolism in manic-melancholic disorder. *Acta Psychiatr. Scand.* 53:360–370, 1976.

133. Christenson, T.A.T. Lithium, hypercalcemia, and hyperparathyroidism. *Lancet* 2:144, 1976.
134. Cervi-Skinner, S.J. Lithium-carbonate-induced hypercalcemia. *West. J. Med.* 127:527–528, 1977.
135. Davis, B.M.; Pfefferbaum, A.; Krutzik, S.; and Davis, K.L. Lithium's effect on parathyroid hormone. *Am. J. Psychiat.* 138:489–492, 1981.
136. Shopsin, B., and Gershon, S. Cogwheel rigidity related to lithium maintenance. *Am. J. Psychiat.* 132:536–538, 1973.
137. Branchey, M.; Charles, J.; and Simpson, G. Extrapyramidal side effects in lithium maintenance therapy. *Am. J. Psychiat.* 133:444–445, 1976.
138. Kane, J.; Rifkin, A.; Quitkin, F.; and Klein, D.F. Extrapyramidal side effects with lithium treatment. *Am. J. Psychiat.* 135:851–853, 1978.
139. Asnis, G.B.; Asnis, D.; Dunner, D.L.; and Fieve, R. Cogwheel rigidity during chronic lithium therapy. *Am. J. Psychiat.* 136:1225–1226, 1979.
140. Cohen, W.J., and Cohen, N.H. Lithium carbonate, haloperidol, and irreversible brain damage. *JAMA* 230:1283–1287, 1974.
141. Baastrup, P.C.; Hollnagel, P.; and Sorensen, R. Adverse reactions in treatment with lithium carbonate and haloperidol. *JAMA* 236:2645–2646, 1976.
142. Spring, G.K. Neurotoxicity with combined use of lithium and thioridazine. *J. Clin. Psychiat.* 40:135–138, 1979.
143. Spring, G.K. EEG observations in confirming neurotoxicity (letter to editor). *Am. J. Psychiat.* 136:1099–1100, 1979.
144. Spring, G.K., and Frankel, M. New data on lithium and haloperidol incompatibility. *Am. J. Psychiat.* 138:818–821, 1981.
145. Sullivan, J.L.; Maltbie, A.; Cavenar, J.O., Jr.; and Stanfield, C. Platelet monoamine oxidase activity predicts response to lithium in manic-depressive illness. *Lancet* 2:1325–1327, 1977.
146. Nurnberger, J.I.; Gershon, E.S.; Murphy, D.L.; Buchsbaum, M.S.; Goodwin, F.K.; Post, R.M.; Lake, C.R.; Guroll, J.J.; and McGinnis, M.H. Biological and clinical predictors of lithium response in depression. In *Lithium: Controversies and Unresolved Issues*, Cooper, T.B., Gershon, S., Kline, N.S., and Scou, M., eds. Amsterdam: Excerpta Medica, 1979, pp. 241–256.
147. Sullivan, J.L.; Sullivan, P.D.; Davidson, J.; Maltbie, A.A.; Mahorney, S.; Taska, R.J.; and Cavenar, J.O. Biological risk factor assessment in lithium treatment of alcoholism. *Psychopharmacology Bull.* 17:37–40, 1981.
148. Ballenger, J., and Post, R. Carbamazepine in manic-depressive illness: A new treatment. *Am. J. Psychiat.* 137:782–790, 1980.
149. Okuma, T.; Kishimoto, A.; and Inoue, K. Anti-manic and prophylactic effects of carbamazepine (Tegretol) on manic depressive psychosis. *Folia Psychiatrica et Neurologica Japonica* 27:283–297, 1973.
150. Okuma, T. Therapeutic and prophylactic effects of carbamazepine in bipolar disorders. In *Psychiatric Clinics of North America*, vol. 6, no. 1, Akiskal, H., ed. Philadelphia: Saunders, 1983.
151. Okuma, T.; Inanaga, K.; and Otsuki, S. Comparison of antimanic efficacy of carbamazepine and chlorpromazine: A double blind controlled study. *Psychopharmacology* 66:211–217, 1979.
152. Brooks, S.C., and Lessin, B.E. Treatment of resistant lithium-induced nephrogenic diabetes insipidus and schizoaffective psychosis with carbamazepine. *Am. J. Psychiat.* 140:1077–1078, 1983.

153. *Physicians Desk Reference,* 37th ed. Oradell, N.J.: Medical Economics Company, 1983.
154. Keisling, R. Carbamazepine and lithium carbonate in the treatment of refractory affective disorders. *Arch. Gen. Psychiat.* 40:223, 1983.
155. Blumer, D. Temporal lobe epilepsy and its psychiatric significance. In *Psychiatric Aspects of Neurological Disease,* Benson, D., and Blumer, D., eds. New York: Grune and Stratton, 1975.
156. Lipinski, J., and Pope, H. Possible synergistic action between carbamazepine and lithium carbonate in the treatment of three acutely manic patients. *Am. J. Psychiat.* 139:948–949, 1982.
157. Gelenberg, A.J. (ed.). Innovative treatments for mania. *Massachusetts General Hospital Newsletter-Biological Therapies in Psychiatry* 6:35, 1983.
158. Chouinard, G.; Jones, B.D.; Young, S.N.; and Annable, L. Potentiation of lithium by tryptophan in a patient with bipolar illness. *Am. J. Psychiat.* 136:719–720, 1979.

CHAPTER 3

Chemotherapy of Schizophrenia

Jonathan Davidson,
John L. Sullivan,
Paula D. Sullivan,
and
Martha M. Letterie

One of the most important developments that has taken place within psychiatry since the 1950s has been the introduction of effective drug treatment for schizophrenia (1). At the present time, the etiology and pathogenesis of schizophrenia are still not fully understood, but evidence for disturbed central nervous system dopaminergic activity is strong. Thus, substances that activate the neurotransmitter dopamine (e.g., amphetamine, L-dopa, and MAO inhibitors) can provoke schizophrenic-like episodes, while drugs that are effective in treating the illness possess dopamine-blocking properties, for which their potency corresponds to the doses used in clinical practice (i.e., high-potency dopaminergic blockers are effective at low doses).

Antipsychotic drugs (neuroleptics or major tranquilizers) do not cure schizophrenia and usually need to be administered over the long term. A number of drugs are available, differing primarily in their side effect profile and potency. Although individual patients will respond more effectively to one particular drug and be refractory to others, there is no overall difference in efficacy among the various neuroleptics. However, there is some reason to believe that various neuroleptics may exert selective action against elements of the central dopamine neuronal systems, such that certain neuroleptics may prove to be differentially useful in specific cases.

TREATMENT GOALS

In using an antipsychotic drug, the first aim of treatment is often to control disturbing or disruptive behavior and to reduce the associated intense affective disturbance, whether this be fear, anger, bewilderment, grandiosity, or depression. Reduction or elimination of delusions and cognitive impairment takes somewhat longer. Our experience is that return of social skills and improved interaction with others takes even longer and is also affected by whether or not

Table 3.1 Commonly Used Antipsychotic Drugs

Group	Generic Name	Oral Dosage Range (mg/day)
Aliphatic phenothiazines	Chlorpromazine	25 to 1,600
	Trifluopromazine	50 to 200
Piperidine phenothiazines	Thioridazine	25 to 800
	Mesoridazine	25 to 400
Piperazine phenothiazines	Trifluoperazine	10 to 80
	Perphenazine	4 to 64
	Fluphenazine hydrochloride	2 to 20
	Fluphenazine enanthate	3.125 to 50 mg every 1 to 2 weeks IM
	Fluphenazine decanoate	3.125 to 50 mg every 1 to 4 weeks IM
Butyrophenones	Haloperidol	1 to 60
Thioxanthines	Thiothixene	5 to 60
Dibenzoxazepines	Loxapine	10 to 100
Dihydroindolones	Molindone	10 to 225

the medication is producing unpleasant side effects (for example, sexual difficulty, involuntary movement, dizziness).

Treatment can be administered by mouth. Except in acutely disturbed patients, all medication can be initially given at night. Advantages include greater compliance, especially in outpatients, minimization of side effects, and enhancement of sleep, without loss of efficacy when compared to administration two or three times a day. However, acutely disturbed or violent patients, those with clinically significant cardiovascular disease or cerebrovascular disease, and elderly patients where the risk of nighttime confusion is high, represent exceptions to this rule. Even in these cases, it is often possible to administer all antipsychotic medication at night once treatment has been stabilized.

TREATMENT REGIMENS

Effective treatment requires avoiding both suboptimal doses and an overly aggressive approach. An average starting dose for chlorpromazine is 300 mg per day by mouth, and for haloperidol it is 10 mg per day by mouth. If adequately tolerated, this dose may be doubled within two or three days and subsequent dose adjustments made on the basis of clinical improvement or the emergence of side effects. In very agitated, violent, noisy patients, a more vigorous approach may be needed. The use of IM medication may be helpful since the drug effect will be more rapid without any increased risk of acute extrapyramidal effects (2). This technique of rapid tranquilization is best accomplished with a high-potency drug such as haloperidol, fluphenazine, or thiothixene. Autonomic effects are unusual and extrapyramidal symptoms are not usually a serious problem with these medications in this context. An initial dose of haloperidol 10 mg can be repeated every two hours until there is evidence of therapeutic benefit. A total dose of 30 to 80 mg over twenty-four hours will usually suffice, and IM medication can be switched to the oral route using IM to oral ratio varying from 1:1 to 1:2. The use of IM medication may also prove valuable when a patient has proved refractory to high oral doses of different antipsychotics. In such a case, nonresponse may be due to noncompliance, poor absorption, or extensive first-pass metabolism. Although the practice of rapid neuroleptization has been questioned (3), a subgroup probably exists in whom this is a useful treatment. However, in order to prevent unnecessary side effects, the use of high doses should be avoided unless a patient has clearly not responded to conservative doses.

Repeated noncompliance or failure to attend clinic appointments represents a further indication for the use of IM medication. Long-acting esters of the piperazine phenothiazine fluphenazine (fluphenazine decanoate or fluphenazine enanthate) often improves compliance, and the existence of a special clinic often heightens the rapport and therapeutic relationship between patient and staff. As the decanoate has a longer duration of action than the enanthate, it is usually preferred by clinicians. It is also important to individualize the dose for a particular patient. For example, individuals who develop intolerable side effects on 6.25 mg of fluphenazine decanoate every four weeks often respond well to 3.1 mg (1/8 cc) every four weeks. Dosage requirements greater than 50 mg every four weeks are unusual, although some chronic schizophrenic patients respond to high doses of depot fluphenazine decanoate. While a patient is being stabilized on fluphenazine decanoate, oral doses of fluphenazine hydrochloride may be required as a supplement.

Noncompliance should always be suspected if the patient is not responding or has deteriorated unaccountably. Here the use of liquid medication with a supervising staff member will ensure that the patient swallows the medication. The reasons for noncompliance should always be addressed since they are frequently valid and have to do with discomforting side effects of medication. These can frequently be avoided, either by adjusting the dose, changing medication, or coprescribing an antiparkinsonian medicine.

Following resolution of the acute illness, and once rehabilitation has been well established, pharmacotherapy may be seen as having entered the maintenance phase. While much work has been conducted, it is by no means clear how to recognize those patients who do not require long-term antipsychotic therapy. Some evidence suggests that unmarried men living with families who express much hostility or overprotectiveness benefit particularly well from antipsychotic drugs (4). An important issue in maintenance therapy is to weigh the risks of discontinuing medication with the possibility that permanent side effects will emerge. In many cases, it may be judged that the risk of producing a relapse after medication withdrawal is not worth taking under any circumstances. In other cases, the patient may decide himself or herself that the risk of relapse is better than the possibility of delayed onset of (tardive) dyskinesia. The decision in regard to maintenance pharmacotherapy for schizophrenia must be an individual decision based upon dialogue between the physician and the patient. In all cases, however, an effort needs to be made to reduce medication gradually to the lowest level compatible with symptom remission, and it is hard to justify routine prescription refills month after month without making an assessment of the patient's condition.

SIDE EFFECTS

Choice of drug will depend to some extent upon an individual physician's experience with particular medications. Since the advent of high-potency drugs, there is no need to use chlorpromazine, thioridazine, or mesoridazine routinely as first-line treatment. High-potency drugs are superior because of fewer potentially catastrophic or disabling side effects—in particular, autonomic effects such as dizziness, hypotension, sexual dysfunction, and interference with bowel or bladder function. With high-potency drugs there is also less disturbance of cardiac conduction as well as a lowered risk of seizures and ocular, liver, and skin toxicity. Extrapyramidal disorders such as dystonia and akathisia are more common with high-potency drugs and occur early in treatment. Akinesia, tremor, and drug-induced parkinsonism are seen alike with high- and low-potency drugs. Longer-term risks of tardive dyskinesia apply to all antipsychotics.

Neurological

The most life-threatening neurological complication of antipsychotic medications, the neuroleptic malignant syndrome (NMS), appears to be relatively uncommon. However, infrequent recognition of this syndrome due to a lack of awareness on the part of physicians may also play a role in incidence figures. NMS is characterized primarily by stupor, extrapyramidal rigidity, involuntary movements, dysarthria, dysphasia, hyperthermia, and autonomic dysfunction, including pallor, blood pressure instability, and diaphoresis (5). Dehydration is also common and may progress to acute renal failure. All neuroleptics have been implicated in neuroleptic malignant syndrome, and symptoms usually begin soon after starting treatment or increasing the dosage. A variety of laboratory abnormalities have been reported, including concomitants of dehydration, although laboratory findings are frequently normal. Although the pathogenesis of NMS is unknown, the primary neurochemical disturbance appears to be in the central nervous system and involves dopamine hypoactivity or receptor blockade (6). When the condition is recognized, neuroleptic treatment should be discontinued and anticholinergic agents such as benztropine or trihexyphenidyl should be administered. Amantadine hydrochloride or bromocriptine mesylate may be helpful in this condition.

Tardive dyskinesia (TD) is another serious side effect of neuroleptic treatment. It is an involuntary movement disorder which may appear after as little as 3 months of treatment with an antipsychotic medication. It is characterized by choreic and choreoathetoid movements of the orofacial and lingual musculature, the hands and extremeties, and may also involve the trunk and the diaphragm. As with other movement disorders, it may be diminished by drowsiness and sleep and may be exacerbated by emotional stress. It has been reported in patients who have received virtually any form of antipsychotic medication (oral or intra-muscular), though less so with reserpine (a dopamine-depleting drug) and molindone (7,8). While data on the prevalence of TD vary with the population studied, roughly 10 to 20 percent of inpatients and 40 percent of elderly, chronic patients (inpatient or outpatient) manifest signs of this syndrome, pointing to an increased risk with age and/or length of exposure (7,8).

TD may present insidiously during the use of the drug, but more often becomes "unmasked" by a reduction in dosage or discontinuation of the drug. Upon discontinuing the drug altogether a transient dyskinesia may emerge, lasting days to weeks, but this entity is self-limiting, a "withdrawal dyskinesia". This may or may not be directly related to the more persistent dyskinesia, tardive dyskinesia.

Consideration of the differential diagnosis of these involuntary movements is critical. TD must be distinguished from other extrapyramidal side effects of antipsychotic medication, including acute dystonic reactions, neuroleptic-induced parkinsonism, akathisia, and tremor. Dyskinesias unrelated to medication may appear in chronic schizophrenics, the elderly, and in those with organic brain damage, confounding the diagnosis. Furthermore, one must consider other neurological diseases such as Huntington's chorea or Wilson's disease which may initially present with psychiatric symptomatology and subsequently be treated with antipsychotic medication.

Although the pathophysiology of TD remains uncertain, there is evidence which supports a denervation hypersensitivity in post-synaptic dopamine receptors as a contributing factor. Some evidence also implicates abnormalities presynaptically in the dopamine system. The cholinergic and GABA systems have been implicated as well. These theories have been both the result of and the basis for therapeutic strategies in the treatment of tardive dyskinesia. This work is reviewed meticulously by Jeste and Wyatt (9) and summarized in Table 3.2.

Once the diagnosis has been reasonably established, one should reduce or discontinue the antipsychotic medication, whenever this is clinically feasible. This is the treatment of choice. Despite an initial exacerbation of the dyskinesia, fully one-third of the patients show improvement in their tardive dyskinesia.

However, when the patient's psychiatric symptoms or the severity of TD preclude withdrawal of the antipsychotic medication, other treatment modal-

Table 3.2 Improvement Rates with Various Treatments for Tardive Dyskinesia

Method of Treatment	No. of Studies	No. of Patients	Patients Improved, %*		
			Open Studies†	Double-blind Studies‡	All Studies
Neuroleptics	50	501	69.0	63.0	66.9
Other dopamine antagonists	32	323	43.8	50.0	46.3
Cholinergic drugs	68	379	47	30.0	39
GABA-ergic drugs	19	204	58.6	42.6	53.8
Dopaminergic drugs	25	146	31	8.1	24.8
Anticholinergic drugs	14	177	7.3	. . .	7.3
Neuroleptic withdrawal	23	1,005	36.0	. . .	36.0
Miscellaneous	57	364	42.7	34.3	40.5
Totals§	285	3,099	44.5	41.7	43.8

*Improvement was defined as a reduction in manifestations of TD of at least 50%.

†The overall distribution of improvement rates with various treatments was significantly different ($X^2 = 114.78$; $P < .001$). Paired comparisons using simultaneous confidence intervals (see text) showed that neuroleptics had a significantly greater improvement rate than every other treatment except γ-aminobutyric acid (GABA)-ergic drugs; GABA-ergic drugs had a significantly higher improvement rate than dopaminergic drugs, anticholinergic drugs, and neuroleptic withdrawal. Anticholinergic drugs had a significantly lower improvement rate than every other treatment except dopaminergic drugs.

‡The overall distribution of improvement rates with various treatments was significantly different ($X^2 = 54.43$; $P < .001$). Paired comparisons (see text) showed that neuroleptics were significantly superior to cholinergic drugs, dopaminergic drugs, and miscellaneous treatments. Nonneuroleptic dopamine antagonists were significantly superior to cholinergic drugs. Dopaminergic drugs had a significantly lower improvement rate than every other treatment for which results of double-blind studies were reported.

§Totals include some repeats with different treatments.

Reprinted with permission of the publisher from Jeste, D.V., and Wyatt, R.J. Therapeutic strategies against tardive dyskinesia. *Arch. Gen. Psych.* 39:806, 1982.

ities may be introduced. Standard neuroleptic medications have been shown to suppress the manifestations of TD and have been advocated by some for the treatment of TD. Some workers have suggested raising the dose of the neuroleptic in use, while others have suggested adding a second neuroleptic. These agents are presumably effective in this manner as a consequence of their direct dopamine receptor blocking activity, further acting on the overly sensitive dopamine receptors. While different workers have promoted one neuroleptic over another for superior efficacy, no significant differences have held up consistently (9). While the "atypical" antipsychotic clozapine looked promising for the treatment of TD, its hematologic side effects (i.e. agranulocytosis) may eclipse its usefulness. Dopamine-depleting antipsychotic medications, including reserpine (0.7-2.5 mg per 24 hours) and tetrabenazine (90-186 mg per 24 hours) have also been used with some success. Whether any of these medications have a specific antidyskinetic property apart from their action on the dopaminergic system remains unclear.

Nonneuroleptic dopamine agonists have been studied, including apomorphine (in the range of 0.5-3.1 mg per 24 hours) and bromocriptine (in the range of 7-31 mg per 24 hours). In moderate and large doses, these drugs are agonistic to dopamine. However, in these relatively small doses, these drugs exert a dopamine effect. Therefore, these drugs have been found to be most useful in small, separated doses to suppress the manifestations of TD. Other dopamine agonists, such as amantadine hydrochloride (in the range of 200-400 mg per 24 hours), have been tried but have not been found to be consistently beneficial.

Cholinergic agents have also been tried for the treatment of TD. Choline (4-20 grams per 24 hours) itself has had equivocal results as has lecithin, a natural source of dietary choline. Anticholinergic drugs have been explored and have been found to either have little effect or worsen TD. Therefore efforts should be made to avoid the chronic use of anticholinergic drugs.

Recent evidence that the GABA-ergic system has inhibitory effects on the dopaminergic system has led to the investigation of such agents as the benzodiazepines and sodium valproate. A number of patients have shown suppression of their TD following use of these agents, but it is difficult to tell whether this improvement results from nonspecific anxiolytic or sedative effects or a specific antidyskinetic effect.

A number of miscellaneous agents have also been explored, including lithium and pyridoxine, without consistent therapeutic benefit. Nonpharmacologic interventions such as biofeedback and prosthodontic work have been reported to be somewhat helpful in specific cases.

In summary, neuroleptic withdrawal is the treatment of choice. In patients for whom this is not clinically possible, other approaches may be necessary. Increasing the dose of the existing neuroleptic or adding small doses of a second neuroleptic may transiently suppress the manifestations of TD, but may also worsen the dyskinesia in the long-run. Switching to another neuroleptic medication to which the patient has not previously been exposed may be helpful. After this has been accomplished, the addition of a benzodiazepine, titrated to induce mild sedation, may prove useful. If these measures fail, the clinician may want to try other strategies described above, although their efficacy is still uncertain. Clinicians should also bear in mind that non-tardive dyskinesia extrapyramidal side effects that are responsive to more gradual tapering and/or antiparkinson agents may occur following reduction of the dosage of antipsychotic medication in some patients who have received prolonged treatment (10).

The syndrome of neuroleptic-induced parkinsonism is strikingly similar to other forms of this disorder and usually appears after the first or second week of treatment and within the first month. Some degree of tolerance appears to develop to this extrapyramidal side effect, and the neurological signs and symptoms usually disappear within several months. Antiparkinson agents (e.g., benztropine, 1 to 6 mg/day; trihexyphenidyl, 5 to 15 mg/day) in divided doses are effective in controlling clinical manifestations of neuroleptic-induced parkinsonism, although these agents should be used judiciously for the shortest possible period of time. When neuroleptic and antiparkinson drugs are both discontinued, there are generally fewer side effects if the neuroleptic is withdrawn first and the antiparkinson compound one to several weeks later, as this affords protection against the basal ganglia effects of the more slowly excreted neuroleptic. Alcohol usage should also be carefully monitored because it has been implicated in the facilitation of neuroleptic-induced tremor, rigidity, and dystonia (11).

A myasthenia gravis-like reaction with profound muscular weakness has also been observed in some patients receiving neuroleptic medication (12). Antiparkinson agents are usually rapidly effective in alleviating this condition.

There is some evidence that neuroleptics may increase the incidence of seizures, particularly in epileptic patients, although haloperidol and molindone appear to have less of a tendency to do this compared to other antipsychotic agents (13,14). Thus, anticonvulsant medication should be monitored in epileptics who concurrently receive neuroleptics since the dosage of anticonvulsant medication may need to be increased for some individuals.

Behavioral

The behavioral side effects of neuroleptics are unclear, and the development of restlessness, excitement, and aggression in some patients may be the result of the mental and muscular unrest that accompanies akathisia associated with postsynaptic dopamine blockade in the mesocortical system (15). Akathisia normally responds to reduction in the dosage of neuroleptic medication. It has been suggested that a 10 mg IM test of procyclidine hydrochloride may be helpful in assessing the effects of reducing the dosage of neuroleptic medication since akathisia usually responds within one hour. However, the therapeutic effect of the procyclidine wears off within several hours.

Other cases of behavioral changes resulting from neuroleptic administration may result from enhancement of presynaptic release of neurotransmitters, including dopamine, at high neuroleptic concentration or anticholinergic toxicity (16). (See Chapter 2 for treatment of anticholinergic delirium or psychosis.) After resolution of the anticholinergic syndrome, it is appropriate to institute a high-potency drug with minimum anticholinergic effect.

The relationship between depression and schizophrenia has been discussed in the literature (17). While high doses of antipsychotic drugs may produce a depressionlike state (akinesia), often as part of a neuroleptic-induced parkinsonism, major depression as a consequence of drug treatment is rare; in fact, significant depressive symptoms present in schizophrenic states generally improve with judicious antipsychotic drug treatment (18). (See Chapter 2 for a discussion on the use of lithium in schizophrenia.)

Cardiac

The clinical significance of cardiovascular effects of the neuroleptics remains controversial (19). However, certain physiologic effects of antipsychotic drugs, particularly the phenothiazines, are similar to the effects of several cardioactive drugs, including quinidine and digitalis, as well as anticholinergic and antihypertensive agents.

The quinidinelike properties include an antiarrhythmic potential, ECG changes, a negative inotropic effect, and supraventricular and ventricular arrhythmias. The inhibition of potassium ATPase by neuroleptics, as well as digitalis, is believed to result in membrane changes, resulting in certain ECG variations in patients receiving neuroleptics. The anticholinergic effects of the antipsychotic agents may produce tachyarrhythmias that can potentially exacerbate angina pectoris. Hypotensive effects of the neuroleptics are correlated with their α-adrenergic blocking as well as their anticholinergic properties.

The most commonly reported cardiovascular changes associated with neuroleptic administration are ECG variations. These include a prolonged P-R interval (first-degree AV block), widening of the QRS complex, prolongation of the Q-T interval, depression of the ST segment, and nonspecific T wave changes.

An important point in this regard is the possible association with ECG changes and sudden death, although considerable controversy exists in regard to this issue. Although sudden death is a rare side effect of neuroleptic administration, the studies reported in the literature indicate that it does occur more frequently in patients receiving neuroleptics than individuals not treated with these drugs (19). It is interesting that the predominant occurrence is in the younger age groups.

The following arrhythmias have also been associated with antipsychotic drug administration: sinus tachycardia, premature atrial contractions, variable degrees of heart block, premature ventricular contractions, ventricular tachycardia, and ventricular fibrillation. The ventricular arrhythmias are potentially the most life threatening and are thought to be primarily associated with the quinidinelike properties of the antipsychotic agents (principally the phenothiazines), resulting in facilitation of re-entrant excitation.

Vascular

Hypotensive side effects are usually of the orthostatic type but can be present in the supine position in the severest cases. Parenteral administration of a neuroleptic drug is particularly associated with the abrupt onset of hypotension. Hypotensive side effects can be a particularly serious problem in the geriatric population, particularly with the phenothiazine derivatives. Although some reduction of blood pressure is common, frank hypotension is rare. Symptomatic hypotension usually responds to conservative measures or fludrocortisone acetate (Florinef), 0.05 mg to 0.20 mg daily. However, acute, life-threatening hypotensive episodes may require IV fluids and norepinephrine (presumably to counteract α-adrenergic receptor blockade). Epinephrine should not be used to treat neuroleptic-induced hypotension (20).

Ocular and Cutaneous

Numerous ocular and cutaneous reactions have been reported with the clinical use of antipsychotic agents, particularly the phenothiazine derivatives (21). Most of these reactions are transient and of limited clinical consequence although a few have led to significant changes in the affected tissues.

Chlorpromazine and thioridazine are associated most clearly with ocular lesions, and the possibility of drug-induced visual impairment must be considered whenever phenothiazines are prescribed. Although little visual loss appears to be associated with corneal or lenticular opacification, impaired vision as a consequence of toxic retinopathy can be a serious problem. Thioridazine is most often associated with pigmentary retinopathy, with dosage level and duration of therapy operating as critical factors. Retinopathy secondary to thioridazine is most likely to occur when the daily dosage exceeds 800 mg. The impact of duration of treatment is more variable, although visual changes have been reported after several weeks of treatment (22). However, pigmentary retinopathy is reversible to some degree, particularly when identified at an early stage. Since prompt discontinuation of the offending phenothiazine and titration of the neuroleptic dosage to the lowest effective level, if chronic medication is warranted, can prevent further deterioration and may permit some recovery of visual function, early recognition and diagnosis of retinal pathology are important. Unfortunately, progression of retinal pigmentation has been reported in some cases even after discontinuation of drug treatment (23). Whenever feasible, patients should be screened ophthalmologically before receiving neuroleptics in order to provide a baseline for future assessment.

Melanosis induced by chronic phenothiazine treatment has been reported in a number of studies, and chlorpromazine (in daily doses of 300 mg or more for at least two years) is most commonly implicated as the offending agent. Melanosis is considered to be a phototoxic reaction; it may contribute to cardiac problems; and severe cases (fewer than 1 percent of phenothiazine-treated patients) may exhibit a blue-gray or purplish skin pigmentation, especially on the nose and cheeks.

Effective treatment measures in melanosis and the blue-gray phenomenon include limitation of drug dosage, drug holidays, use of alternate neuroleptic agents (e.g., haloperidol), avoidance or limitation of sunlight exposure with the use of appropriate sun-screening agents, and in the most serious cases, use of the copper-chelating agent penicillamine. Routine use of penicillamine is not advisable because it has been associated with serious adverse effects (e.g., leukopenia, thrombocytopenia nephrotoxicity, and pemphigus). Treatment of melanosis also has been reported to decrease drug-induced ocular pigmentation and to improve visual acuity in patients with both ocular and cutaneous side effects (21,24).

During neuroleptic (or antidepressant) treatment of psychiatric patients, granulocytopenia and, rarely, agranulocytosis may occur. While these side effects may be serious enough to require cessation of treatment with the offending drug, many patients may need continuation of medication for maintaining remission or for controlling psychopathology. However, if neutropenia continues to be a persistent problem with alternate neuroleptic agents, addition of lithium carbonate may be useful in combating neuroleptic-induced neutropenia (25). Lithium has been reported to stimulate granulopoiesis, and improvement is associated with a blood level of 0.25 to 0.80 mEq/L. Thus, lithium-associated side effects can be minimized because lithium treatment for psychotropic-drug-induced neutropenia usually requires a lower dosage than is conventionally used for treatment of manic-depressive illness.

Clinical signs and symptoms are the best indexes of neuroleptic-induced granulocytopenia or agranulocytosis. Routine blood counts before and during treatment are unnecessary because they are rarely helpful and can foster a false sense of security.

Reports of severe anemia associated with neuroleptic administration are quite rare and are most often associated with chlorpromazine (26). The mechanism appears to be a drug-induced autoimmune hemolytic anemia that quickly resolves when the offending drug is withdrawn.

Endocrine

The role of endocrine response to psychotropic drugs is also of interest in regard to the neuroleptics. For example, the rise in plasma prolactin concentration following dopamine receptor blockade in the central nervous system with antipsychotic drug administration may prove to have useful clinical applications. However, there are also reports of an exaggerated prolactinemic response to neuroleptic administration with consequent galactorrhea and amenorrhea or menstrual irregularity accompanied by normal roentgenograms of the sella, computerized tomography (CT) scan, and visual fields (27). Diminished potency and libido in men are also long-recognized side effects of the neuroleptics. These alterations in reproductive and sexual functioning point to a neuroleptic effect on the pituitary-gonadal system.

Although alterations in reproductive and sexual functioning can occur with all neuroleptic agents, thioridazine is most frequently associated with sexual dysfunctions, perhaps because men receiving long-term thioridazine treatment have significantly lower testosterone and luteinizing hormone (LH) levels than men taking other neuroleptics (28). As previously discussed, higher-potency antipsychotic agents appear to have the lowest incidence of impotence and sexual dysfunction. Delay in, or inability to ejaculate, and retrograde ejaculation also appear to be more frequently associated with thioridazine administration. Inability to ejaculate may be associated with a sympatholytic effect on peripheral α-adrenergic receptors in the pelvic plexus, whereas retrograde ejaculation may be associated with relaxation of the bladder detrusor muscle as a consequence of impaired cholinergic transmission.

Neuroleptics have also been implicated in the syndrome of inappropriate secretion of ADH (SIADH), although psychogenic polydipsia and renal, adrenal, hepatic, and thyroid disorders also need to be considered in the differential diagnosis of mental confusion, low serum creatinine, albumin, sodium, and hypertonic urine (29). Mild to moderate water intoxication normally responds to discontinuation of the antipsychotic agent and restriction of fluid intake to about 800 to 1,000 ml daily. Occasionally, the intravenous administration of 200 to 300 ml of 5 percent saline solution over several hours is necessary to raise the serum sodium to a level at which symptoms improve. Simultaneous administration of furosemide may also be necessary when the possibility of congestive heart failure due to fluid overload exists.

Fetal

Although neuroleptics do cross the placenta, their effects on the fetus are largely unknown. Conflicting reports of their teratogenicity have been recorded; however, there does appear to be some risk of transient behavioral and neurological disturbances for the neonate, including irritability as well as choreiform and dystonic movements. In at least one case, these signs and symptoms may have responded to diphenhydramine (Benadryl), although a nine-month treatment course was necessary (30). Consistent handling of the neonate in an upright position and reduction of environmental stimulation may also be helpful.

Gastrointestinal

A number of psychiatric patients experience bowel disorders, most often constipation; ileus is fortunately a rare occurrence. Most of these bowel disturbances appear to be related to deterioration in the patient's general psychobiological status during psychotic episodes or to the anticholinergic properties of the neuroleptics, primarily the phenothiazines. Although the butyrophenone and thioxanthene classes of neuroleptics are associated less frequently with bowel disturbances (presumably as a consequence of their less-potent anticholinergic properties), the use of high doses of these medications may be accompanied by an increased incidence of gastrointestinal side effects. For example, Maltbie and colleagues have reported a case of ileus complicating haloperidol therapy in a patient receiving relatively high dosage levels of the medication (31). Since ileus is potentially life threatening, physicians should be particularly alert to the possibility of its occurrence in patients receiving neuroleptic medication. Unfortunately, in some cases, prolonged paralytic ileus has progressed to intestinal pseudo-obstruction with bowel perforation (32).

Hepatic

Antipsychotic-induced jaundice is an uncommon entity that has most often been associated with the phenothiazine derivatives (33). The clinical onset of neuroleptic-induced jaundice is usually within the first two to six weeks after exposure, considering chlorpromazine as the prototype drug. The tissue reaction to chlorpromazine is characterized by a hepatic inflammation and cholestasis that does not appear to be dose dependent. The disease is more lengthy histologically than clinically. Many patients remain anicteric, although jaundice may last for several years in some cases. However, it appears that cirrhosis does not develop as a consequence of the drug-induced liver abnormalities (34). The incidence of hepatotoxicity with the butyrophenone and thioxanthene classes of antipsychotics appears to be significantly less than with the phenothiazine derivatives. Differential diagnosis of jaundice associated with neuroleptic administration includes acute cholestasis, obstructive jaundice (e.g., gallstones), viral hepatitis, neoplastic bile duct obstruction, and primary biliary cirrhosis.

The offending antipsychotic medication should be discontinued when jaundice initially appears following drug administration, and if necessary, a thioxanthene or butyrophenone neuroleptic may be used cautiously. Jaundice usually remits within the ensuing month, although death has been reported as a rare complication of persistent hepatocellular damage. Corticosteroids are not indicated and most authorities recommend elimination of all medications except those that are essential. Although bed rest is advocated as part of the treatment regimen, no controlled studies have been done to verify its effectiveness. Routine liver function screening to detect cholestatic jaundice does not appear to be useful.

If there is a suggestion of active or past liver disease, liver function tests should be ordered since the liver is the primary route of metabolism of the neuroleptics. Although there is no contraindication to the use of antipsychotic agents in patients with hepatic disease, dosage adjustment may be required because impairment of hepatic function may reduce metabolic degradation of the neuroleptics. Weight gain can also be a problem with long-term antipsychotic drug treatment. In this situation, molindone may have an advantage since it has been associated with no weight gain or actual weight loss.

THERAPEUTIC BLOOD LEVELS

The current state of the art with respect to therapeutic monitoring of neuroleptic blood levels is discussed in the chapter on use of the clinical laboratory. In general, wide dosage ranges exist for antipsychotic drugs, a fact that has stimulated efforts to find a relationship between plasma drug level and clinical response. Haloperidol, which has no active metabolites, has been extensively studied, and it appears likely that a therapeutic window does exist for this drug (35). Many of the other compounds have several active metabolites, and at the present time data are inconclusive regarding therapeutic blood levels. A promising development is the radioreceptor assay that measures total in vitro dopamine-blocking activity, whether due to parent drug or active metabolites. Using this technique, preliminary data indicate that a therapeutic range may exist for many antipsychotics (36). At the present time, however, measuring blood levels of antipsychotic drugs, or their dopamine-blocking activity, is of limited value to the practicing clinician.

SUMMARY

While the general efficacy of presently available antipsychotics is clearly established, the search for more effective and less toxic compounds continues. Alternative treatments currently under investigation, and less likely to produce extrapyramidal side effects, include propranolol, sulpiride, drugs of the carboline and carbazole groups, and clozapine. Drugs that block the action of calcium in the nervous system, such as spiroperidol, and dopamine may be even more effective than standard neuroleptics in the treatment of schizophrenia. The calcium channel-blocking action appears to be related to the reported efficacy of these compounds in decreasing social and emotional withdrawal and language problems, as well as exerting the more traditional actions of lessening hallucinations, delusions, and thought disorders which are associated with dopamine-receptor blockade. Further studies into which calcium channels in the nervous system are affected by drugs that prevent calcium from binding to receptor sites in the brain promise to advance our understanding of the psychobiology of schizophrenic illnesses, as well as basic mental functions.

The brain imaging technologies, including imaging of dopamine and dopamine receptors, also provide more sensitive methods to improve our understanding of biological processes critical to the pathophysiology of schizophrenic illnesses, with implied practical applications in regard to diagnosis, prognosis, and treatment (37). These developments are discussed more fully in Chapter 12.

REFERENCES

1. May, P.R.A.; Tuma, A.H.; and Dixon, W.J. Schizophrenia. *Arch. Gen. Psychiat.* 38:776–784, 1981.

2. Donlon, P.T.; Hopkin, J.; and Tupin, J. Overview: Efficacy and safety of the rapid neuroleptization method with injectable haloperidol. *Am. J. Psychiat.* 136:273–278, 1979.
3. Kirkpatrick, B., and Burnett, G.B. Observations on neuroleptic use in acutely psychotic patients. *J. Clin. Psychopharmacol* 3:205–207, 1982.
4. Vaughn, C.E., and Leff, J.P. The influence of family and social factors on the course of psychiatric illness. *Br. J. Psychiat.* 129:125–137, 1976.
5. Morris, H.H.; McCormick, W.F.; and Reinarz, J.A. Neuroleptic malignant syndrome. *Arch. Neurol.* 37:462–463, 1980.
6. Henderson, V.W., and Wooten, G.F. Neuroleptic malignant syndrome: A pathogenetic role for dopamine receptor blockade? *Neurology* 31:132–137, 1981.
7. American Psychiatric Association Task Force on Tardive Dyskinesia. Task Force Report 18. Washington, D.C.: American Psychiatric Association, 1980.
8. Symposium on Tardive Dyskinesia. *Clinical Neuropharmacology* 6:77–167, 1983.
9. Jeste, D.V., and Wyatt, R.H. Therapeutic strategies against tardive dyskinesia. *Arch. Gen. Psych.* 39:803–816, 1982.
10. Inoue, F., and Janikowski, A.M. Withdrawal akinesia. *J. Neurol. Neurosurg. Psychiat.* 44:958, 1981.
11. Freed, E. Alcohol-triggered-neuroleptic-induced tremor, rigidity and dystonia. *Med. J. Aust.* 2:44–45, 1981.
12. Crews, E.L., and Daw, J. Neuroleptic-induced syndrome mimicking myasthenia gravis. *Psychosomatics* 22:67–68, 1981.
13. Baldessarini, R.J. *Chemotherapy in Psychiatry.* Cambridge: Harvard University Press, 1977.
14. Oliver, A.P.; Luchins, D.J.; and Wyatt, R.J. Neuroleptic-induced seizures. *Arch. Gen. Psychiat.* 39:206–209, 1982.
15. Guirguis, W.R., and Bowden, S.E. Disturbed behavior induced by high-dose antipsychotic drugs. *Br. Med. J.* 282:312–313, 1981.
16. Barnes, T.R., and Bridges, P.K. Disturbed behavior induced by high-dose antipsychotic drugs. *Br. Med. J.* 281:274–275, 1980.
17. McGlashan, T.H., and Carpenter, W.T. Postpsychotic depression in schizophrenia. *Arch. Gen. Psychiat.* 33:231–239, 1976.
18. Knights, A., and Hirsch, S.R. "Revealed" depression and drug treatment for schizophrenia. *Arch. Gen. Psychiat.* 38:806–811, 1981.
19. Levenson, A.J.; Beard, O.W.; and Murphy M.L. Major tranquilizers and heart disease: To use or not use. *Geriatrics* 35:55–61, 1980.
20. Friend, D. Adverse cardiovascular and hematologic effects of psychotropic agents. In *Clinical Handbook of Psychopharmacology*, DiMascio, A., and Shader, R.I., eds. New York: Science House, 1970, pp. 195–204.
21. Bond, W.S., and Yee, G.C. Ocular and cutaneous effects of chronic phenothiazine therapy. *Am. J. Hosp. Pharm.* 37:74–78, 1980.
22. Hagopian, V.; Stratton, D.B.; and Busick, R.D. Five cases of pigmentary retinopathy associated with thioridazine administration. *Am. J. Psychiat.* 123:97–100, 1966.
23. Davidorf, F.H. Thioridazine pigmentary retinopathy. *Arch. Ophthalmol.* 90: 251–255, 1973.
24. Gibbard, B.A., and Lehmann, H.E. Therapy of phenothiazine-produced skin pigmentation, a preliminary report. *Am. J. Psychiat.* 123:351–352, 1966.
25. Yassa, R., and Anath, J. Treatment of neuroleptic-induced leucopenia with lithium carbonate. *Can. J. Psychiat.* 26:487–489, 1981.
26. Stein, P.B., and Inwood, M.J. Hemolytic anemia associated with chlorpromazine therapy. *Can. J. Psychiat.* 25:659–661, 1980.

27. Ash, P.R., and Bouma, D. Exaggerated hyperprolactinemia in response to thio-thixene. *Arch. Neurol.* 38:534–535, 1981.
28. Brown, W.A.; Laughren, T.P.; and Williams, B. Differential effects of neuroleptic agents on the pituitary-gonadal axis in men. *Arch. Gen. Psychiat.* 38:1270–1272, 1981.
29. Husband, C; Mai, F.M.; and Carruthers, I. Syndrome of inappropriate secretion of anti-diuretic hormone in a patient treated with haloperidol. *Can. J. Psychiat.* 26:196–197, 1981.
30. O'Connor, M.; Johnson, G.A.; and James, D.I. Intrauterine effect of phenothia-zines. *Med. J. Aust.* 1:416–417, 1981.
31. Maltbie, A.A.; Varia, I.G.; and Thomas, N.U. Ileus complicating haloperidol ther-apy. *Psychosomatics* 22:158–159, 1981.
32. Kemeny, W.M.; Martin, E.C.; Lane, F.C.; and Stillman, R.M. Abdominal disten-tion and aortic obstruction associated with phenothiazines. *JAMA* 243:683–714, 1980.
33. Snyder, S. Fluphenazine jaundice. *Am. J. Gastroenterology* 73:336–340, 1980.
34. Sherlock, S. Drugs causing cholestasis. In *Drugs and the Liver*, Sickinger, G.W., ed. Stuttgaart: Schattauer, 1975, pp. 349–350.
35. Magliozzi, J.R.; Hollister, L.E.; Arnold, K.V.; Earle, G.M. Relationship of serum haloperidol levels to clinical response in schizophrenic patients. *Am. J. Psychiat.* 138:365–367, 1981.
36. Tune, L.E.; Creese, I.; DePaulo, J.R.; Slavney, P.R.; Snyder, S.H. Neuroleptic serum levels measured by radioreceptor assay and clinical response in schizo-phrenic patients. *J. Nerv. Ment. Dis.* 169:60–63, 1981.
37. Wagner, H.A., Jr.; Burns, H.D.; Dannals, R.F.; Wong, D.F.; Langstrom, B.; Duelfer, T.; Frost, J.J.; Ravert, H.T.; Links, J.M.; Rosenbloom, S.B.; Lukas, S.E.; Kramer, A.V.; and Kuhar, M.J. Imaging dopamine receptors in the human brain by position tomography. *Science* 221:1264–1266, 1983.

CHAPTER 4

Electroconvulsive Therapy
Richard D. Weiner

The psychiatric use of electrically induced seizures, known as electroconvulsive therapy (ECT), is a treatment modality that has been widely used in the treatment of severe psychiatric illnesses, particularly major depressive episodes and schizophrenia. Despite the fact that ECT continues to be controversial and is attacked by some members of the lay community along with a small minority of mental health professionals as being ineffective, outmoded, and dangerous, the practice of ECT in recent years has been growing, as have research activities. This chapter covers both the efficacy and the safety of ECT and, in addition, discusses how this treatment modality may be carried out in optimum fashion. For a more in-depth review of the ECT literature, we refer the reader to several book-length publications that have become available (1,2,3,4,5).

HISTORY OF ECT

During the early decades of this century, psychiatry was severely limited with respect to what it had to offer in the way of treatments for most of the prevalent severe psychiatric illnesses, particularly schizophrenia and depression. Breakthroughs were established in the 1930s with the advent of insulin coma and metrazol induction of seizures. Soon thereafter, Cerletti and Bini, working in Italy to develop an animal model for experimental epilepsy, were able to establish that seizures could be induced much more efficiently utilizing an electrical stimulus passed across the head (6). Within the space of a very few years, ECT became the established somatic treatment for schizophrenia and depressive illnesses, remaining thus until the advent of effective pharmacologic alternative treatments in the 1950s.

CURRENT USAGE PATTERNS

Although the use of ECT declined with the advent of antidepressive and antipsychotic drugs, this decline appears to have leveled out within the last several years. This is likely due to several factors. First, as we discuss later, many patients do not respond to alternative treatments. Second, some patients will not tolerate a lengthy drug trial—e.g., those who are actively suicidal or those who are grossly debilitated. Third, many patients, particularly those with cardiovascular disease, cannot tolerate the side effects anticipated from pharmacologic agents.

In 1976, an estimated 88,000 patients received ECT in the United States (1). Most of these were suffering from a major depressive disorder, with schizophrenia being the second most common diagnosis, followed by mania. Very few patients with other diagnoses appear to be receiving ECT. The fraction of psychiatric inpatients who receive ECT appears to be within the range of 3 to 5 percent, which is similar to the rate reported for Sweden. Despite allegations that ECT is preferentially utilized with the poor or underprivileged, it appears to be the case, at least in contemporary times, that the typical ECT patient is middle class in background and is receiving his or her treatment in a private psychiatric hospital.

EFFICACY OF ECT

Affective Disorders

ECT is clearly the most effective treatment for major depressive episodes available to psychiatry at the current time. This is particularly the case when melancholia or psychosis is involved. With such patients, the remission rate ranges between 80 and 90 percent in most studies (2).

In 1979, Avery and Lubrano (7) presented the results of a prospective Italian study done by DeCarolis et al. (8) fifteen years previously. DeCarolis and his collaborators initially treated 437 depressed patients with 200 to 350 mg per day of imipramine. All patients who did not respond to this regimen by thirty days were then given ECT. DeCarolis et al. were wise enough, even in the early 1960s, to break down the diagnoses of their depressed patients into a number of areas, and from this we can select those who would now most likely be diagnosed as having a major depressive episode via DSM-III criteria. In doing so, we are still left with 282 patients. DeCarolis et al. found that 61 percent of these individuals showed a significant improvement with imipramine, a finding which is very consistent with that reported by others. The remaining 39 percent—i.e., the imipramine failures—were then given ECT. Eighty-five percent of these then showed significant improvement. The results for depressed patients with delusional ideation were even more striking, with only 40 percent responding to imipramine but with 83 percent of the imipramine failures still responding to ECT.

A report by West (9) compared ECT to sham ECT—i.e., the use of general anesthesia to convince the patient and his or her treating psychiatrist that a real course of ECT had been given. Twenty-two severely depressed patients were randomly assigned to either of these two groups. West reported a highly significant and clinically important improvement in the ECT-treated group, whether rated by the psychiatrist, nurses, or the patients themselves. . . . However, the patients treated by simulated ECT showed little clinical change. As ten of the eleven patients who had received simulated ECT remained severely depressed, they were then given a course of real ECT, to which they then had a therapeutic response at a significance level better than the $p = .005$ level.

In a major critical review of ECT efficacy, Scovern and Kilmann (10) concluded that the most methodologically sophisticated studies are remarkably consistent in demonstrating the superiority of ECT for treating depression.

Although not widely used for such a purpose, ECT also appears to be as effective as lithium in inducing remissions in cases of mania (2). This fact is certainly useful to keep in mind with some patients with bipolar affective disorder who do not respond to lithium or who may not be able to tolerate either the side effects of lithium or of neuroleptics, the latter of which are sometimes necessary during the acute phase of mania.

Schizophrenia

In acute schizophrenic syndromes, ECT appears to work as well as neuroleptics and, in cases of catatonic or schizoaffective schizophrenia, may even be more effective. With chronic schizophrenia, however, ECT is markedly less effective, with approximately only a 5 to 10 percent remission rate (11). Still, when faced with a profoundly disturbed schizophrenic patient who is not responding to pharmacologic intervention, even such a low response rate may have an appeal. Balanced against such use, however, should be the fact that schizophrenics often require twice as many ECT treatments to reach maximum benefit, thereby exposing them to a greater risk of adverse sequelae.

The use of regressive ECT—i.e., the daily or even twice daily application of a large number of ECT treatments in order to produce a severe organic regression—has in the past been touted as an effective means of producing a remission in chronic schizophrenics (12). Unfortunately, the methodologic aspects of these data leave them far from convincing, and most psychiatrists do not believe that the greatly enhanced level of central nervous system impairment is worth the risk.

Other Diagnoses

As alluded to earlier, ECT is minimally utilized for conditions other than affective disorders and schizophrenia (1). This is with good reason since ECT has never been clearly established to be effective for conditions other than these.

There are, however, several possible exceptions to this rule. The first has to do with certain types of atypical depression, where the predominant symptomatology is somatic—e.g., a pain syndrome or hypochondriasis. The second type of such indication deals with certain types of organic psychoses—e.g., drug withdrawal state or typhoid catatonia—where ECT may be effective even in the absence of a functional disease entity. Finally, the neurochemical alteration evoked by the seizure activity may prove to be beneficial for some organic disorders—e.g., panhypopituitarism or the on-off phenomenon associated with Parkinson's disease (13). ECT has even been suggested as a treatment for diabetes mellitus but, at least for severe cases, is more likely to make the syndrome worse (14).

How Does ECT Work?

The number of research investigations into the mechanisms of ECT range into the hundreds. Still, as with virtually all areas of psychiatric treatment, our understanding of how ECT works remains grossly incomplete.

The potentiation by ECT of monoaminergic systems, particularly norepinephrine, makes it quite tempting to hypothesize mechanisms that could be seen as analogous to those of the actions of antidepressant drugs (2). Such a hypothesis could be structured as follows. First, the electrical stimulation induces a diencephalically mediated synchronization of generalized seizure activity. This then potentiates monoaminergic pathways to the hypothalamus, thereby affecting many of the vegetative features known to accompany depressive disorders. In addition, monoaminergic pathways to the limbic areas of the temporal lobe and elsewhere are also potentiated, resulting in direct effects upon mood.

An exact understanding of biochemical effects of ECT awaits the application of more sophisticated neurochemical techniques, including those related to receptor activity. Studies addressing this issue continue to be a major focus in a number of laboratories worldwide.

At a neurophysiologic level, however, certain aspects of how ECT works are well understood. Studies involving subconvulsive or sham ECT have clearly demonstrated that the application of electricity alone does not have a beneficial effect (9,15). This is entirely consistent with the comparable therapeutic results of chemically induced seizures (16). Furthermore, we now know that seizures that are too brief or are not sufficiently generalized likewise have a diminished therapeutic effect (17). While some investigators have suggested that the precise amount of time spent in seizure activity may be important therapeutically (18), there is now reason to believe that, within a broad range of seizure duration, one suprathreshold seizure may be functionally equivalent to another (19).

ADVERSE EFFECTS OF ECT

Systemic Morbidity and Mortality

The systemic risks of ECT are at a level comparable to that of the brief level of general anesthesia that is utilized. Deaths occur at a rate of approximately 1 per 10,000 patients and are usually due to cardiovascular collapse (2). ECT does produce a profound, although quite transient, series of stresses in the cardiovascular system, with large fluctuations in heart rate and blood pressure/ typically encountered during and immediately following the seizure (1). Still, the only relatively common sequela of this consists of the occasional mild transient cardiac arrhythmia. The use of oxygenation, anesthesia, and muscular relaxation along with anticholinergic premedication have acted to decrease considerably the cardiovascular morbidity associated with ECT.

Rarely, one may encounter a prolonged apneic state, due either to an insufficiency in the ability to metabolize the muscle relaxant agent or to a grossly prolonged seizure. Other sorts of toxic or allergic reactions to muscle relaxants or anesthetic agents have been reported (1) but, again, on a rare basis.

The Central Nervous System

A series of generalized seizures, whether evoked by ECT or occurring on a spontaneous basis, are associated with some degree of organic brain syndrome, typically building up over the course of treatments. This is characterized mainly by confusion and amnesia (20) on a behavioral basis and by generalized slowing in the electroencephalogram (EEG) on a physiologic basis (21). The amnesia, about which the patients typically appear most concerned, consists of three types. The first type is a difficulty in remembering newly learned material. This is termed *anterograde* amnesia. The second type is a difficulty in remembering material learned prior to the initiation of ECT. This is termed *retrograde* amnesia. The third type is a difficulty in remembering material learned during the course of ECT. The first two types of amnesia have been the subject of numerous anecdotal reports and various types of experimental investigations. The third has not been well studied, but researchers acknowledge that some degree of amnesia for the period of ECT remains fixed, probably due to the accompanying transient confusional state.

The EEG slowing associated with ECT is a nonspecific form of encephalopathic impairment, and as with the level of memory impairment, it varies considerably among individuals and, as we discuss later, is dependent upon certain treatment parameters such as electrode placement and stimulus waveform (22). Other types of EEG abnormalities—e.g., the occurrence of spontaneous epileptiform activity—appear to be quite rare (23).

All of the elements of the organic brain syndrome associated with ECT begin to diminish in severity immediately upon completion of the ECT course. Again, the persistence of pertinent signs and symptoms is quite variable, but in most individuals it ranges from days to weeks (24).

Does ECT Cause Brain Damage?

From the early days of ECT use, anecdotal reports appeared of patients who complained of permanent impairment in cognitive capabilities following ECT. Particularly insofar as contemporary treatment modifications such as oxygenation, anesthesia, and muscular relaxation were not utilized, and since many of these patients were exposed to many applications of ECT sometimes given over brief time intervals, these studies may not be pertinent to ECT as it is currently utilized. Still, it should be noted that such complaints never appeared to have been widespread.

Studies investigating the long-term persistence of amnestic symptomatology have tended not to reveal the presence of long-term effects, except for some suggestive spotty loss of autobiographic material related to the period of weeks and occasionally months prior to the ECT treatments (25). Even there, the validity of such findings has not been established.

A number of ECT patient surveys have established that a sizable fraction of such patients do complain of persistent memory difficulties (26). While this certainly would be consistent with the presence of an actual organic deficit, a variety of functional etiologies must also be considered. These include the presence of residual depressive symptomatology, which is known to have a clear dysamnestic effect, along with a sensitization to the problems of normal forgetting. In addition, surveys of ECT patients have also indicated that these individuals do not tend to be concerned with the level of any amnestic impairment they feel exists (27).

The situation with regard to the persistence of EEG slowing is somewhat better described inasmuch as it is readily quantifiable. Evidence of such slowing occurs occasionally by a month following completion of the ECT course but is only rarely seen past three months (28).

A number of efforts to investigate the neuropathologic substrate of ECT have been accomplished. Unfortunately, most of these were done prior to the era of contemporary treatment modifications, and in addition, they suffered from a wide variety of severe methodologic insufficiencies. The findings of these studies range from no pathologic changes to severe and widespread irreversible effects. On careful examination of the data, however, one does not find any clear evidence that ECT is associated with irreversible structural alterations (24). The most elegant research investigation, that of Hartelius (29), is widely quoted by those who argue against the use of ECT. While some irreversible neuropathologic changes were felt to occur in the experimental animals by Hartelius, he also pointed out that they were extremely rare and of questionable significance.

Studies that attempted to look at the effects of stimulus intensity upon the occurrence of pathologic changes within the brain substance found that only with stimuli that reflected intracerebral current densities much greater than that occurring with ECT did irreversible changes occur (30). Similarly, investigations of the effects of chemically induced prolonged seizure activity have indicated that the length of seizure activity necessary for irreversible central nervous system changes is many times that encountered with ECT (31). Nevertheless, it is unfortunate that methodologically adequate studies using contemporary ECT and neuropathologic techniques have not been thus far accomplished.

A few reports of human autopsy findings exist for patients who have died during or immediately after a course of ECT (2). While the occurrence of certain types of intracerebral hemorrhages initially suggested a direct role for ECT, more complete analysis suggests that such findings more likely relate to antemortem changes associated with cardiovascular collapse.

RISK-BENEFIT CONSIDERATIONS

The choice of any given treatment modality depends upon an analysis of its anticipated effectiveness and risks as compared with those of the available treatment alternatives. Given the factors described earlier, for many patients it may be most prudent to try pharmacologic intervention before attempting a course of ECT. As already alluded to, however, an actively suicidal or physically debilitated patient, particularly if delusional, may not be appropriate for a lengthy drug trial and should instead be immediately considered for ECT. Similarly, patients for whom the clinically appropriate drugs may be medically contraindicated also fit into this category. The concerns regarding long-term risks with psychopharmacologic agents, such as sudden death with antidepressant drugs and tardive dyskinesia with neuroleptic agents, have in particular contributed to a milieu in which ECT is being looked at more favorably by psychiatrists.

THE ECT WORKUP

Patients receiving ECT should have the standard medical history, physical exam, and laboratory evaluations associated with a hospital admission. In addition, an ECG is indicated. If any significant underlying cardiovascular, pulmonary, orthopedic, or metabolic disorder exists that may interfere with the use of the various drugs used during ECT treatments or with the occurrence of a seizure, the appropriate medical or surgical consultation should be obtained.

There are no absolute contraindications to the use of ECT. However, a number of conditions do exist for which one would be advised not to utilize this treatment modality until either the underlying condition has been dealt with or it has been made clear that any increased risk is tolerable given the underlying risk-benefit considerations. These situations include the presence of an intracranial mass, a recent myocardial infarction, and a recent cerebrovascular accident. In some of these cases, it may be possible to decrease morbidity pharmacologically—e.g., the use of steroids in cases of brain tumor. The presence of a coexisting organic brain syndrome, particularly that of senile dementia, is not a contraindication for ECT. Such patients should be monitored particularly closely for the development of a severe exacerbation in their level of central nervous system impairment, but this is not usually a problem. If this does occur, increased spacing between the ECT treatments can often be utilized to minimize the severity of such impairment.

Many patients referred for ECT are taking a variety of psychopharmacologically active substances. At least for patients receiving ECT for the treatment of depression, no evidence indicates that concurrent psychopharmacologic use increases the therapeutic efficacy of ECT, and there is some reason to believe that it may increase the morbidity. This is particularly the case for lithium, where the presence of severe organic brain syndromes and even spontaneous seizure activity has been reported (32). The use of sedative hypnotics during a course of ECT may also be ill advised because these agents tend to increase the seizure threshold, thereby making it difficult for some patients to develop adequate seizures (33). One should also take into mind that some psychotropic drugs—e.g., phenelzine and lithium carbonate—may diminish the capacity to metabolize succinylcholine, which is the most common muscular relaxant agent used with ECT (34).

The last, but certainly not the least, component of the ECT workup is the psychologic preparation of the patient, which includes the establishment of informed consent. One should always describe to the patient, and usually to the major available significant other, the reason why ECT is being recommended, what the treatment involves, and enough information regarding both efficacy and adverse effects so that a reasonable decision can be made (1). The conveyance of this information should be noted in the chart, along with the consent form. In addition, it is often helpful to leave an information sheet regarding ECT with the patient and/or his or her family. Procedures like those outlined here are, of course, not always possible. Severely depressed and schizophrenic patients may not be sufficiently in contact with reality and/or otherwise able to deal with such preparations in a voluntary, competent fashion. In such cases, it may be prudent for additional psychiatric consultation and also for access to legal counsel for the patient (35). A variety of state laws across the country relate to informed consent for ECT. The more stringent of these seriously impinge upon the ability of the psychiatrist to provide safe and effective treatment, even at times when such treatment would be truly lifesaving (36).

ECT TECHNIQUE

Premedication, Anesthesia, and Muscular Relaxation

The use of anticholinergic premedication, usually with atropine, has been universally adopted as an ECT modification for two reasons. The first has to do with the capacity to decrease the risk of aspiration, and the second is due to its antiarrhythmic effects. The development of effective anticholinergic agents that do not act centrally, like methscopolamine, has led to suggestions that these supplant the use of atropine, which has a significant central effect. A typical dose of atropine is 0.8 mg injected subcutaneously or intramuscularly approximately thirty minutes before the ECT treatment. One can, of course, get a much more exact effect by giving the drug intravenously at the time of the treatment, before anesthesia, and titrating it to the occurrence of a mild tachycardia.

The use of general anesthesia was adopted largely because conscious patients do not well tolerate the experience of ECT without such agents, particularly when muscle relaxants are utilized. Unfortunately, the use of general anesthesia has also produced an increase in the intensity of the electrical stimulus necessary to produce an effective seizure, although this appears to be less of a problem with methohexital (Brevital) than with thiopental or other barbiturate agents. In those patients for whom effective seizures cannot be produced, ketamine may be utilized as an anesthetic that does not raise the seizure threshold (37). With ketamine, the patient takes approximately twice as long to wake up postictally as with methohexital, and occasional patients will experience frightening hallucinations as they are coming out from under its effect. The amount of methohexital given should be only enough to achieve a mild level of anesthesia. This tends to occur in a dosage range of 30 to 160 mg given by IV push, with a mean starting dose of 60 mg for an average-sized man. With successive treatments, the dosage should be titrated to the level of anesthesia necessary.

The use of muscular relaxant agents such as succinylcholine has led to a virtual disappearance of the risk of musculoskeletal complications with ECT. A lesser recognized, though possibly as important, effect of such agents is their ability to reduce the risk of anoxic changes by suppressing muscular activity during the seizure. The optimal dose of succinylcholine is that for which a very mild movement of the toes or feet is the only behavioral manifestation of the seizure. This can be accomplished with 30 to 120 mg of this agent, with a mean typical starting dose of 60 mg, given IV push immediately upon achievement of the anesthetic state. With the succinylcholine, one will see muscle fasciculations that begin rostrally and move caudally, ending in the calves and feet. For patients with significant orthopedic disease, particularly in the spinal area, or who complain of muscle aches following ECT, premedication with curare may be indicated. This is accomplished by IV push of 3 to 6 mg of curare given approximately three minutes before anesthesia is to be induced. This amount of curare will not compromise respiration but will be noticeable to the patient as a heaviness of the eyelids. With curare, no fasciculations are seen, and one should wait approximately 90 seconds before providing the electrical stimulus.

Oxygenation has been shown both in animals and in humans to diminish the central nervous system metabolic imbalance that is associated with generalized seizure activity (31). It should be provided at least as soon as muscular relaxation is achieved and, except for the passage of the electrical stimulus, should be continued until normal respiration resumes after the seizure. Patients with a history of cardiac ischemia should receive oxygen for a minute or two before muscular relaxation is given in order to exert a more protective effect. When ventilating the patient, care should be taken not to hyperventilate because this may prolong both the seizure excessively and the apnea due to the lowering of pCO_2.

Stimulus Electrode Placement

The ECT modification that has generated the most space in the psychiatric literature, along with the most controversy, is the matter of where to place the stimulus electrodes on the patient's head. The standard fashion is to place these electrodes over the frontotemporal areas bilaterally, but as early as 1942, researchers were moving these electrodes over the surface of the head in order to find out where one could get the most effect with the least amount of electrical stimulus (38). Not until a landmark paper by Lancaster et al. (39) in 1958, however, was it clearly established that stimulation over the nondominant cerebral hemisphere was associated with the least confusion and amnestic changes.

Although there is no question at this time that unilateral ECT is associated with fewer side effects (40), there has been a great deal of heated discussion in the literature and elsewhere about whether it is as therapeutically effective as the standard bilateral treatments (2). In general, however, the data indicate that unilateral ECT is in fact as effective as bilateral, but only if it is performed in a technically adequate fashion (41). I stress this point because unilateral ECT is a more difficult technique, and many of those who have tried it and gone back to bilateral ECT have not paid proper attention to factors such as the precise placement of the electrodes and the preparation of the scalp. It should also be pointed out that occasional patients appear to require more treatments with unilateral ECT, and there is a possibility that an undefined subgroup exists of patients who may not respond to unilateral ECT at all (42). For this reason, bilateral ECT should still be available. Some centers around the country now routinely start patients on unilateral ECT and switch to bilateral if no response occurs after a certain number of treatments.

One problem with unilateral ECT is that even though one of the two stimulus electrodes is still placed at the standard position over the frontotemporal cortex on the nondominant hemisphere, there have been a number of different opinions as to where to place the second electrode. The initial placement described by Lancaster et al. (39) utilizes a low central position for the second electrode. D'Elia (43) has advocated a higher centroparietal position, with which generalized seizures can be more easily evoked with a less intense electrical stimulus. The frontal position for the second electrode, advocated by Muller (44) and others, requires a much higher intensity of electrical stimulus to produce an adequate seizure, while the various parieto-occipital positions suggested by some English psychiatrists (45) appear to be associated with a higher incidence of autonomic side effects, probably due to the closer positioning to brain stem areas.

Precise measurement of electrode position is not necessary due to the widespread diffusion of the stimulus current throughout the scalp (46). The classic description of stimulus placement for bilateral ECT is with the right and left electrodes positioned with their midpoints located approximately 2.5 cm above the middle of an imaginery line drawn between the upper tragus of the ear and the external canthus of the eye. For unilateral ECT as described by d'Elia (43), the second electrode should be located approximately 11.5 cm posteriorly and rostrally to the frontotemporal electrode, at a point just homolateral to the vertex of the head. It should be kept in mind that placement of stimulus electrodes too closely together will result in increased seizure threshold and the possibility of skin burns. As mentioned earlier, it is important that the stimulus electrode sites be prepared by removal of skin oil, sweat, and hair. In addition, good electrode contact is aided by the use of mild abrasion of the superficial skin layer by a rough gauze and the rubbing in of a small amount of electrode jelly or saline into the skin. If EEG-monitoring electrodes are to be placed, it is important that the conductive electrode jelly or paste does not form a bridge across the path of the stimulus electrodes since this would cause an alternative current path, resulting in no induced seizure. One should also be careful not to stimulate over a skull defect inasmuch as the current density within the brain substance would be considerably higher.

When using unilateral ECT, it is always important to establish which side of the brain is dominant so that the nondominant hemisphere can be stimulated. For strongly right-handed individuals, it is safe to assume that the left hemisphere is dominant. The situation is more complex with patients who are left-handed, where approximately half are right-hemisphere dominant. In such cases, one suggested procedure is to give the first treatment bilaterally then to follow this with a right unilateral and a left unilateral ECT in successive treatments, with the time to awakening and the time at which the patient can give his or her correct surname and is able to answer a few simple naming questions, contrasted for the three sessions. In such cases, the nondominant hemisphere is that associated with the most rapid responses. In patients whose livelihood depends on the function of the nondominant hemisphere—e.g., artists—it is still appropriate to use nondominant unilateral ECT since the degree of nondominant hemispheric impairment with this is still less than with bilateral ECT and since there is some reason to believe that dominant hemispheric ECT may not be as effective.

The Electrical Stimulus

As soon as the stimulus electrodes have been placed, muscle fasciculations from the succinylcholine have dissipated, and a mouthpiece has been inserted in the oral cavity, the ECT stimulus should be delivered. During the passage of the ECT stimulus, any other electrical equipment, particularly any that is connected to a wall socket, should be temporarily disconnected for safety reasons. If no seizure, to be described later, or only a brief abortive seizure of not more than five or ten seconds occurs, restimulation at a higher stimulus intensity should be accomplished within twenty to thirty seconds. Waiting longer than this may produce a situation in which the anesthesia or muscular relaxation is metabolized before the seizure is over.

The two major types of stimulus waveforms utilized by devices currently marketed in the United States are the sine wave and the pulse. The sine wave was the original waveform used for ECT and was chosen not because of any scientific rationale but because of convenience, since this is what comes out of a wall socket. Liberson (47) and others, beginning in the early 1940s, began to experiment with alternative types of stimulus waveforms in order to produce seizures with less electrical energy and, thereby, possibly to decrease central nervous system morbidity. They found that the brief pulse stimulus, which is an interrupted pattern of very short-duration electrical discharges, was relatively optimum in this regard. With the pulse stimulus, one can produce seizures with about one-third the electrical energy output of the sine wave stimulus (48). Some evidence suggests that the seizures produced by the pulse stimulus may be qualitatively different than those produced by the sine wave stimulus, but in general it appears that the pulse stimulus is just as effective (19). Some evidence indicates that EEG slowing is significantly less with the use of the pulse stimulus, probably due to differences in the seizures produced, and there may also be less amnesia with the use of these low energy stimuli, although the difference is not as great as that between unilateral nondominant and bilateral ECT (22).

The two most popular ECT devices of those currently marketed in this country are the Medcraft B-24 Mark III (Hittman Medical Systems, Inc.) and the MECTA (MECTA Corp.). The Medcraft B-24 device is a sine wave device with a variable voltage ranging from 70 to 170 volts rms and variable stimulus duration from 0.1 to 1 second. A typical starting set of stimulus parameters is 140 volts at 0.6 second. It should be noted that elderly patients usually require a higher stimulus intensity, probably due to both greater skin resistance and a lower cerebral excitability. The amount of stimulus intensity necessary to produce an adequate seizure also is known to increase over a course of ECT, almost as a reverse kindling effect. The Medcraft B-24 also contains what is termed a *glissando* control that represents a slowly rising increase in stimulus intensity interposed immediately before the delivery of the stimulus set by the user. This is a vestigial control, present from the days before the use of muscular relaxation, where it was helpful to avoid the initial muscular contraction associated with the passage of stimulus current.

The MECTA ECT device is a bidirectional pulse device that puts out a constant current of 800 milliamperes and has a variable pulse frequency, pulse width, and stimulus duration. A typical starting set of stimulus parameters is 60 Hz pulse frequency, 0.75 msec pulse width, and 1.25 second stimulus duration. Other features of the MECTA device include an impedance check to establish the electrical continuity of the entire machine-to-patient pathway before each stimulation, single-channel EEG and ECG monitors, and a coded chart output that allows the calculation of electrical energy delivered to the patient. This latter information is helpful in that regardless of whatever an ECT device is set to deliver, the stimulus energy that relates to the seizure threshold will vary with the impedance across the stimulus electrodes.

The Seizure Produced with ECT

In the absence of EEG monitoring, only the behavioral manifestations of the seizure are available for the determination of whether a seizure has occurred and, if so, for how long it lasts. Electromyographic (EMG) monitoring can also be utilized, but as with the behavioral signs, it is often briefer in duration than the EEG signs of seizure activity (49). With the passage of the stimulus current, one can see a brief period of muscular contraction, followed at a latency of 1 to 15 seconds by the onset of the clonic phase of the seizure, which is typically characterized by plantar extension and muscular rigidity. This phase lasts for approximately 5 to 20 seconds and gradually is replaced by generalized clonic contractions that decrease in frequency until they finally disappear. A variety of autonomic signs such as flushing in the face and chest, piloerection, and systemic hypertension are also seen. Following the seizure, the patient is typically rather confused as he or she wakes up from the anesthesia, with this confusion normally lifting within the first hour. Occasionally, with unilateral ECT, there may only be unilateral convulsive movements. This indicates a poorly generalized seizure that is probably less effective.

Since behavioral manifestations do not give an adequate reflection of seizure duration, and sometimes may not even indicate whether or not the seizure has occurred, it is optimal to carry out EEG monitoring. It should be pointed out, however, that interpretation of the EEG activity is not always a trivial matter since the anesthetic agent also has an effect upon the EEG and since a variety of artifacts may also be present. The EEG changes associated with the seizure can be divided into a number of phases. The first consists of a gradual buildup of fast rhythmic activity that is often not seen and that only lasts for a second or two. This then develops into a high-frequency discharge, consisting of polyspikes, that is concurrent with the tonic phase of the seizure. The polyspike activity eventually breaks up into an interrupted pattern of polyspike and slow wave activity that is synchronous with the clonic behavioral manifestations noted previously. The end of the seizure is indicated electrographically by either an abrupt termination of the epileptiform activity into a pattern reminiscent of a flat line, indicating gross EEG suppression, or may be seen as a slow fading out of the epileptiform activity over a period of even tens of seconds. Particularly with unilateral ECT, the gross postictal EEG suppression may not be seen, and the activity may present as mixed fast and slow activity that is probably related to the effect of the anesthesia.

As already mentioned, in case of missed or very brief seizures, the patient should be restimulated rapidly. If the seizure, as monitored by EEG, is in the range of 15 to 35 seconds, a larger stimulus intensity should be used at the next treatment session. For a seizure greater than 60 seconds, a decrease in stimulus intensity should be utilized at the next treatment session, although it should be noted that some patients have a very narrow threshold range and will go from a seizure of, say, 90 seconds to no seizure at all with even a small decrease in the stimulus intensity. Extremely prolonged seizures rarely occur. Should the seizure continue past five minutes, intubation and artificial termination of the seizure with intravenous valium and/or diphenylhydantoin should be carried out with neurological consultation. If the patient is waking up, it is unlikely that he or she is still seizing, regardless of what one thinks is occurring on the EEG.

Choice of Number and Spacing of Treatments

Most ECT facilities in the United States give ECT three times a week with treatments separated by two days. Occasionally, a patient with an urgent need for a rapid remission may require daily treatments for the first two or three sessions. The typical number of treatments for depressed patients ranges between six and ten and, for schizophrenics, between six and twenty. It is much better to decide when to end the treatments by the individual response of the patient rather than to give a fixed number. Most psychiatrists give treatments until the patient appears to have reached a therapeutic plateau and then two more treatments past that point, although the scientific justification for this is rather limited (50). In patients who become very confused over the course of ECT, the treatments can be spaced out to two a week. Some evidence indicates that unilateral ECT, with its much lesser degree of central nervous system impairment, may be given four or five times a week without the presence of a large amount of confusion or amnesia in most patients.

Multiple-monitored ECT is a modified ECT technique by which at least several seizures are induced during a single ECT session, during which time the patient is kept anesthetized and relaxed via an IV drip (51). Multiple-monitored ECT allows a remission to be established within a fewer number of sessions, but usually a larger number of seizures are necessary. While neuropsychological impairment is usually not greater than with ECT delivered with the standard time intervals, this is not always the case, and there is an increased risk of prolonged seizures (52).

It has been suggested that the total cumulative seizure duration can be used as a means to decide when the treatments can be discontinued (18), but this is presently highly controversial. A more promising technique, however, is the following of the results of the dexamethasone suppression test (53). For those patients who pre-ECT are nonsuppressors, a normalization of the dexamethasone suppression test response during the course of ECT appears to indicate an early response and may eventually be useful in deciding when treatments can be terminated.

The Need for Maintenance Therapy

It is important to realize that, when effective, ECT induces a therapeutic remission rather than a cure. Following successful treatment with ECT, the likelihood of relapse with time is the same as if psychotropic drugs had been discontinued after successful pharmacologic treatment of the episode. Maintenance ECT, typically one treatment per month for an extended period, though apparently effective in reducing the risk of relapse (54), has not been adequately studied and, at any rate, is only infrequently used at present. In patients with depressive disorders, the use of antidepressant drug maintenance post-ECT has been studied more carefully and has been found to decrease the likelihood of relapse significantly. Seager and Bird reported, for example, in a double-blind placebo-controlled study, that 75 mg per day of imipramine was associated with a relapse rate at six months of 17 percent versus 69 percent for placebo (55). This finding has since been corroborated by others, and, in addition, evidence supporting a potential role for lithium in post-ECT maintenance therapy in patients with depressive disorders has been presented (56). For patients receiving ECT treatment for acute mania or schizophrenia, maintenance chemotherapy with lithium or neuroleptic medication is also beneficial.

SUMMARY

ECT is the most potent means presently available to produce a therapeutic remission in cases of major depressive disorder. It also appears to have some efficacy in schizophrenic and manic disorders. For the most part the use of ECT in the U.S.A. has diminished to the point where it is used principally in the treatment of psychotic depressive conditions, when patients have not responded to available alternatives, or when chemotherapy cannot be used because of clinical urgency (e.g., suicide) or potential side effects. While the therapeutic mechanism underlying ECT is still unclear, the potentiating effects of induced seizures upon central noradrenergic activity may be involved. The major morbidity related to ECT is associated with the occurrence of organic CNS changes, notably confusion and amnesia. These appear to be transient, and can be diminished by the use of a variety of treatment modifications.

REFERENCES

1. American Psychiatric Association Task Force on ECT. Task Force rep. no. 14. Washington, D.C.: American Psychiatric Association, 1978.
2. Fink, M. *Convulsive Therapy–Theory and Practice.* New York: Raven Press, 1979.
3. Palmer, R.L., ed. *Electroconvulsive Therapy: An Appraisal.* Oxford: Oxford University Press, 1981.
4. Maletzky, B.M. *Multiple-Monitored Electroconvulsive Therapy.* Boca Raton: CRC Press, 1981.
5. Abrams, R., and Essman, W.B., eds. *Electroconvulsive Therapies: Biological Foundations and Clinical Applications.* New York: SP Books, 1982.
6. Cerletti, U., and Bini, L. Un nuevo metodo di shockterapie "L'elettro-shock." *Boll. Acad. Med. Roma* 64:136–138, 1938.
7. Avery, D., and Lubrano, A. Depression treated with imipramine and ECT: The DeCarolis study reconsidered. *Am. J. Psychiat.* 136:559–562, 1979.
8. DeCarolis, V.; Gibertz, F.; Roccatagliata, G.; Rossi, R.; and Venutti, G. Imipramine and electroshock in the treatment of depression. *Syst. Nerv.* 16:29–42, 1964.
9. West, E.D. Electric convulsion therapy in depression: A double-blind controlled trial. *Br. Med. J.* 282:355–357, 1981.
10. Scovern, A.W., and Kilmann, P.R. Status of ECT: A review of the outcome literature. *Psychol. Bull.* 87:260–303, 1980.
11. Salzman, C. The use of ECT in the treatment of schizophrenia. *Am. J. Psychiat.* 137:1032–1041, 1980.
12. Murillo, L.G., and Exner, J.E. The effects of regressive ECT with process schizophrenia. *Am. J. Psychiat.* 130:269–273, 1973.
13. Balldin, J.; Eden, S.; Granerus, A.K.; Modigh, K.; Svanborg, A.; Walinder, J.; Wallin, L. Electroconvulsive therapy in Parkinson's syndrome with "on-off" phenomenon. *J. Neural. Trans.* 47:11–21, 1980.
14. Yudofsky, S.C., and Rosenthal, N.E. ECT in a depressed patient with adult onset diabetes mellitus. *Am. J. Psychiat.* 137:100–101, 1980.
15. Fink, M.; Kahn, R.L.; and Green, M. Experimental studies of electroshock process. *Dis. Nerv. Syst.* 19:113–118, 1958.
16. Small, J.G., and Small, I.F. Clinical results: Indoklon vs. ECT. *Seminars in Psychiatry* 4:13–26, 1972.
17. Ottosson, J.O. Experimental studies on the mode of action of electroconvulsive therapy. *Acta Psychiat. Neurol. Scand.* 35 (suppl. 145) :1–141, 1960.
18. Maletzky, B.M. Seizure duration and clinical effect in psychiatry. *Compr. Psychiat.* 19:541–550, 1978.
19. Welch, C.A.; Weiner, R.D.; Weir, D.; Cahill, J.F.; Rogers, H.J.; Davidson, J.; and Mandel, M.R. Efficacy of ECT in the treatment of depression: Waveform and electrode placement considerations. *Psychopharm. Bull.* 18:31–34, 1982.
20. Squire, L.R. ECT and memory loss. *Am. J. Psychiat.* 134:997–1001, 1977.

21. Small, J.G.; Small, I.F.; and Milstein, V. Electrophysiology of EST. In *Psychopharmacology: A Generation of Progress*, Lipton, M.A., DiMascio, A., and Killam, K.F., eds. New York: Raven Press, 1978, pp. 759–769.
22. Weiner, R.D.; Rogers, H.J.; Davidson, J.; and Miller, R.D. Evaluation of the central nervous system's risks of ECT. *Psychopharm. Bull.* 18:29–31, 1982.
23. Blackwood, D.H.R.; Cull, R.E.; Freeman, C.P.L.; Evans, J.I., and Mawdsley, C. A study of the incidence of epilepsy following ECT. *J. Neurol. Neurosurg. Psychiat.* 43:1098–1102, 1980.
24. Weiner, R.D. Electroconvulsive therapy: Do persistent changes occur? *J. Psychiat. Treatment Eval.* 3:309–313, 1981.
25. Squire, L.R.; Slater, P.C.; and Miller, P.L. Retrograde amnesia following ECT: Long term follow-up. *Arch. Gen. Psychiat.* 38:89–95, 1981.
26. Squire, L.R., and Chace, P.M. Memory functions six to nine months after ECT. *Arch. Gen. Psychiat.* 32:1557–1564, 1975.
27. Hughes, J.; Barraclough, B.M.; Reeve, W. Are patients shocked by ECT? *J. Royal Soc. Med.* 74:283–285, 1981.
28. Weiner, R.D. Persistence of ECT-induced EEG changes. *J. Nerv. Ment. Dis.* 168:224–228, 1980.
29. Hartelius, H. Cerebral changes following electrically induced convulsions: An experimental study on cats. *Acta Psychiatr. Scand.* (suppl.) 77:3–128, 1952.
30. Alexander, L., and Lowenbach, H. Experimental studies on ECT: The intracerebral vascular reaction as an indicator of the path of the current and the threshold of early changes within the brain tissue. *J. Neuropath. Exp. Neurol.* 3:139–171, 1944.
31. Meldrum, B.S.; Papy, J.J.; Toure, M.F.; and Brierley, J.B. Four models for studying cerebral lesions secondary to epileptic seizures. In *Primate Models of Neurological Disorders (Advances in Neurology)*, Meldrum, B.S., and Marsden, C.D., eds. New York: Raven Press, 1975, pp. 147–167.
32. Small, J.G.; Kellamy, J.J.; and Milstein, V. Complications with electroconvulsive treatment combined with lithium. *Biol. Psychiat.* 15:103–112, 1980.
33. Stromgren, L.; Dahl, J.; Fjeldbrog, N.; and Thomsen, A. Factors influencing seizure duration and number of seizures applied in unilateral electroconvulsive therapy: Anesthetics and benzodiazepines. *Acta Psychiatr. Scand.* 62:158–165, 1980.
34. Packman, M.; Meyer, M.A.; and Verdun, R.M. Hazards of succinylcholine administration during electrotherapy. *Arch. Gen. Psychiat.* 35:1137–1141, 1978.
35. Culver, C.M.; Ferrell, R.B.; and Green, R.M. ECT and special problems of informed consent. *Am. J. Psychiat.* 137:586–591, 1980.
36. Roy-Byrne, P., and Gerner, R.H. Legal restrictions on the use of ECT in California: Clinical impact on the incompetent patient. *J. Clin. Psychiat.* 42:300–303, 1981.
37. Lunn, R.J.; Savageau, M.M.; Beatty, W.W.; Gerst, J.W.; Staton, R.D.; and Brumback, R.A. Anesthetics in electroconvulsive therapy seizure duration: Implications for therapy from a rat model. *Biol. Psychiat.* 16:1163–1175, 1981.
38. Friedman, E., and Wilcox, P.H. Electrostimulated convulsive doses in intact humans by means of unidirectional currents. *J. Nerv. Ment. Dis.* 96:56–63, 1942.
39. Lancaster, N.P.; Steinert, R.R.; and Frost, I. Unilateral electroconvulsive therapy. *J. Ment. Sci.* 104:221–227, 1958.
40. Squire, L.R., and Slater, P.C. Bilateral and unilateral ECT effects on verbal and nonverbal memory. *Am. J. Psychiat.* 135:1316–1320, 1978.
41. d'Elia, G., and Raotma, H. Is unilateral ECT less effective than bilateral ECT? *Br. J. Psychiat.* 126:83–89, 1975.

42. Price, T.R.P. Unilateral electroconvulsive therapy for depression. *N. Engl. J. Med.* 304:53, 1981.
43. d'Elia, G., and Perris, C. Seizure and post-seizure electroencephalographic pattern. *Acta Psychiatr. Scand.* (suppl.) 215:9–29, 1970.
44. Muller, D.J. Unilateral ECT. *Dis. Nerv. Syst.* 32:422–424, 1971.
45. Halliday, A.M.; Davison, K.; Brown, M.W.; and Kreeger, L.C. A comparison of the effects on depression and memory of bilateral ECT and unilateral ECT to the dominant and nondominant hemispheres. *Br. J. Psychiat.* 114:997–1012, 1968.
46. Weaver, L.; Williams, R.; and Rush, S. Current density in bilateral and unilateral ECT. *Biol. Psychiat.* 11:303–312, 1976.
47. Liberson, W.T. Brief stimulus therapy: Physiological and clinical observations. *Am. J. Psychiat.* 105:28–39, 1948.
48. Weiner, R.D. ECT and seizure threshold. *Biol. Psychiat.* 15:225–241, 1980.
49. Sorensen, P.S.; Bolwig, T.G.; Lauritsen, B.; and Bengtson, O. Electroconvulsive therapy: A comparison of seizure duration as monitored with electroencephalograph and electromyograph. *Acta Psychiatr. Scand.* 64:1193–1198, 1981.
50. Snaith, R.P. How much ECT does the depressed patient need? In *Electroconvulsive Therapy: An Appraisal*, Palmer, R.L., ed. Oxford: Oxford University Press, 1981 pp. 61–64.
51. Blachley, P., and Gowing, D. Multiple monitored electroconvulsive treatment. *Compr. Psychiat.* 7:100–109, 1966.
52. Weiner, R.D.; Volow, M.R.; Gianturco, D.T.; and Cavenar, J.O. Seizures terminable and interminable with ECT. *Am. J. Psychiat.* 11:1416–1418, 1980.
53. Papakostas, Y.; Fink, M.; Lee, J.; Irwin, P.; and Johnson, L. Neuroendocrine measures in psychiatric patients: Course and outcome with ECT. *Psychiatric Res.* 4:55–64, 1981.
54. Stevenson, G.H., and Geoghegan, J.J. Prophylactic electroshock—A five-year study. *Am. J. Psychiat.* 107:743–748, 1951.
55. Seager, C.P., and Bird, R.L. Imipramine with electrical treatment and depression—A controlled trial. *J. Ment. Sci.* 108:704–707, 1962.
56. Coppen, A.; Abou-Saleh, M.T.; Milln, P.; Bailey, J.; Metcalfe, M.; Burns, B.H.; and Armond, A. Lithium continuation therapy following electroconvulsive therapy. *Br. J. Psychiat.* 139:284–287, 1981.

CHAPTER 5

Use of the Clinical Laboratory

Lynn E. DeLisi

LABORATORY DIAGNOSIS OF PHYSICAL ILLNESS PRESENTING AS A PSYCHIATRIC DISORDER

Estimated incidences of hospitalized psychiatric patients with medical illness range from 10 to 80 percent (1). These illnesses may include depression, anxiety states, apathy, aggressive outbursts, personality changes, sexual dysfunctions, delusions, hallucinations, and manic or schizophreniform psychotic states. One study determined that 36 out of 100 consecutive psychiatric admissions between the ages of 18 and 52 had significant medical problems causing or exacerbating their mental symptoms (2). While a physical examination missed most of these cases, laboratory procedures including routine blood chemistry profiles, differential blood cell counts, urinalysis, ECG and EEG after sleep deprivation detected over 90 percent. Statistics from other similar studies are reviewed in Table 5.1.

The following primarily physical disorders need to be distinguished from functional psychiatric disorders and require specific medical treatment (for review, see references 10,11,12). While tests to screen for all of them are not routinely prescribed for every patient with psychiatric symptoms, obtaining a good history of concurrent physical symptoms or environmental exposures will suggest further medical and diagnostic laboratory evaluations.

Infections

Neurosyphilis at one time accounted for 10 to 20 percent of state hospital admissions. Due to the advent of antibiotic treatment and programs for

---

*Drs. J.L. Sullivan and T.N. Wise are thanked for their helpful suggestions.

Table 5.1   Studies of the Incidence of Medical Illness in Psychiatric Populations

Study	Causing or Exacerbating Psychiatric Symptoms (percent)	Total (percent)
Hall et al., 1980 (2)	46	80
Koranyi, 1979 (3)	30	43
Burke, 1972 (4)	—	43
Johnson, 1968 (5)	—	60
Maguire & Granville-Grossman, 1968 (6)	—	33.5
Davies, 1965 (7)	30.5	44.4
Herridge, 1960 (8)	34	50
Marshall, 1949 (9)	—	44

rigorous control of syphilis in its early stages, it is now a rare entity. Diagnosis can be made by positive Wasserman reactions in both blood and cerebrospinal fluid. Cells and protein are increased in the cerebrospinal fluid, and a characteristic colloidal gold curve can be identified.

Encephalitis, although relatively rare, may present as an acute psychosis. Herpes simplex encephalitis, which has a high mortality rate, usually involves the temporal and/or frontal lobes. The rare, Russian-tick-borne encephalitis, in its chronic form, may also evolve with progressively severe psychiatric symptoms.

Some viruses may be cultured from the cerebrospinal fluid and can be identified in the laboratory within several days. Early diagnosis is important because antiviral agents may be useful in these cases.

Chronic (slow) virus infections of the central nervous system have been associated with some psychoses. Subacute sclerosing panencephalitis is now known to fall into this category. It usually affects persons under the age of twenty and produces gradual intellectual impairment, loss of interest in usual activities, restlessness, and behavior changes. Increased gamma-globulin levels as well as a paretic-type colloidal gold curve are found in the cerebrospinal fluid. Increased serum measles antibody titers have also been associated with this illness.

Creutzfeldt-Jakob disease is another slow viral illness, the first signs of which may be intellectual impairment, behavioral disturbances, and apathy. These progress to easy fatigability and eventual mutism. While cerebrospinal fluid total protein may be elevated and cerebral atrophy may be shown by CT scans, at present, no viral titer or isolation is useful and no treatment is available for this disorder.

Endocrine Disorders

Hyperthyroidism (Graves disease) may be associated with memory and judgment impairment, disorientation, and manic or schizophreniform symptoms. Older patients show apathy and mental confusion but lack the characteristic tremor and overactivity. Hypothyroidism has been associated with depression and lethargy. In severe cases, so-called myxedema madness is present, involving psychomotor retardation, depression, delusions, and auditory or visual hallucinations (13). The disease may go undetected without a comprehensive thyroid evaluation and determination of serum levels of thyroid hormones. The earliest biochemical evidence of hypothyroidism is the demonstration of an augmented thyrotropin-releasing-hormone (TRH) induced thyroid-stimulating hormone (TSH) response (14).

Adrenal cortical insufficiency, Addison's disease, is characterized by apathy, easy fatigability, irritability, and depression and occasionally by psychotic symptoms. Patients with Cushing's syndrome, excessive cortisol secretion, may have insomnia, anxiety, and depression and may exhibit a variety of psychotic behaviors.

Other adrenal disorders such as primary aldosteronism (excess aldosterone secretion) and pheochromocytoma (a tumor of the adrenal medulla that secretes large amounts of epinephrine) may also produce diffuse psychiatric symptoms. Obtaining twenty-four-hour urinary excretion of adrenal steroids and catecholamine metabolites, diurnal serum cortisols, serum electrolyte concentrations and testing for dexamethasone suppression are among the procedures necessary to clarify the presence and nature of adrenal pathology.

Serum alterations in both calcium and phosphorus concentrations suggest parathyroid dysfunction. Either increased or decreased parathyroid hormone, which leads to alterations in calcium and phosphorus metabolism, can cause anything from anxiety to psychosis to severe depression.

Disturbances of glucose metabolism, either hyperglycemic or hypoglycemic, also have psychiatric manifestations and may not be detected during routine admission evaluation of psychiatric patients, particularly if only one fasting blood glucose concentration is obtained. A glucose tolerance test may be necessary and may yield abnormal results in these cases.

Intracranial Neoplasms or Vascular Alterations

Personality changes or other psychiatric symptoms are often the earliest and only symptoms of central nervous system tumors. Temporal arteritis, a disease of the elderly, frequently is misdiagnosed as depression. It should be suspect in any depressed patient over the age of sixty with an elevated sedimentation rate (15).

A variety of psychiatric symptoms have been described in patients with lupus erythematosus who have central nervous system changes. These reportedly are due to cerebrovascular basement membrane deposition of immune complexes and include progressive dementia, classical major affective disorder, delusions, hallucinations, and catatonic or paranoid behavior (16).

Nutritional Disorders

Many nutritional disorders accompany chronic alcoholism and may be directly related to several of the psychiatric symptoms associated with this disease. Thiamine deficiency, which is commonly seen in alcoholics, may manifest as apathy, depression, irritability, and generalized nervousness. Severe deficiency can lead to memory and intellect changes as well. Beriberi, Wernicke-Korsakoff syndrome, and Korsakoff's psychosis respond to thiamine treatment. Marchiafava-Bignami disease (primary degeneration of the corpus callosum) is another, although rare, complication of alcoholism and is attributed to the crude red wine used by alcoholics in Italy. Neurological signs and mental changes are almost always present. Treatment consists of abstinence from alcohol and establishment of good nutrition.

Pellagra, a deficiency of nicotinic acid and tryptophan, typically produces headaches, insomnia, apathy, confused states, delusions, and dementia. Pernicious anemia, due to vitamin B_{12} deficiency, affects the central nervous system and produces irritability, memory disturbances, mild depression, or psychotic symptoms. It is normally diagnosed by initially obtaining serum B_{12} levels. A macrocytic anemia may or may not be present prior to central nervous system involvement. Vitamin B_{12} deficiency, due to malabsorption, is distinguished by an abnormal Shilling test that detects failure to absorb orally administered radioactive vitamin B_{12}. Laboratory screening for specific vitamin and mineral deficiencies of chronic alcohol or drug abusers and other patients exhibiting a lack of self-care may lead to a determination of the treatment necessary to reverse some of the major psychiatric signs.

Inherited Syndromes and Inborn Errors of Metabolism

Hartnup's disease, an inherited defect in intracellular transport of tryptophan, is somewhat similar in symptomatology to pellagra and is detected by an increase in urinary excretion of indole metabolites.

Huntington's chorea, an autosomal dominant trait present in 6 of 100,000 people may develop in midlife. The initial sign is gradual personality change that progresses to choreiform movements and dementia. At present, no laboratory test is readily available to predict the occurrence of this disorder.

Acute intermittent porphyria, also an autosomal dominant trait, appears in the third or fourth decade of life and may present with anxiety and emotional instability accompanied by abdominal pain. It is caused by a defect in δ-amino levulinic acid synthetase and is detected by elevations of δ-amino levulinic acid in the urine.

Wilson's disease, which is an inherited defect in copper transport, is diagnosed by decreased concentrations of ceruloplasmin, decreased serum copper, and increased urinary copper excretion. Copper deposits appear in the brain, kidneys, liver, and other organs. Its first signs may be personality alterations, irritability, difficulty concentrating, memory and intellectual impairment, and psychotic behavior including delusions and hallucinations. It is a progressive disease that may be aborted by treatment with the chelating agent D-penicillamine.

Phenylketonuria (PKU) is another autosomal recessive syndrome detectable in infancy although on rare occasions it may remain undetected until adulthood and present as an acute psychosis (17). The initial presentation of such cases may be through a schizophreniform illness. Screening of suspected cases can be accomplished with a urine ferric chloride test, fasting plasma phenylalanine, and oral phenylalanine loading procedures similar to glucose tolerance tests.

Chromosomal Abnormalities

No specific chromosomal abnormality has been associated with any of the psychiatric disorders. Increased prevalence, however, of certain chromosomal abnormalities, particularly of the X chromosome, exists in certain psychiatric disorders. For example, Klinefelter's syndrome (XXY) and the XXX configuration are found in an increased frequency among populations of schizophrenic patients. The XYY and XXYY syndromes are prevalent in approximately 2 percent of inmates in mental-penal institutions. Turner's syndrome (XO) is associated with deficits in perceptual organization, as well as with personality changes (18,19,20). Nevertheless, studies employing new banding techniques fail to find more subtle changes in chromosomal structure in most psychiatric patients, and at present, there is no indication that these should be a part of routine psychiatric evaluations (21). Perhaps future research based on a recombinant DNA approach may isolate areas of genetic material that appear altered in subgroups of psychiatric patients and give one information on the genetics of these disorders.

Environmental Intoxications

The determination of blood or urinary concentrations of toxic metals or chemicals may be necessary in cases of suspected exposure to environmental toxins.

Manganese madness—emotional lability, pathological laughter, nightmares, and hallucinations—is an early symptom of manganese intoxication. This is usually a result of manganese dust inhalation. Most cases are seen in miners of manganese ore and in manufacturers of batteries or other manganese-containing products.

Behavioral changes including paranoia and depression have occurred with exposure to thallium, a compound found in rat poisons and depilatory agents. Chronic intoxication with arsenic, also a chemical in rat poisons and insecticides, can result in intellectual impairment and apathy.

Mercury intoxication, resulting from inhalation of mercury nitrate vapors, previously was found among workers in factories where mercury nitrate was used to process hair for hats. Depression, insomnia, irritability, and hallucinations have been attributed to mercury.

Chronic lead intoxication may also cause a variety of psychiatric symptoms. Organophosphate insecticide exposure, particularly when chronic, may cause memory impairment and episodic psychotic behavior.

Miscellaneous

Serum and cerebrospinal fluid creatinine phosphokinase (CPK) activity has been studied extensively in hospitalized psychotic patients (22,23). In particular, newly hospitalized psychotic patients, regardless of diagnosis, frequently appear to have elevations in serum CPK activity. Chronic hospitalized psychotic patients may also, although less frequently, have elevated CPK activity (22). Isoenzyme studies relate these elevations to increases in the muscle rather than the brain isoenzyme. Subsequent histological studies on muscle biopsies from psychotic patients have revealed abnormalities such as an excess of atrophic fibers, Z-band streaming, and abnormal branching patterns of subterminal motor nerves—all strong evidence for motor neuron abnormalities (24). These abnormalities are correlated with elevated serum CPK activity. Genetic studies further suggest that there may be an inherited basis to these elevations (25).

Since increased serum CPK activity occurs in some acute medical emergencies such as myocardial infarctions and cerebrovascular accidents, clinicians should be aware of the increased frequency of this abnormal laboratory value in psychotic patients. In such patients, it does not represent an acute physical emergency but a nonspecific response to psychiatric stress that warrants further research but not specific clinical action.

DETECTION OF DRUG ABUSE OR OVERDOSE

Initial evaluation of an acutely psychotic individual, if drug abuse is at all suspected, should include a blood and/or urine drug screen. In an emergency room situation, when acute overdose of a psychopharmacological substance is suspected, immediate blood, urine, or gastric content analyses should be made.

Methods now in use in commercial laboratories can reliably and specifically identify many classes of street and prescription drugs in the plasma and urine of patients. These include phencyclidine (PCP), methaqualone, methadone, morphine, cocaine and its metabolites, the benzodiazepines and their metabolites, amphetamines, methamphetamine (methadrine), 2,5-dimethoxy-4-methylamphetamine (DOM), mescaline, and the indole hallucinogens (26).

Abuse of over-the-counter medications for anxiety, many of which contain bromides (e.g., Narvane), may lead to bromide intoxication. Most commonly, this is manifested by a predominantly paranoid psychosis. It is important to test for this condition by obtaining a blood bromide level (150 mg/100 ml is considered necessary to produce symptoms of intoxication, but this is variable). Sodium chloride is used effectively as a treatment.

Psychiatric symptoms may also be iatrogenic. Prescribed antihypertensives such as reserpine, alpha-methyldopa, and MAO inhibitors, can cause depressive or other symptoms (27). While psychiatric symptoms are associated with the monoamine metabolic properties of these drugs, distinguishing from previous premorbid manifestations, as well as manifestations of the hypertension itself, may be difficult.

LABORATORY ASSESSMENT OF PSYCHOPHARMACOLOGIC TREATMENT

Blood monitoring of pharmacological treatment has enabled clinicians to adjust doses of medication in order to achieve optimal clinical response with minimal toxicity. It also has been useful in determining patient compliance with treatment. Since individuals vary in rate and degree of gut absorption of oral medications, blood concentrations have become useful for determination of medication adjustments, particularly in patients who are clinically unresponsive to the medication.

In psychiatry, blood concentrations of all major classes of drugs have been studied extensively. While monitoring of lithium blood concentrations is accepted as a necessary part of lithium pharmacotherapy, the practice of monitoring tricyclic and neuroleptic blood concentrations is not established, and commercial laboratories only recently have made these assays available for use.

Lithium Treatment

Pretreatment Evaluation

Pretreatment evaluations of patients selected for lithium therapy emphasize factors that might enhance the potential for toxicity. In addition to the physical examination, laboratory tests of renal, electrolyte, and thyroid function; a fasting blood sugar; complete blood cell counts; and an ECG should be performed (Table 5.2). Particular caution should be observed in the treatment of the elderly or other patients who may be subject to electrolyte imbalance or decreased renal clearance. These patients should receive lower initial doses and have blood concentrations monitored more frequently.

Lithium Blood Levels

Lithium serum concentrations are routinely used for adjustment of dose at start of treatment, manipulation of concentration to determine minimum effective dose, control of disturbing side effects, and guarding against progressive toxicity. Once patients are stabilized on an appropriate dose schedule, bimonthly checks may be sufficient. In acute concomitant medical or surgical illnesses, monitoring lithium serum concentrations is a necessity. Since the range of blood concentrations achieved by ingestion of a given dose of lithium is wide and depends on absorption, tissue sequestration, and renal clearance, obtaining lithium serum concentrations is a necessity in clinical practice both to ensure optimal response and to prevent toxicity (28).

Maximum patient response with minimal toxicity occurs when the serum lithium concentration is in the range of 0.6 to 1.2 mEq/L. An initial administration of 1,200 mg/24 hours in divided doses has resulted in optimal blood concentrations for a large proportion of manic patients. Dosage adjustments are made after allowing five to seven days for equilibration. Blood concentrations should be monitored every two to three days during this phase of

Table 5.2 Lithium Treatment: Laboratory Recommendations

Test	Frequency
Plasma lithium	2 to 3 days, weeks 1 to 2; weekly, weeks 3 to 4; bimonthly, when stabilized
Complete blood count	6 months
Sedimentation rate	6 months
Whole blood urea nitrogen, Creatinine	Bimonthly
T_3, T_4, TSH (if TSH is raised)	6 months (monthly)
Twenty-four-hour urine volume	6 months
ECG	Annually
Physical examination	Annually

treatment. For the purpose of interlaboratory standardization, blood should be drawn in the morning eight to twelve hours following the last dose of lithium.

An alternative method for determining a maintenance lithium dose has been proposed by Cooper et al. (29). A single loading dose of 600 mg is given orally, and the selection of a dose regimen is based on the serum lithium concentration twenty-four hours later. Serum lithium concentrations are then repeated the fourth and seventh days after the start of treatment. This method, however, should be used with caution because it is not always reliable and may produce concentrations either in the toxic or subtherapeutic range (30).

Some controversy still exists with regard to the range of optimal blood concentrations for the treatment of mania. Earlier studies suggested that all manic patients who responded favorably to lithium did so at blood concentrations below 1.3 to 1.4 mEq/L (31,32). Others (33,34), however, have reported that nonresponders at the 1 to 1.5 mEq/L range may become responders at higher concentrations. Therefore, it seems reasonable to increase plasma concentrations until either remission of symptoms or significant toxicity occurs. Plasma concentrations above 1.5 mEq/L should be carefully monitored in a hospital setting with frequent observations for signs of toxicity. Once mania remits, many patients require lower maintenance doses. Failure to recognize this can lead to toxicity. Therapeutic concentrations between 0.9 and 1.2 mEq/L should be maintained at least six months if no intolerable side effects exist. Patients should not be considered to be lithium refractory until they have received at least a three-week trial at optimal blood concentrations.

During lithium maintenance, blood concentrations of lithium, whole blood urea nitrogen (BUN), and creatinine should be obtained monthly, and a full blood count, T_3, T_4, TSH, twenty-four-hour urine volume, and creatinine clearance should be obtained every six months. If plasma TSH is elevated, a sign of impending hypothyroidism, then thyroid function should be rechecked more closely.

Using salivary lithium for monitoring dosage has been investigated quite extensively since it was first suggested as a convenient alternative to obtaining serum concentrations. Many difficulties are inherent in this method, including variability among patients in saliva/plasma ratios, alterations in ratios associated with length of time lithium has been administered, and variations in saliva flow rate and its electrolyte composition. Further work is needed to establish the weights of these variables and to compare serum and saliva concentrations before this measure may be used in clinical practice.

Tricyclic Antidepressant Plasma Levels

Although the routine clinical practice of assessing and monitoring plasma tricyclic concentrations is still controversial, it is recommended for evaluating a lack of therapeutic response after several weeks of treatment with conventional doses, for monitoring compliance, and for preventing acute overdose. Since, for a given dose, plasma concentrations of tricyclics increase with the age of the patient and since higher concentrations are associated with cardiotoxicity, tricyclic concentrations should also be monitored in the elderly and in patients with cardiovascular problems.

The relationship between plasma concentrations and therapeutic response has been established for at least three major tricyclics: imipramine, amitriptyline, and nortriptyline, while investigations of the others are in progress. This relationship, however, has been established most consistently only for nondelusional endogenously depressed patients (for review of the literature, see references 35–39).

The rate of plasma elimination of tricyclic antidepressants varies considerably among individuals. Thus, the same daily dose results in widely differing steady-state concentrations in individual patients. Although no absolute consensus has been reached, optimal clinical response appears to be obtained with nortriptyline at plasma concentrations between 50 and 150 ng/ml, with doxepin and protriptyline between 100 and 200 ng/ml, with desipramine between 100 and 300 ng/ml, and with amitriptyline and imipramine between 180 and 300 ng/ml. While a curvilinear relationship between therapeutic response and plasma concentrations exists for nortriptyline, a linear relationship with no upper limit appears to be present for imipramine and desipramine. Toxicity may occur in some patients with plasma concentrations above 500 ng/ml and usually occurs above 1,000 ng/ml for all tricyclic antidepressants.

Steady-state plasma concentrations of the drugs are reached when daily elimination of drug equals the amount ingested and plasma and tissue concentrations are approximately the same at similar times on successive days. This usually occurs seven to twenty-one days after the commencement of treatment, and therefore, it is recommended that plasma concentrations be monitored at appropriate intervals after two weeks of regular drug ingestion. Cooper and Simpson (38) have found plasma concentrations of tricyclics after a single dose to be predictive of steady-state plasma concentrations, and they endorse this method of predicting the dose necessary for therapeutic response.

Plasma tricyclics are usually measured in the clinical laboratory using gas-chromatographic techniques. The most specific is the most expensive method—combined gas chromatographic–mass spectrometry (GC–MS). Both high performance liquid chromatographic and radioimmunoassay methods have also been introduced (reviewed in reference 39).

The blood for tricyclic concentrations must not be drawn into glass Vacutainer tubes because a compound that is eluted from the rubber stoppers in these tubes decreases the plasma binding of tricyclic antidepressants to varying degrees and, thus, results in artifactually lowered values. Blood samples obtained through indwelling needles flushed with heparinized saline may also show changes in plasma drug concentrations due to indirect interaction with the heparin. In addition, at least one study (40) suggests a variable ratio of erythrocyte to plasma drug content for individuals, which may necessitate measuring whole blood samples instead of plasma.

When obtaining tricyclic antidepressant plasma concentrations, time of day as well as time since last dose must be standardized. It is recommended that samples be drawn in the morning prior to the first dose and approximately twelve hours after the last dose.

Neuroleptic Levels

Although new assay methods have made the measurement of neuroleptic blood concentrations available to clinicians, its clinical utility is not presently well established. Whether these values can help clinicians improve clinical response or prevent side effects in their patients remains questionable. Nevertheless, since tardive dyskinesia is a frequent and potentially irreversible side effect, monitoring the administration of these drugs in some way is of considerable importance. Some research studies find correlations of neuroleptic concentrations with clinical response, while others fail to find this (reviewed in reference 41). Difference in assay methods and type of neuroleptic used may explain this discrepancy. It is also unclear which is more relevant to clinical response: neuroleptic concentrations in erythrocytes and other blood cells or plasma concentrations.

The main procedures found to be most reliable and specific for neuroleptic determinations have been GC-MS, radioreceptor assays, and radioimmunoassays. Like radioimmunoassays, radioreceptor assays are based on the principle that the amount of radioactive substance specifically attached to a binding site is a quantitative function of the amount of unlabeled substance present. For radioimmunoassays, the labeled substance is an antigen that attaches to a corresponding antibody; while for radioreceptor assays, the labeled substance is a radioactive ligand that attaches to a specific neurotransmitter or drug receptor site on a biologic membrane (42). High correlations have been found between these two assay procedures (41). While radioreceptor and radioimmunoassays have the advantage over other methods of actually measuring binding to neuroleptic receptors and thus to any active drug, most other methods measure specific neuroleptics and may not take into account their activities. Nevertheless, reliance on the radioreceptor assay has also been criticized because it assumes that replacement of spiroperidol from receptors will be the same for all neuroleptics.

The dose of medication needed to treat psychotic symptoms decreases with age, partly as a result of the increase in neuroleptic plasma concentrations per given dose with age (43). Thus, in treatment of the elderly, neuroleptic serum level monitoring is frequently helpful. In addition, the elderly are particularly prone to toxic and uncomfortable side effects. Clinically efficacious concentrations for the numerous antipsychotics have not yet been established, however, and a direct relationship between increased concentrations and increased side effects, like tardive dyskinesia, has not been clearly established. Clinical wisdom justifies using only the minimal amount necessary to produce clinical response.

Other conditions such as of noncompliance or gastrointestinal malabsorption may specifically indicate random checks of neuroleptic blood concentrations during the course of treatment. Much research is needed to establish criteria for the use of this procedure.

Prolactin

The pituitary-hypothalamic tuberoinfundibular dopaminergic tract has been of interest in schizophrenia because the effect of various drugs affecting dopamine receptors can be monitored by measuring serum prolactin concentrations. The pituitary dopamine receptors that influence prolactin secretion respond to antipsychotic drugs in a manner similar to those of the mesolimbic and mesocortical dopamine receptors believed to mediate the antipsychotic response to neuroleptic drugs. The dopaminergic influence on prolactin excretion is thought to be inhibitory, and thus, after the commencement of treatment with most neuroleptic drugs (clozapine excluded), increases in serum prolactin concentrations are seen (44,45).

The prolactin response appears to be correlated with clinical response to neuroleptics. Lack of a characteristic rise in serum prolactin concentration should suggest either subtherapeutic dose use, inadequate drug absorption, or rapid metabolism and excretion of the drug. Prolactin concentrations during the course of treatment may also be predictive of relapse in schizophrenic patients maintained on neuroleptics (46).

BIOLOGIC SUBTYPING AND PREDICTIONS OF RESPONSE TO MEDICATION

Established clinical signs and symptoms characteristic of an endogenous depressive disorder such as sleep disturbances, appetite loss, and motor retardation have normally been used as indications for a pharmacological approach to treatment. The risks, however, of short- and long-term use of tricyclic medications are significant—as indeed they are for the use of all psychotropic medication—and the need for judicious use cannot be overestimated. Advances in psychiatric research during the past decade have led to promising biological approaches to prediction of responsiveness to antidepressant medications. Such measures, while not presently accepted for routine use, may be clinically indicated on an individual basis, especially as they become more readily available to practicing clinicians. Some will become important adjuncts to a good initial psychiatric evaluation. Prediction of response to neuroleptic medications, as well as to lithium, however, has not been possible using any presently available laboratory measures. While some initial studies show promise, additional research is needed in these areas.

Dexamethasone Suppression Test (DST)

Conventional methods of psychiatric evaluation have, in many instances, failed to distinguish subtypes of depression from other clinical syndromes. Moreover, many patients with endogenous depression do not receive effective somatic treatment, and likewise, many patients with nonendogenous depressions are treated inappropriately with antidepressive medications. Therefore, the dexamethasone suppression test, a relatively simple procedure, has been used as a laboratory procedure to aid in the diagnosis of endogenous (major) depression (47). Dexamethasone is a synthetic corticosteroid several times more potent than cortisol. When administered to the majority of healthy subjects, it turns off the endogenous secretion of adrenocorticotrophic hormone (ACTH) and, thus, cortisol.

A relationship between depression and the hypothalamic-pituitary-adrenal axis has long been recognized. Several studies have shown increased cortisol secretion in some depressed patients, particularly during the late evening hours (48,49,50,51). It also has been shown that the dexamethasone suppression test is abnormal almost exclusively in hypersecretors although hypersection is not enough to distinguish endogenous from nonendogenous depressives (52).

The dexamethasone suppression test is important in the diagnosis of Cushing's disease in that it distinguishes a primary adrenal from a pituitary etiology. While patients with adrenal pathology are typically dexamethasone resistant, about 50 to 60 percent of patients with major depressive disorders are also dexamethasone resistant or at least show early escape from suppression within twenty-four hours of a dexamethasone dose. The test appears to distinguish endogenous from exogenous depressions with a sensitivity of approximately 67 percent and a specificity of about 95 percent (47,53).

The most validated and sensitive procedure for administering the dexamethasone suppression test is as follows: 1 mg of dexamethasone is given orally at 11:30 PM. Blood samples for plasma cortisol determinations are then obtained the following day at 8:00 AM, 4:00 PM, and 11:00 PM. If it is possible to obtain only one sample, the 4:00 PM sample is thought to be the most crucial (54,55), although abnormalities will be missed if the 11:00 PM sample is omitted (53). Suppression by dexamethasone is shown if the plasma cortisol concentration is 5 μg/dl or less for twenty-four hours (Figure 5.1).

Although some of the literature suggests that good response to tricyclic treatment is associated with escape from suppression, the dexamethasone suppression test is not considered an established method for prediction of treatment response (56,57). Further research and evaluation are needed to

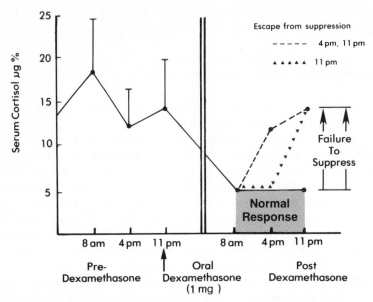

Figure 5.1 Serum Cortisol Concentration Versus Time in the Dexamethasone Suppression Test. One Milligram of Dexamethasone is Administered Orally at 11 PM. Blood Samples are Drawn at 8 AM, 4 PM, and 11 PM Prior to and Post Dexamethasone. The Solid Line Depicts the Maximum Normal Response.

determine whether escape from suppression is related to lithium or specific tricyclic and/or electroconvulsive therapy (ECT) responsiveness. Clarification of the pathological significance of abnormal dexamethasone suppression tests could also be important to our understanding of the biochemical mechanisms involved in the pathogenesis of depressive illnesses (see Chapter 2).

While some practitioners are now using the dexamethasone suppression test routinely, there is significant controversy over its specificity. Contrary to Carroll's studies (47), Amsterdam et al. (58) reported a high percentage of escape from suppression in normal controls and failed to find the test useful as a distinguisher in outpatient populations. In addition, others have found a relatively high incidence of abnormal test suppression in elderly demented patients who do not have a major depressive illness (59), as well as patients suffering from alcoholism, anorexia, or taking certain medication. There is also a concern that some agitated and distressed patients, including an unknown proportion of acutely psychotic, manic, and schizophrenic patients, may also yield positive test results. Some investigators now believe that a positive test reflects a more general central nervous system limbic dysfunction, which is seen in a variety of psychiatric conditions.

Finally, a few case reports have surfaced concerning the coincidence of the administration of the dexamethasone suppression test with suicide attempts (60,61). Although the data are not adequate to connect dexamethasone with suicidal ideation, caution is advised.

Thyrotrophin Releasing Hormone (TRH) Stimulation Test

The release of thyroid stimulating hormone (TSH) from the anterior pituitary is mediated by the hypothalamic tripeptide, TRH; release of TRH is stimulated by norepinephrine and dopamine and is inhibited by serotonin (62,63). The measurement of the release of TSH by the pituitary after the IV infusion of TRH is an established diagnostic procedure for thyroid disease. In the absence of overt thyroid disease, however, abnormal response to this challenge has been associated with major affective disorders (64,65,66,67).

TSH undergoes a circadian rhythm in which basal values are greatest at midnight and lowest at noon or early afternoon. In order to standardize results among institutions, the TSH response test is routinely performed in the morning. Five hundred micrograms of synthetic TRH is infused over 30 seconds into an antecubital vein. Blood specimens are collected before the infusion. Serum TSH can be measured in commercial laboratories by radioimmunoassay. The change in TSH concentration (ΔTSH)—from baseline to peak subsequent to the infusion—is used to interpret the results, regardless of the rate of change (although this may be found to be of future importance). Patients who have a maximum ΔTSH of less than 7 μIU/ml are considered to have a blunted TSH response, while patients with a ΔTSH of greater than 21 μIU/ml are considered to have an augmented response (68) (see Figure 5.2).

Both blunted and augmented responses to TRH have been associated with endogenous depression (69). This test appears to distinguish with a high degree of specificity endogenous from reactive depressions and schizophrenia (65,70). While researchers disagree about the findings in bipolar versus unipolar depression (67,69,71,72), some suggest that a blunted response may be predictive of unipolar depression and an augmented response of bipolar depression. The TRH challenge also may be useful in distinguishing mania and schizoaffective illness (which may be closely related to or synonymous with manic-depressive illness) from chronic schizophrenia (73,74). While initial reports are promising (66,71,72,74), further studies are needed to determine if this provocative challenge will be useful as a predictor of response to tricyclics, lithium, and/or ECT. Furthermore, it appears that abnormal TSH response is independent of abnormal dexamethasone suppression test response so that both tests together can perhaps help define depression in as many as 80 to 90 percent of cases (69,75,76). Little is known of the relationship of TSH response to the so-called low 3-methoxy-4-hydroxyphenylglycol and low 5-hydroxyindoleacetic acid subgroups of depressive disorders, although some relationship might be expected given the dependence of the hypothalamic-pituitary axis on the monoamine neurotransmitters (76).

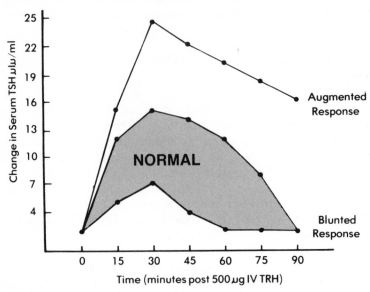

Figure 5.2 The Change in Serum Thyroid-Stimulating Hormone (TSH) with Time Post IV Thyrotrophin-Releasing Hormone (TRH) (500 μg) in the TRH Stimulation Test. The Shaded Area Depicts the Range of the Normal Response.

3-Methoxy-4-hydroxyphenylglycol

3-Methoxy-4-hydroxyphenylglycol (MHPG) is the major metabolite of nor-epinephrine in the brain (77), although the amount of MHPG excreted in the urine that is derived from metabolism of brain norepinephrine remains controversial (78,79). Reports of MHPG excretion in unipolar depressed patients are inconsistent. While some investigators have reported increases in twenty-four-hour urinary MHPG (80), others have reported decreases (81,82). Some also have reported that bipolar patients have decreased concentrations during depression (83) but that these are increased during mania (84).

Further investigations have shown that mixed clinical subtypes of depressed patients with relatively low pretreatment twenty-four-hour urinary MHPG concentrations respond more favorably to imipramine than those with higher concentrations, while the reverse is true for those responding favorably to amitriptyline (83,85,86,87). On the basis of these studies, researchers have hypothesized that unipolar depression may be subclassified into at least two biological subtypes (87,88): Subtype I is characterized by low pretreatment MHPG concentrations and thus is low norepinephrine depression. Subtype I patients may especially benefit from drugs acting predominantly on the noradrenergic system. Those in subtype II are unipolar depressed patients with normal MHPG concentrations but with other abnormalities like alterations in serotonin metabolism, such as low cerebrospinal fluid 5-HIAA. Drugs that affect serotonergic neuronal systems, like amitriptyline, may be more effective for them. A third group contains patients with high pretreatment MHPG excretion and high urinary free cortisol. Specifics of treatment response in this group have not been defined.

Regardless of biological subtype, changes in MHPG concentrations have been associated with clinical improvement (86,89). Despite the already accumulated evidence in support of these hypotheses, further studies are necessary before MHPG becomes a routine pretreatment laboratory measure. The effect of inadequately controlling for nutritional differences between patient and control populations in previous studies needs to be explored further.

In addition, measurement of twenty-four-hour urinary metabolites may be deceiving if careful directions for complete collection are not followed by patients. Some investigators try to circumvent this issue by either collecting a few consecutive twenty-four-hour collections or discounting any collection with a volume below 900 ml. At present, this remains an interesting research finding that awaits further clinical validation.

5-Hydroxyindoleacetic Acid

It has been hypothesized that abnormal indoleamine metabolism is relevant both to depression (90) and schizophrenia (91). 5-Hydroxyindoleacetic acid (5-HIAA), the major metabolite of the indole neurotransmitter serotonin (5-HT), has been measured in the cerebrospinal fluid, blood, and urine of patients with affective and schizophrenic disorders. The cerebrospinal fluid measures are considered the most relevant since sufficient evidence shows that at least some of the 5-HIAA in the lumbar spinal fluid is derived from brain 5-HT metabolism and that most of the 5-HIAA excreted appears to come from peripheral sources (92,93).

Cerebrospinal fluid 5-HIAA concentrations were found to be lower in depressed patients than in normal controls (94). Identification of a subgroup of unipolar depressives with cerebrospinal fluid 5-HIAA below 15 ng/ml and of another with normal cerebrospinal fluid 5-HIAA has been significantly associated with treatment response. Responders to chlorpromazine had lower concentrations of 5-HIAA in the cerebrospinal fluid, while responders to nortriptyline had higher 5-HIAA concentrations (95,96). There is a clear relationship involving the level of 5-HIAA in cerebrospinal fluid, the degree of 5-HT activity of the treatment drug, and the subsequent drug response.

It has also been shown that concentrations of 5-HIAA are reciprocally related to concentrations of urinary MHPG, suggesting the existence of low 5-HIAA/high MHPG and high 5-HIAA/low MHPG subgroups of depressed patients (97). Finally, 5-HIAA concentrations have been found to be lower in suicides than controls, and it has been hypothesized that a 5-HT deficiency may indicate a high risk for suicide attempts (98).

Studies of indole metabolism in schizophrenic patients have been less conclusive. While some investigators have found decreased cerebrospinal fluid and urine 5-HIAA, others have found no difference than controls (99,100,101,102,103). Furthermore, it appears that at least peripherally, blood 5-HT may be elevated in a subgroup of chronic schizophrenics (104,105). It is not known whether these findings relate directly to the illness or if they are predictive of response to treatment with various drugs that deplete 5-HT. Initial use of a 5-HT synthesis inhibitor (Fenclonine) in schizophrenic patients, however, has failed to show any promise (106). Further studies are needed to determine the usefulness of 5-HIAA as a predictive marker in psychiatric practice.

Prediction of Lithium Response

Red Cell/Plasma Lithium Ratio

When possible to determine, the red blood cell/plasma lithium ratio may be of value. Depressed patients who respond to lithium have consistently higher red cell/plasma lithium ratios than nonresponders (greater than 0.5), and this difference appears to be independent of the dose of lithium and of the plasma-lithium concentration (107,108). If this procedure can be consistently validated and is standardized for clinical use, it promises to be of predictive value.

The Lithium Excretion Test

Serry (109) first hypothesized that high lithium excretors do not respond to lithium therapy. He studied lithium excretion in patients for four hours subsequent to a 1,200 mg oral lithium loading dose. He found that twenty-four of thirty manic patients excreted less than 11 mg of lithium in four hours (lithium retainers) and that all twenty-four responded to lithium carbonate within ten days. Those who excreted more than 20 mg did not respond to lithium. Other investigators, however, have failed to confirm this finding (110,111), and at present, results with this test are equivocal and subject to considerable variance. Thus, it is not recommended as an effective screening measure for lithium responsiveness.

Divalent Cation Measurements

Carman et al. (112) used serum calcium and magnesium to predict the antidepressant effect of lithium carbonate in thirty-three patients. They found that the calcium/magnesium ratio related significantly to subsequent antidepressant response to lithium. Those patients who had a baseline ratio of calcium to magnesium greater than 2.62 were responders, whereas those with a baseline ratio less than 2.62 were nonresponders. The most accurate prediction came from an analysis of the changes that took place during the first five days of lithium treatment.

Platelet MAO Activity

MAO is a major enzyme that catalyzes the conversion of the neuroamines dopamine, norepinephrine, phenylethylamine, and serotonin to their inactive metabolites. As platelets share a number of physicochemical properties in common with neurons and are an easily obtainable source of MAO, MAO activity in platelets has been extensively studied in psychiatric research (113,114,115,116,117). Platelet MAO activity appears to be useful as a predictor of pharmacologic response to some of the MAO inhibitors and, perhaps, to lithium as well (see Chapter 2). Its possible role as a biological marker for a specific subtype of psychopathology and/or predictor of neuroleptic treatment response for schizophrenic patients is still under investigation. (See Chapter 2 for a further discussion of laboratory tests associated with lithium and MAO inhibitor therapies.)

Amphetamine Infusions

Plasma cortisol response to IV administration of amphetamine (methamphetamine at 0.2 mg/kg) or dextroamphetamine (0.15 mg/kg) is a promising procedure for differential diagnosis of endogenous depression. Sachar et al. (118) reported that while normal individuals have a sharp increase in plasma cortisol 30 minutes after the infusion, two-thirds of endogenously depressed patients, paradoxically, have a suppression. (See Chapter 2 for a discussion of the dextroamphetamine challenge test for predicting HCA treatment response.)

Apomorphine Infusions

The rationale for the use of an apomorphine challenge is derived from the observation that central dopaminergic neurons are involved in stimulating growth hormone (GH) release (119). Apomorphine is a known direct dopamine receptor agonist and, thus, a stimulator of GH release (120,121).

Initial studies suggest that the GH response to a subcutaneous apomorphine infusion may be predictive of treatment response in schizophrenic patients (122,124). Rotrosen et al. (122,123) examined the GH response to apomorphine in acute and chronic schizophrenics. Patients who had a blunted GH response to apomorphine were neuroleptic responders, while those who had an exaggerated GH response were nonresponders to neuroleptics. The patients with exaggerated GH responses to 0.5 ng of subcutaneous apomorphine had increases in GH concentrations to 40 to 60 ng/ml. Hirschowitz and Garver (124) examined schizophrenic patients' GH response to 0.75 ng of subcutaneous apomorphine and found that those with a mean postinjection peak of 38.7 ng/ml were responders to lithium therapy. Initial data on affective disorders seem less promising (125). Other stimuli used to elicit GH release that may be predictive tools include insulin-induced hypoglycemia; IV amphetamine, IV TRH, and IV clonidine; oral levodopa; and oral 5-hydroxy-tryptophan (126,127,128,129,130,131).

Urinary Phenyl Acetate (PAA)

2-Phenylethylamine (PEA) is a neuroamine which may play a role in initiating and sustaining wakefulness, excitement, and alertness by modulating central nervous system catecholaminergic activity. A decrease in brain concentrations or turnover of endogenous PEA may therefore play a pathophysiological role in certain forms of depression. As PEA is structurally and functionally closely related to amphetamine, it is sometimes referred to as an "endogenous amphetamine." There is also data which support the hypothesis that an increase in the concentrations of brain PEA or the activation of specific brain PEA receptors may be at least partly responsible for the actions of antidepressant and stimulant drugs (132). PEA is principally metabolized by MAO type B to form phenyl acetate.

In a careful study where the twenty-four-hour urinary excretion of PAA was measured, inpatients with major depressive disorder (unipolar type) excreted significantly less PAA compared with healthy volunteers of both sexes (133). Fifty-five percent of the depressives excreted less than 70 mg per 24 hours. Although there were no significant differences in the PAA excretion between untreated patients and those treated with antidepressants that were ineffective, effective antidepressant treatment appeared to increase PAA excretion. However, both increases and decreases in urinary excretion of PAA have been reported to be associated with a number of psychiatric diagnostic categories, as well as individuals under severe stress. Consequently, the role of PAA as a marker for psychiatric diagnosis and treatment awaits further evaluation.

EEG Studies

The availability of a laboratory equipped to monitor all-night sleep EEG responses is the limiting factor in determining the usefulness of this procedure. It may, for practical purposes, be limited to inpatient psychiatric services.

Sleep EEG (polysomnography) recordings of endogenously depressed individuals, when compared to those of normal individuals, have shown significantly shorter rapid-eye-movement (REM) latency (time between falling asleep and the first period of the REM, or dreaming, phase of sleep) as well as increased REM activity throughout the night. Two nights of recordings, one before the onset of medication and the other after the administration of one dose of medication, have been used for evaluation of the future effectiveness of pharmacological treatment. In one study of depressed patients, with the administration of just 50 mg of amitriptyline, the REM percentage decreased by 44 percent, the REM activity decreased by 33 percent, and the REM latency increased by 118 percent (134). Nonresponders to the antidepressant effects of the drug had significantly less change in REM latency and average REM activity compared to responders. (Difficulty in sleep onset and REM latency were strong predictors of final Hamilton scale scores of depression.) Currently available data indicate that the sleep EEG test is one of the most reliable clinical laboratory tests in diagnosing major depressive disorders.

While sleep EEGs have been less extensively studied in schizophrenia, baseline EEG abnormalities have been reported in some schizophrenic patients (135).

Averaged Evoked Responses

Averaged evoked responses (AER) are EEG measurements of responses to visual or auditory stimuli. Individual differences have been found to a gradual increase in stimulus intensity. With increasing stimulus intensity, some patients have a decrease in the amplitude of their evoked response (reducers), while others reveal an increase (augmenters). Men tend to be reducers and women tend to be augmenters. Schizophrenics and unipolar patients tend to be reducers, and bipolar patients tend to be augmenters. These appear to be heritable and replicable findings and do not appear to be state dependent (136,137,138). Future studies may find these parameters useful in defining meaningful treatment subgroups or in determining risk of subsequent development of overt mental disorders.

Nocturnal Penile Tumescence Studies (NPT)

Nocturnal penile tumescence studies are derivatives of electroencephalographic investigations. Thirty years ago, sleep EEG reseachers discovered rapid eye movement as a specific phase of the sleep EEG. REM sleep is characterized by high metabolic activity and autonomic instability of physiologic parameters such as blood pressure and pulse (139). The concurrence of penile erection during REM sleep has allowed development of this investigative strategy (140). Utilization of a string gauge to measure penile circumferential changes allows documentation of erectile function. Simultaneous monitoring with EEG and electrooculogram (EOG) concurrently validates electrophysiologic levels of sleep (141). In addition to increased penile circumference, the length of the penis as well as buckling strength of the bulbocavernosus-ischiocavernosus muscles allows further documentation of erectile strength (142). This technology is used to ascertain erectile ability for men complaining of impotence. In individuals with a non-psychiatric medical etiology for such complaints, whether due to vascular, neurologic or endocrine dysfunction, there will be minimal or no erections during REM stages of sleep. Analogous phenomena occur in female populations (143). Utilization of a vaginal plethysmograph to measure vaginal ballooning during REM sleep may allow further understanding of physiologic elements that contribute to anorgasmic states. The role of diagnosable psychiatric disorders in modifying REM stage erections is unclear, but such disorders may modify REM erectile functioning resulting in an intermediate response between normal REM stage tumescence and no response in documented non-psychiatric medical conditions.

Molecular and Receptor Markers

Several potentially useful markers have been identified for affective disorders, including HLA (major histocompatibility gene complex) linkage, increased platelet α_2-receptor activity, and decreased platelet imipramine-binding sites. Although the significance and clinical implications of these findings are still unclear, these developments augur important new strategies for both treatment and enhanced understanding of the pathophysiology of affective disorders.

The segregation of HLA antigens and depressive illness in some families suggests that early screening for family members at high risk may be possible for certain types of affective disorder. This phenomenon is also intriguing because many other illnesses previously shown to be linked to the HLA system have an important immunological basis (144).

Changes in sensitivity of neurotransmitter-linked receptors also appear to be relevant to psychiatric disorders and to the pharmacologic treatment of these conditions, as discussed in previous chapters. In patients with major depression, α_2-receptors, which presynaptically inhibit norepinephrine release, appear to be increased on the platelet membrane and decreased after successful pharmacologic treatment (145). A decreased platelet membrane binding of tritiated imipramine has also been associated with major depression, and there is evidence that these binding sites are functionally and perhaps structurally associated with serotonin uptake (transport) sites in brain and other tissues (146). However, further study will be required to assess whether this phenomenon represents an inherited or acquired deficiency rather than an artifact associated with pharmacologic treatment, as well as its potential value for identifying individuals at risk and evaluating treatment response.

SUMMARY

Adjunct use of the clinical laboratory is as necessary to clinical psychiatry as it is to other fields of medicine. Determining differential diagnoses and predicting and monitoring treatment response can be assisted with appropriate use of the laboratory. While much of biological psychiatric evaluation and treatment remains an area for future research, important strides toward more empirical and scientific decision making have been made in the last several decades which depend, in part, upon proper utilization of the clinical laboratory.

REFERENCES

1. Hall, R.C.W.; Gardner, E.R.; Stickney, S.K.; LeCann, A.F.; and Popkin, M.K. Physical illness manifesting as psychiatric disease. *Arch. Gen. Psychiatry* 37:989–995, 1980.

2. Hall, R.C.W.; Gardner, E.R.; Popkin, M.K.; LeCann, A.F.; and Stickney, S.K. Unrecognized physical illness prompting psychiatric admission: A prospective study. *Am. J. Psychiatry* 138:629–635, 1981.

3. Koranyi, E.K. Morbidity and rate of undiagnosed physical illnesses in a psychiatric clinic population. *Arch. Gen. Psychiatry* 36:414–419, 1979.

4. Burke, A.W. Physical illness in psychiatric hospital patients in Jamaica. *Br. J. Psychiatry* 121:321–322, 1972.

5. Johnson, D.A.W. Evaluation of routine physical examination in psychiatric cases. *Practitioner* 200:686–691, 1968.

6. Maguire, G.P., and Granville-Grossman, K.L. Physical illness in psychiatric patients. *Br. Med. J.* 114:1365–1369, 1968.

7. Davies, W.D. Physical illness in psychiatric outpatients. *Br. J. Psychiatry* 111:27–37, 1965.

8. Herridge, C.F. Physical disorders in psychiatric illness: A study of 209 consecutive admissions. *Lancet* 2:949–951, 1960.

9. Marshall, H. Incidence of physical disorders among psychiatric inpatients. *Br. Med. J.* 2:468–470, 1949.

10. Freedman, A.M.; Kaplan, H.I.; and Sadock, B.J. *Comprehensive Textbook of Psychiatry*, 2nd ed., 2 vols., volume 1. Baltimore: Williams and Wilkins Co., 1975.

11. Koranyi, E.J. *Physical Illness in Psychiatric Patients.* New York: Plenum Press, 1982.

12. Jefferson, J.W., and Marshall, J.F. *Neuropsychiatric Features of Medical Disorders.* (Critical Issues in Psychiatry Series). New York: Plenum Press, 1981.

13. Asher, R. Myxedematous madness. *Br. Med. J.* 2:555–562, 1949.

14. Gold, M.S.; Pottash, A.C.; Mueller, E.A.; and Extein, I. Grades of thyroid failure in 100 depressed and anergic psychiatric inpatients. *Am. J. Psychiatry* 138:253–255, 1981.

15. Sandok, B.A. Temporal arteritis. *JAMA* 222:1405–1406, 1972.

16. O'Connor, J.F., and Musher, D.M. Central nervous system involvement in systemic lupus erythematosus: A study of 150 cases. *Arch. Neurol.* 14:157–161, 1966.

17. Perry, T.L.; Hansen, S.; Tischler, B.; Richards, R.M.; and Sokol, M. Unrecognized adult phenylketonuria: Implications for obstetrics and psychiatry. *N. Engl. J. Med.* 289:395–398, 1973.

18. Hoaken, P.C. Schizophrenia and Klinefelter's syndrome. *Can. J. Psychiatry* 26:519–521, 1981.

19. Waber, D.P. Neuropsychological aspects of Turner's syndrome. *Dev. Med. Child Neurol.* 21:58–70, 1979.

20. Hook, E.B. Behavioral implications of the human XYY genotype. *Science* 179:139–151, 1973.

21. Dorus, E. Application of chromosome banding techniques in psychiatric research. In *Physico-Chemical Methodologies in Psychiatric Research,* Hanin, I., and Koslow, S.H., eds. New York: Raven Press, 1980, pp. 179–197.

22. Zweig, M.H.; van Steirteghem, A.C.; and Torrey, E.F. Creatinine kinase isoenzymes in the serum and CSF of schizophrenic patients. *Arch. Gen. Psychiatry* 38:1107–1109, 1981.

23. Meltzer, H.Y.; Ross-Stanton, J.; and Schlessinger, S. Mean serum creatinine kinase activity in patients with functional psychoses. *Arch. Gen. Psychiatry* 6:650–655, 1980.

24. Ross-Stanton, J., and Meltzer, H.Y. Motor neuron branching patterns in psychotic patients. *Arch. Gen. Psychiatry* (in press).

25. Meltzer, H.Y. Neuromuscular abnormalities in the major mental illnesses: I. Serum enzyme studies. *Res. Publ. Assoc. Res. Nerv. Mental Dis.* 54:165–188, 1975.

26. Foltz, R.L.; Fentinian, A.F.; and Foltz, R.B. *GC/MS Assays for Abused Drugs in Body Fluids.* NIDA Research Monograph series 32. Rockville, Md. 1980; 1-202.

27. Pottash, A.L.C.; Black, H.R.; and Gold, M.S. Psychiatric complications of antihypertensive medications. *J. Nerv. Ment. Dis.* 169:430–438, 1981.

28. Johnson, F.N., ed. *Handbook of Lithium Therapy.* Baltimore: University Park Press, 1980.

29. Cooper, T.B.; Bergner, P.E.E.; Simpson, G.M. The 24 hr serum lithium level as a prognosticator of dosage requirements. *Am. J. Psychiatry* 130:601–603, 1973.

30. Naiman, I.F.; Muniz, C.E.; Stewart, R.B.; and Yost, R.L. Practicality of a lithium dosing guide. *Am. J. Psychiatry* 138:1369–1371, 1981.

31. Spring, G.; Schweid, D.; Gray, L.; Steinberg, J.; and Harwitz, M. A double blind comparison of lithium and chlorpromazine in the treatment of manic states. *Am. J. Psychiatry* 126:1306–1310, 1970.

32. Prien, R.F.; Coffey, E.M., Jr.; and Klett, C.J. A comparison of lithium, carbonate and chlorpromazine in the treatment of excited schizoaffectives. *Arch. Gen. Psychiatry* 27:182–189, 1972.

33. Stokes, J.W.; Kocsis, J.H.; and Arcuni, O.J. Relationship of lithium chloride dose to treatment response in acute mania. *Arch. Gen. Psychiatry* 33:1080–1084, 1976.

34. Himmelhoch, J.M.; Forrest, J.; Neil, J.F.; and Detre, T.P. Thiazide lithium synergy in refractory mood swings. *Am. J. Psychiatry* 134:149–152, 1977.

35. Baldessarini, R.J. Status of psychotrophic drug blood level assays and other biochemical measurements in clinical practice. *Am. J. Psychiatry* 136:1177–1180, 1979.

36. Amsterdam, J.; Brunswick, D.; and Mendels, S. The clinical application of tricyclic antidepressant pharmacokinetics and plasma levels. *Am. J. Psychiatry* 137:653–662, 1980.

37. Ban, T.A. *Psychopharmacology of Depression: A Guide for Drug Treatment.* Karger, S., ed. New York: Basal, 1981.

38. Cooper, T.B., and Simpson, G.M. Prediction of individual dosage of nortriptyline. *Am. J. Psychiatry* 135:333–335, 1978.

39. Scoggins, B.A.; Maguire, K.P.; Norman, T.R.; and Burrows, G.D. Measurement

of tricyclic antidepressants Part I. A review of methodology. *Clin. Chem.* 26:5–17, 1980.

40. Linnoila, M.; Dorrity, F.; and Jobson, K. Plasma and erythrocyte levels of tricyclic antidepressants in depressed patients. *Am. J. Psychiatry* 135:557–561, 1978.

41. Rosenblatt, J.E.; Pary, R.J.; Bigelow, L.B.; DeLisi, L.E.; Wagner, R.L.; Kleinman, J.E.; Weinberger, D.R.; Potkin, S.G.; Shiling, D.; Jeste, D.V.; Alexander, P.; and Wyatt, R.J. Measurement of serum neuroleptic concentrations by radioreceptor assay: Concurrent assessment of clinical response and toxicity. In *Neuroreceptors—Basic and Clinical Aspects*, Usdin, E., Bunney, W.E., and Davis, J.M., eds. New York: John Wiley and Sons, 1981.

42. Enna, S.J. Radioreceptor assays. In *Physico-Chemical Methodologies in Psychiatric Research*, Hanin, I., and Koslow, S.H., eds. New York: Raven Press, 1980, pp. 83–101.

43. Jeste, D.V.; Rosenblatt, J.E.; Wagner, R.L.; and Wyatt, R.J. High serum neuroleptic levels in tardive dyskinesia. *N. Engl. J. Med.* 301:1184, 1979.

44. Meltzer, H.Y.; Goode, D.J.; and Fang, V.S. The effect of psychotropic drugs on endocrine function. In *Psychopharmacology: A Generation of Progress*, Lipton, M.A., DiMascio, A., and Killam, K.F., eds. New York: Raven Press, 1978, pp. 509–529.

45. de la Fuente, J.R., and Rosenbaum, A.H. Prolactin in psychiatry. *Am. J. Psychiatry* 138:1154–1160, 1981.

46. Laughren, T.P.; Brown, W.A.; and Williams, B.W. Serum prolactin and clinical state during neuroleptic treatment and withdrawal. *Am. J. Psychiatry* 136:108–110, 1979.

47. Carroll, B.J.; Feinberg, M.; Greden, J.F.; Tareka, J.; Albala, A.A.; Haskett, R.F.; James, N.M.; Kronfol, Z.; Lohr, N.; Steiner, M.; Vigne, J.P.; and Young, E. A specific laboratory test for the diagnosis of melancholia: Standardization, validation and clinical utility. *Arch. Gen. Psychiatry* 38:15–22, 1981.

48. Carroll, B.J.; Curtis, G.C.; and Mendels, J. Neuroendocrine regulation in depression. I. Limbic system-adrenocortical dysfunction. *Arch. Gen. Psychiatry* 33:1039–1044, 1976.

49. Ettigi, P., and Brown, G.M. Psychoneuroendocrinology of affective disorders: An overview. *Am. J. Psychiatry* 134:493–501, 1977.

50. Sachar, E.J.; Hellman, L.; and Fukushima, D.K. Cortisol production in depressive illness. *Arch. Gen. Psychiatry* 23:289–298, 1970.

51. Sachar, E.J.; Hellman, L.; and Roffwarg, H.P. Disrupted 24-hour patterns of cortisol secretion in psychotic depression. *Arch. Gen. Psychiatry* 28:19–24, 1973.

52. Asnis, G.M.; Sachar, E.J.; Halbreich, U.; Nathan, R.S.; Ostrow, L.; and Halpern, F.S. Cortisol secretion and dexamethasone response in depression. *Am. J. Psychiatry* 138:1218–1221, 1981.

53. Carroll, B.J.; Curtis, G.C.; and Mendels, J. Neuroendocrine regulation in depression: Discrimination of depressed from nondepressed patients. *Arch. Gen. Psychiatry* 33:1051–1057, 1976.

54. Carroll, B.J. Neuroendocrine function in psychiatric disorders. In *Psychopharmacology: A Generation of Progress*, Lipton, M.A., DiMascio, A., and Killam, K.F., eds. New York: Raven Press, 1978.

55. Carroll, B.J., and Mendels, J. Neuroendocrine regulation in affective disorders. In *Hormones, Behavior and Psychopathology*, Sachar, E.J., ed. New York: Raven Press, 1976.

56. Brown, W.A.; Johnston, R.; and Mayfield, D. The 24-hour dexamethasone suppression test in a clinical setting: Relationship to diagnoses, symptoms and response to treatment. *Am. J. Psychiatry* 136:543–547, 1979.

57. Brown, W.A.; Haier, R.J.; and Qualls, C.B. The dexamethasone suppression test in the identification of subtypes of depression differentially responsive to antidepressants. *Psychopharmacol. Bull.* 17:88–89, 1981.

58. Amsterdam, J.D.; Winokur, A.; Caroff, S.N.; and Conn, J. The dexamethasone suppression test in outpatients with primary affective disorder and healthy control subjects. *Am. J. Psychiatry* 139:287–291, 1982.

59. Spar, J.E., and Gerner, R. Does the dexamethasone suppression test distinguish dementia from depression? *Am. J. Psychiatry* 139:238–240, 1982.

60. Beck-Friis, J.; Aperia, B.; Kjellman, B.; Llringgren, J.G.; Petterson, U.; Sara, V.; Sjolin, A.; Unden, F.; and Welkerberg, L. Suicidal behavior and the dexamethasone suppression test. *Am. J. Psychiatry* 138:993–994, 1981.

61. Asberg, M.; Varpila-Hansson, R.; Tomba, P.; Aminoff, A.K.; Martensson, B.; Thoren, P.; Traskman-Bendz, L.; Eneroth, P.; and Astron, G. Suicidal behavior and the dexamethasone suppression test. *Am. J. Psychiatry* 138:993–994, 1981.

62. Martin, J.B.; Reichlin, S.; and Brown, G.M. *Clinical Neuroendocrinology.* Philadelphia: F.A. Davis Co., 1977.

63. Kirkegaard, C.; Bjorum, N.; Cohn, D.; Faber, J.; Lauridsen, U.B.; and Nerup, J. Studies on the influence of biogenic amines and psychoactive drugs on the prognostic value of the TRH stimulation test in endogenous depression. *Psychoneuroendocrinology* 2:131–136, 1977.

64. Kirkegaard, C.; Norlem, N.; Lauridsen, U.B.; Bjorum, N.; and Chustiansen, C. Protirelin stimulation test and thyroid function during treatment of depression. *Arch. Gen. Psychiatry* 32:1115–1118, 1975.

65. Kirkegaard, C. The thyrotropin response to thyrotropin releasing hormone in endogenous depression. *Psychoneuroendocrinology* 6:189–212, 1981.

66. Extein, I.; Pottash, A.L.C.; Gold, M.S.; Cadet, J.; Sweeney, D.R.; Davies, R.K.; and Martin, D.M. The thyroid stimulating hormone response to thyrotropin releasing hormone in mania and bipolar depression. *Psychiatry Res.* 2:199–204, 1980.

67. Linkowski, P.; Brauman, H.; and Mendlewuicz, J. Thyrotropin response to thyrotropin releasing hormone in unipolar and bipolar affective illness. *J. Affect. Dis.* 3:9, 1981.

68. Loosen, P.T., and Prange, A.J. Thyrotropin releasing hormone (TRH): A useful tool for psychoneuroendocrine investigation. *Psychoneuroendocrinology* 5:63–80, 1980.

69. Targum, S.D.; Sullivan, A.C.; and Byrnes, S.M. Neuroendocrine interrelationships in major depressive disorder. *Am. J. Psychiatry* 139:282–286, 1982.

70. Extein, I.; Pottash, A.L.C.; and Gold, M.S. The thyrotropin-releasing hormone test in the diagnosis of unipolar depression. *Psychiatry Res.* 5:311–316, 1981.

71. Papakostas, Y.; Fink, M.; Lee, J.; Irwin, P.; and Johnson, L. Neuroendocrine measures in psychiatric patients: Course and outcome with ECT. *Psychiatry Res.* 4:55–64, 1981.

72. Gold, M.S.; Pottash, A.L.C.; Davies, R.K.; Ryan, N.; Sweeney, D.R.; and Martin, D.M. Distinguishing unipolar and bipolar depression by thyrotropin release test. *Lancet* 2:411–412, 1979.

73. Extein, I.; Pottash, A.L.C.; Gold, M.S.; and Martin, D.M. Differentiating

mania from schizophrenia by the TRH test. *Am. J. Psychiatry* 137:981–982, 1980.

74. Extein, I.; Pottash, A.L.C.; Gold, M.S.; and Cowdry, R.W. Using the protirelin test to distinguish mania from schizophrenia. *Arch. Gen. Psychiatry* 391:77–81, 1982.

75. Kirkegaard, C., and Carroll, B.J. Dissociation of TSH and adrenocortical disturbances in endogenous depression. *Psychiatry Res.* 3:253–264, 1980.

76. Davis, K.L.; Hollister, L.E.; Mathe, A.A.; Davis, B.M.; Rothpearl, A.B.; Faull, K.F.; Hsieh, J.Y.K.; Barchas, J.D.; and Berger, P.A. Neuroendocrine and neurochemical measurements in depression. *Am. J. Psychiatry* 138:1555–1561, 1981.

77. Schanberg, S.M.; Schildkraut, J.J.; and Breese, G.R. Metabolism of normetanephrine-H^3 in rat brain—Identification of conjugated 3-methoxy-4-hydroxyphenylglycol as the major metabolite. *Biochem. Pharmacol.* 17:247–254, 1968.

78. Maas, J.W.; Dekirmenjian, H.; Garver, D.; Redmond, D.-E.; and Landis, D.H. Excretion of catecholamine metabolites following intraventricular infection of 6-hydroxy-dopamine in the macaca speciosa. *Eur. J. Pharmacol.* 23:121–130, 1973.

79. Kopin, I.J. Measuring turnover of neurotransmitters in human brains. In *Psychopharmacology: A Generation of Progress*, Lipton, M.A., DiMascio, A., and Killam, K.F., eds. New York: Raven Press, 1978, p. 933.

80. Garfinkel, P.E.; Warsh, J.J.; and Stancer, H.C. Depression: New evidence in support of biological differentiation. *Am. J. Psychiatry* 136:535–539, 1979.

81. Maas, J.W.; Fawcett, J.A.; and Dekirmenjian, H. 3-methoxy-4-hydroxyphenylglycol (MHPG) excretion in depressive states. *Arch. Gen. Psychiatry* 19:129–134, 1968.

82. Fawcett, J.A.; Maas, J.W.; and Dekirmenjian, H. Depression and MHPG excretion. *Arch. Gen. Psychiatry* 26:246–251, 1972.

83. Schildkraut, J.J. Norepinephrine metabolites as biochemical criteria for classifying depressive disorders and predicting responses to treatment. Preliminary findings. *Am. J. Psychiatry* 130:695–699, 1973.

84. Deleon-Jones, F.; Maas, J.W.; and Dekirmenjian, H. Urinary catecholamine metabolites during behavioral changes in patients with manic-depressive cycles. *Science* 179:300–302, 1973.

85. Maas, J.W.; Fawcett, J.A.; and Dekirmenjian, H. Catecholamine metabolism, depressive illness and drug response. *Arch. Gen. Psychiatry* 26:252–262, 1972.

86. Modai, I.; Apter, A.; Golomb, M.; and Wijsenbeek, H. Response to amitriptyline and urinary MHPG in bipolar depressive patients. *Neuropsychobiology* 5:181–184, 1979.

87. Schildkraut, J.J.; Orsulak, P.J.; Schatzberg, A.F.; Cole, J.O.; and Rosenbaum, A.H. Possible pathophysiological mechanisms in subtypes of unipolar depressive disorders based on differences in urinary MHPG levels. *Psychopharmacol. Bull.* 17:90–91, 1981.

88. Maas, J.W. Biogenic amines and depression. Biochemical and pharmacological separation of two types of depression. *Arch. Gen. Psychiatry* 32:1357–1362, 1975.

89. Beckman, H., and Goodwin, F.K. Antidepressant response to tricyclics and urinary MHPG in unipolar patients. *Arch. Gen. Psychiatry* 32:17–21, 1975.

90. Zarcone, V.P.; Berger, P.A.; Brodie, H.K.H.; Sack, R.; and Barchas, J.D. The indoleamine hypothesis of depression: An overview and pilot study. *Dis. Nerv. Syst.* 38:646–653, 1977.

91. Wooley, D.W., and Shaw, E. On the relationship of serotonin to schizophrenia. *Br. Med. J.* 2:122, 1954.

92. Anderson, H., and Roos, B.E. 5-hydroxyindole-acetic acid in cerebrospinal fluid of hydrocephalic children. *Acta Paediat. Scand.* 58:601–608, 1969.

93. Young, S.N.; Garelis, E.; Lal, S.; and Sourkes, T.L. Tryptophan and 5-hydroxyindoleacetic acid in human cerebrospinal fluid. *J. Neurochem.* 22:777–779, 1974.

94. Murphy, D.L.; Cambell, I.C.; and Costa, J.L. The brain serotonergic system in affective disorders. *Prog. Neuropsychopharmacol.* 2:1–31, 1978.

95. van Praag, H.M. Significance of biochemical parameters in the diagnosis, treatment and prevention of depressive disorders. *Biol. Psychiatry* 12:101–131, 1977.

96. Asberg, M.; Bertilsson, L.; Tuck, D.; Cronholm, B.; and Sjoqvist, F. Indoleamine metabolites in the cerebrospinal fluid of depressed patients before and during treatment with nortriptyline. *Clin. Pharmacol. Ther.* 14:277–286, 1973.

97. Goodwin, F.K.; Cowdry, R.W.; and Webster, M.H. Predictors of drug response in the affective disorders: Toward an integrated approach. In *Psychopharmacology: A Generation of Progress*, Lipton, M.A., DiMascio, A., and Killam, K.F., eds. New York: Raven Press, 1978.

98. Asberg, M.; Traskman, L.; and Thoren, P. 5-HIAA in the cerebrospinal fluid: A biochemical suicide predictor. *Arch. Gen. Psychiatry* 33:1193–1197, 1976.

99. Bowers, M.B., Jr.; Heninger, G.R.; and Gerbode, F. Cerebrospinal fluid 5-hydroxy-indoleacetic acid and homovanillic acid in psychiatric patients. *Int. J. Neuropharmacology* 8:255–262, 1969.

100. Ashcroft, G.W.; Crawford, T.B.B.; Eccleston, D.; Sharman, D.F.; MacDougall, E.J.; Stanton, J.B.; and Binns, J.K. 5-hydroxyindole compounds in the cerebrospinal fluid of patients with psychiatric or neurological diseases. *Lancet* 2:1049–1052, 1966.

101. Berger, P.A.; Faull, K.F.; Kilkowski, J.; Anderson, P.J.; Kraemer, H.; Davis, K.L.; and Barchas, J.D. CSF monoamine metabolites in depression and schizophrenia. *Am. J. Psychiatry* 137:174–180, 1980.

102. Domino, E.F. Urinary acid metabolites of biogenic amines in schizophrenic patients. *Schizophrenia Bull.* 6:238–244, 1980.

103. Leckman, J.F.; Cohen, D.J.; Shaywitz, B.A.; Caparulo, B.K.; Henniger, G.R.; and Bowers, M.B. CSF monoamine metabolites in child and adult psychiatric patients: A developmental perspective. *Arch. Gen. Psychiatry* 37:677–681, 1980.

104. DeLisi, L.E.; Neckers, L.M.; Weinberger, D.R.; and Wyatt, R.J. Increased whole blood serotonin concentrations in chronic schizophrenic patients. *Arch. Gen. Psychiatry* 38:647–650, 1981.

105. Freedman, D.X.; Belendivk, K.; Belenduck, G.W.; and Crayton, J.W. Blood tryptophan metabolism in chronic schizophrenics. *Arch. Gen. Psychiatry* 38:655–659, 1981.

106. DeLisi, L.E.; Freed, W.J.; Gillin, J.C.; Kleinman, J.E.; Bigelow, L.B.; and Wyatt, R.J. Parachlorophenylalanine (PCPA) trials in schizophrenic patients: A brief report. *Biol. Psychiatry* 17:471–477, 1982.

107. Elizir, A.; Shopsin, B.; Gershon, S.; and Ehlenberger, A. INTA: Extracellular lithium ratios and clinical course in affective states. *Clin. Pharmacol. Ther.* 13:947–952, 1972.

108. Mendel, J., and Frazer, A. Intracellular lithium concentration and clinical response: Towards a membrane theory of depression. *J. Psychiatr. Res.* 10:9–18, 1973.

109. Serry, M. Lithium retention and response. *Lancet* 1:1967–1968, 1969.

110. Platman, S.R.; Rohrlich, J.; and Fieve, R.R. Absorption and excretion of lithium in manic depressive illness. *Dis. Nerv. Syst.* 29:733–738, 1968.

111. Stokes, J.W.; Mendel, J.; Secunda, S.K.; and Dyson, W.L. Lithium excretion and therapeutic response. *J. Nerv. Ment. Dis.* 154:43–48, 1972.

112. Carman, J.S.; Post, R.H.; Teplitz, T.A.; and Goodwin, F.K. Divalent cations in predicting antidepressant response to lithium. *Lancet* 2:1454, 1974.

113. Wyatt, R.J.; Cutler, N.R.; DeLisi, L.E.; Jeste, D.V.; Kleinman, J.E.; Luchins, D.J.; Potkin, S.G.; and Weinberger, D.R. Biochemical and morphological factors in schizophrenia. In *American Psychiatric Association Annual Review*, Grinspoon, L., ed. Washington, D.C.: American Psychiatric Press Inc., 1982.

114. Murphy, D.L., and Weiss, R. Reduced monoamine oxidase activity in blood platelets from bipolar depressed patients. *Am. J. Psychiat.* 128:1351–1354, 1972.

115. Sullivan, J.L.; Sullivan, P.D.; Davidson, J.; Maltbie, A.A.; Mahorney, S.; Taska, R.J.; and Cavenar, J.O. Biological risk factor assessment in lithium treatment of alcoholism. *Psychopharmacol. Bull.* 17:37–40, 1981.

116. Sullivan, J.L.; Cavenar, J.O.; Maltbie, A.A.; and Stanfields, C.N. Platelet monoamine oxidase activity predicts response to lithium in manic-depressive illness. *Lancet* 2:1325–1327, 1978.

117. Nurnberger, J.I.; Gershon, E.S.; Murphy, O.L.; Buchsbaum, M.S.; Goodwin, F.K.; Post, R.M.; Lake, C.R.; Guroff, J.J.; and McGinnis, M.H. Biological and clinical predictors of lithium response in depression. In *Lithium: Controversies and Unresolved Issues*, Cooper, T.B.; Gershon, S.; Kline, N.S.; and Schou, M., eds. Amsterdam: Excerpta Medica, 1979, pp. 241–256.

118. Sachar, E.J.; Halbreich, U.; Asnis, G.M.; Nathan, R.S.; Halpern, F.S.; and Ostrow, L. Paradoxical cortisol responses to dextroamphetamine in endogenous depression. *Arch. Gen. Psychiatry* 38:1113–1117, 1981.

119. Fuxe, K., and Hokfelt, T. *Frontiers in Neuroendocrinology.* New York: Oxford University Press, 1969.

120. Colpaert, F.C.; van Bever, W.F.M.; and Leysen, J.E.M. Apomorphine, chemistry, pharmacology, biochemistry. *Int. Rev. Neurobiol.* 19:255, 1976.

121. Brown, W.A.; Van Woert, M.H.; and Ambani, L.M. Effect of apomorphine on growth hormone release in humans. *J. Clin. Endocrinol. Metab.* 37:463–465, 1973.

122. Rotrosen, J.; Angrist, B.M.; and Gershon, E. Dopamine receptor alteration in schizophrenia: Neuroendocrine evidence. *Psychopharmacology* 51:1–7, 1976.

123. Rotrosen, J.; Angrist, B.; and Paquin, J. Neuroendocrine studies with dopamine agonists in schizophrenia. *Psychopharmacol. Bull.* 14:14–17, 1978.

124. Edelstein, T.; Schultz, J.R.; Kanter, D.R.; Hirschowitz, J.; and Garver, I.L. Physostigmine and lithium response in the schizophrenias. *Am. J. Psychiatry* 138:1078–1081, 1981.

125. Maany, I.; Mendels, J.; Frazer, A.; and Brunswick, D. A study of growth hormone release in depression. *Neuropsychobiology* 5:282–289, 1979.

126. Sachar, E.J.; Finkelstein, J.; and Hellman, L. Growth hormone responses in depressive illness. I. Response to insulin tolerance test. *Arch. Gen. Psychiatry* 25:263–269, 1971.

127. Langer, D.; Heinze, G.; Reim, B.; and Matussek, N. Reduced growth hormone responses to amphetamine in endogenous depressive patients. *Arch. Gen. Psychiatry* 33:1471–1475, 1976.

128. Maeda, K.; Kato, V.; Ohgo, S.; Chihara, K. Growth hormone and prolactin release after infection of TRH in patients with depression. *J. Clin. Endocrinol. Metab.* 40:501–505, 1975.

129. Matussek, N.; Achenheil, M.; and Hippuis, H. Effect of clonidine on growth hormone release in psychiatric patients and controls. Sixth World Congress of Psychiatry, Honolulu, 1977.

130. Sachar, E.J. Neuro-endocrine responses to psychotropic drugs. In *Psychopharmacology: A Generation of Progress*, Lipton, M.A., DiMascio, A., and Killam, K.F., eds. New York: Raven Press, 1978.

131. Takahashi, S.; Kondo, H.; and Yoshimura, M. Growth hormone response to administration of L-5-hydroxytryptophan (L-5HTP) in manic-depressive psychosis. *Folia Psychiat. Neurol. Jap.* 27:198–205, 1973.

132. Sabelli, H.C., and Mosnaim, A.D. Phenylethylamine hypothesis of affective behavior. *Am. J. Psychiatry* 131:695–699, 1974.

133. Sabelli, H.C.; Fawcett, J.; Gusovsky, F.; Javaid, J.; Edwards, J.; and Jeffriess, H. Urinary phenyl acetate: A diagnostic test for depression? *Science* 220:1187–1188, 1983.

134. Kupfer, D.J.; Spiker, D.G.; Coble, P.A.; Neil, J.F.; Ulrich, R.; and Shaw, D.H. Sleep and treatment prediction in endogenous depression. *Am. J. Psychiatry* 138:429–433, 1981.

135. Itil, T.M. Qualitative and quantitative EEG findings in schizophrenia. *Schizophrenia Bull.* 3:61–81, 1977.

136. John, E.R.; Karmel, B.Z.; Corning, W.C.; Easton, P.; Brown, D.; Ahn, H.; Harmony, J.T.; Prichep, L.; Toro, A.; Gerson, I.; Bartlett, F.; Thatcher, R.; Kaye, H.; Valdes, P.; and Schwartz, E. Neurometrics-Nemerical taxonomy identifies different profiles of brain functions within groups of behaviorally similar people. *Science* 196:1393–1409, 1977.

137. Shagass, C.; Staumans, J.J.; and Roemer, R.A. Evoked potentials of schizophrenics in several sensory modalities. *Biol. Psychiatry* 12:221–235, 1977.

138. Shagass, C. EEG and evoked potentials in the psychoses. In *Biology of the Major Psychoses. A Comparative Analysis*, Freedman, D.X., ed. New York: Raven Press, 1975, pp. 101–127.

139. Fisher, C.; Gross, J.; and Zuch, J. Cycle of penile erection synchronous with dreaming sleep. *Arch. Gen. Psychiatry* 12:29–45, 1965.

140. Fisher, C.; Schiavi, R.; Edwards, A.; and Davis, D. Evaluation of nocturnal penile tumescence in the differential diagnosis of sexual impotence. *Arch. Gen. Psychiatry* 36:431–437, 1979.

141. Karacan, I.; Salis, P.; and Ware, J. Nocturnal penile tumescence and diagnosis in diabetic impotence. *Am. J. Psychiatry* 135:191–197, 1978.

142. Karacan, I., and Salis, P. Diagnosis and treatment of erectile impotence. *Psych. Clinics North Am.* 3:97–111, 1980.

143. Fisher, C.; Cohen, H.D.; and Schiavi, R.C. Patterns of female sexual arousal

during sleep and waking: vaginal thermo-conductance studies. *Arch. Sex. Behav.* 12:97–122, 1983.

144. McDevitt, H.O., and Bodmer, W.F. HLA, immune-response genes and disease. *Lancet* 1:1269–1275, 1974.

145. Freedman, D.X., and Glass, R.M. Psychiatry. *JAMA* 247:2975–2977, 1982.

146. Baldessarini, R.J. *Biomedical Aspects of Depression.* Washington, D.C.: American Psychiatric Press, Inc., 1983, p. 58.

CHAPTER 6

Evaluation of Treatment Results

D. Ted George
and
William W. K. Zung

Since the 1940s, medical science has made a concerted effort to evaluate, describe, and even predict human behavior. As new methods became available for the treatment of emotional disorders, parallel new methods had to be developed to measure the presence and severity of these disorders and the efficacy of the new treatments. Following the discoveries of antipsychotic drugs, antidepressant drugs, and antianxiety drugs came the new science of psychometric scale development to fill the need of evaluating these psychobiological treatments. Just trying to define normal versus abnormal behavior shows the magnitude of the task at hand. However, equal to the task are the potential rewards. We hope, by adequately identifying and defining behavior, then to go on to develop more specific and efficacious treatments for disordered behavior that will allow us to manipulate the psychological component inherent in health and disease. This chapter gives an overview of diagnostic tools available to assess emotional disturbances and the signs and symptoms of the most commonly encountered emotional disorders. By using these measures serially over time, as a repeat measure, it becomes possible to evaluate treatment effects quantitatively.

EVALUATION OF NORMAL

In our physical examination of the patient, we are usually asked by the patient "Is my blood pressure normal?" We are guided in our response to the patient's concern and need to know by at least two factors: (1) Knowing the scientific word hypertension, we can use the values that have been set as clinically significant, and (2) within these values, we need to know how the word *normal* is used by the patient.

In evaluating emotional disorders, as in evaluating physical vital signs, the word *normal* obviously has a number of meanings. Assuming that we have taken a measurement of the patient's emotional pressure by using an anxiety rating scale, how do we interpret the meaning of such a measure? In short, what is normal in this case? Normal has multiple meanings. For example, as used in a statistical sense, it means that when scores of the test from many patients are plotted as a frequency distribution, the resultant curve is bell shaped or a normal distribution curve. Second, normal could mean that a particular score is the most representative value for anxiety ratings obtained from a particular group. Thus, we would have one set of normal values for people who are primarily anxious and another set of normal values for people who are primarily depressed. Third use of the word *normal* is to apply it to a set of values commonly encountered in a specific situation. Here we might expect different normal values for anxiety ratings in different clinical settings or by medical specialties. For instance, a psychiatrist who specializes in treating patients with anxiety disorders would have a different norm for his population of patients than an internist who sees patients with acute infectious diseases. Fourth, a normal value could mean that the value is clinically insignificant, that it was expected under the circumstances, or that it is innocuous and has no treatment implications. Last, normal could mean a consensus by experts and committees that a value is normal or is in the normal range. Unfortunately, in our state of the art today, we can only present reference values for the measurement of anxiety (or of any other psychopathology) because we lack the certainty and finitude to determine health or disease. Reference values represent a set of quantifiable values obtained from measurements using a standard tool from a group of individuals with a specific description and these reference values are the most commonly encountered for that group.

EVALUATION OF ABNORMAL

The application of the psychometric approach to determining what is abnormal or psychopathological can be complex. However, by taking into account what we want to measure, what we know influences these measurements, and what we cannot measure, we can increase the power of our rating tools. We propose the following formula as one approach to the science of diagnosis and measurement:

$$I + i + i + \ldots + i + x + r$$

I is the indicator of the particular abnormality that the scale is purported to measure. The investigator must decide how large or small a unit he or she wants to measure. Starting with the smallest unit of abnormality, he or she can use individual signs and symptoms as indicators. Next, he or she can focus on a symptom complex where groups of two or more symptoms tend to go together in a sizable number of cases but do not necessarily point to a single underlying disease. The investigator may want to set out using the disorder as the indicator of abnormality. For example, if the investigator decides to develop a rating scale for measuring depression as a disorder (the I in the formula), then all the necessary core signs and symptoms of depression would have to be included. Each of these would be one of the is in the formula and with as many is as there are signs and symptoms. For example, the is could include depressed mood, crying spells, sleep disturbance, and so on. If the investigator wanted to develop a scale measuring only the sleep disturbance found in depression, then the I of interest would now be sleep disturbance. The is would be items that measured how long it took to fall asleep, how long the patient stayed in bed, how many times during the night the patient woke up, and so on.

During and before the time these measurements are made, the investigator and the clinician using the rating tool would make every effort to exert controls in order to maximize the measurement made as being a true measure. This means they must be aware of the experimental noise, or x, in our formula, which enters into every evaluation but cannot always be controlled. These variables include intellect—the intelligence of the subject; affect—the emotional set of the subject at the time of evaluation; motivation—the amount of cooperation given; adaptation—the amount of learning, habituation, and practice effect of repeated measurements; introspection—the effect of the subject thinking about the contents of the scale and his or her responses as he or she completes the scale; premorbid personality—what the patient is like before development of the emotional illness; cultural background—influence of the socioeconomic and ethnic background; and external environment—circumstances under which the tests are being conducted.

Even when the investigator or clinician has made attempts to account for the experimental noises, a small residue, or r, always remains unaccounted for and unknown to him or her. Evaluations of psychobiological treatments that take these multifaceted influences into account will yield the most accurate and useful results.

GENERALIZED EVALUATION OF EMOTIONAL DISTURBANCES

Patient-Rated Evaluations

The Minnesota Multiphasic Personality Inventory

Perhaps one of the most familiar of the psychological tests in the medical setting is the Minnesota Multiphasic Personality Inventory (MMPI) (1). This test was published in 1943 by Hathaway and McKinley to provide an objective assessment of major personality characteristics. In its usual form, it consists of 566 true/false questions intended for subjects with at least a seventh-grade education and an I.Q. of 80. The scored test yields numerical values representing profiles for Hs (hypochondriasis), D (depression), Hy (hysteria), Pd (psycho-pathic deviate), Mf (interest scale, or masculinity-femininity), Pa (paranoia), Pt (psychasthenia), Sc (schizophrenia), and Ma (hypomania). For the purpose of this chapter, we focus our attention on the first three scales.

The hypochondriasis scale, or Hs, reflects an individual's concern for health and somatic complaints. The test questions cover many physiological systems and are thus designed to circumvent a false elevation that might arise when a bona fide medical problem is present. Possible diagnostic implications for an elevated score on this scale are suggested by Dahlstrom (2) to be so-matic reactions like hypochondriasis, depressive reaction with an important anxiety component such as reactive depression and agitated depression, hys-teria, and anxiety reaction.

The D (depression) scale focuses on issues such as work, level of interest and happiness. It is important to remember some patients might score high on the D scale yet deny feelings of depression. Such patients need careful evaluation because they may represent a smiling or masked depression and are at an increased risk for suicide.

The Hy (hysteria) scale is designed to identify those individuals who under stress are predisposed to use conversion symptomatology to solve con-flicts. These individuals, when clinically evaluated, may demonstrate no ob-vious personality disorder when not under stress. In the medical context, those scoring high on the hysteria scale often display anxiety attacks, sudden episodes of tachycardia, palpitations, and headaches. When the scale is ele-vated in psychiatric patients, denial and repression are prominent and the individual appears manipulative, self-centered, and superficial.

The literature is replete with studies applying the MMPI test results to clinic situations. For example, Leverenz (3) found in medical and surgical pa-tients in an army hospital that the test results often redirected clinical evalua-tion into previously unsuspected abnormal areas and assisted in the decision regarding a soldier's fitness for military service. Other studies have shown a correlation between high scores on hypochondriasis and hysteria and poor postoperative courses for elective knee surgery (4). Likewise, many studies have used the MMPI to evaluate low back pain patients. Pleasant et al. (5) evaluated 103 patients with low back pain. Functional ratings were made by an orthopedist and a psychologist before and one year following the surgery. Surgery was only employed for gross instability or malalignment of the ver-tebral axis or neurologic deficits judged secondary to neuronal compression and amenable to surgical intervention. Their results showed that high scores on the Hs and Hy scales were inversely related to positive surgical outcome. Such studies suggest that patients scoring high on Hs and Hy scales are poor risks for surgery and that psychotherapy aimed at reducing reinforcement of illness behavior should be instituted before elective surgery.

Hopkins Symptom Checklist

A scale that serves as a generalized psychiatric evaluation and that measures a wide spectrum of psychopathology is the Hopkins Symptom Checklist, or

HSCL (6). There are many versions of this scale, and various versions contain a different number of items—for example, the HSCL-90 contains ninety items, while the HSCL-35 contains thirty-five items. This test has been shown to measure the following nine dimensions: somatization, obsessive-compulsive, interpersonal sensitivity, depression, anxiety, hostility, phobic anxiety, paranoid ideation, and psychoticism. The test consists of ninety items each rated from 0 to 4 on a scale of distress ranging from not at all to extremely and requires approximately 20 minutes to complete. Its applicability ranges from assessing a patient's symptomatic psychiatric profile to measuring objective changes resulting from pharmacological and non-pharmacological interventions. Studies looking at the test-retest reliability showed coefficients of 0.80 and 0.85. Similarly, when comparing test results with evaluations by professional clinicians, investigators found coefficients that ranged from 0.64 for depression to 0.80 for interpersonal sensitivity (7).

Profile of Mood States

This sixty-five-item scale (8) was developed to measure six clearly defined dimensions of mood. It is scored by adding the responses given to adjectives related to that mood and takes three to five minutes for most patients to complete. The mood states rated are tension-anxiety, depression-dejection, anger-hostility, vigor-activity, fatigue-inertia, and confusion-bewilderment. Adding the total raw scores across all six dimensions gives a total mood disturbance score. Using it clinically, the scores on the six mood factors, when standardized by use of a profile sheet, gives the clinician knowledge of how much change has occurred on these dimensions.

Observer-Rated Evaluations

Brief Psychiatric Rating Scale

In 1962 Overall and Gorham described an instrument they called the Brief Psychiatric Rating Scale (BPRS), which consisted of sixteen symptom constructs (9). The rating is based on information and direct observation obtained in a brief semiguided interview that lasts about 20 minutes. Approximately half the rating is based on patient observation, mode of communication, and organization of thought processes, without regard for specific content. Its advantage is to allow the interviewer a flexibility to evaluate the constructs without having to follow a set pattern of questioning. Its intent is to provide an objective classification of patients and to evaluate the nature of therapeutic effect, with an emphasis on psychotic symptomatology. Most studies of efficacy of antipsychotic drugs or other treatment modalities with populations of patients with schizophrenia or other symptom profiles that are considered to be psychotic have used this rating scale. In addition to the separate constructs, the results can be grouped to measure thinking disturbance, anxious depression, paranoid disturbance, and withdrawal retardation factors.

*Nurses' Observation Scale for Inpatient
Evaluation*

The Nurses' Observation Scale for Inpatient Evaluation (NOSIE) is a thirty-item rating scale designed to objectify the behavior of hospitalized schizophrenic patients (10). A trained nurse is asked to evaluate each of the thirty items according to a five-point rating ranging from never to always. The results are then interpreted in relation to the following six broad categories: (1) social competence, (2) social interest, (3) personal neatness, (4) irritability, (5) manifest psychosis, and (6) retardation. It has been found useful in cross-sectional descriptions of psychiatric patients, as well as being sensitive to treatment-induced changes in a patient's clinical condition. Evaluations made by nurses can be invaluable since nurses are able to observe the patient for a longer duration of time than can the patient's physician.

SPECIFIC EVALUATION FOR EMOTIONAL DISTURBANCES

Rating Scales for Depression

Depression is probably the most common of all the emotional disorders, and the ability to quantitate its severity and change with psychobiological treatment has been recognized by a number of investigators. A major depressive disorder as defined by the American Psychiatric Association's *DSM-III* is a constellation of signs and symptoms that reflect somatic complaints (e.g., crying, sleep disturbance, loss of appetite, decreased libido, fatigability, and weight loss) and psychological phenomena (e.g., lowering of mood, pessimism, hopelessness, sense of failure, guilt, and self-accusation). Numerous rating scales have used similar or identical symptomatology as their core psychopathology either to diagnose or quantitate depression and may involve either self-rating scales or evaluation by skilled observers.

Skilled clinical observers have the obvious benefit of being able to capture subtle nonverbal cues, assess the patient's level of denial or exaggeration, and ultimately, integrate the patient's overt behavior and subjective symptoms. However, clinical evaluation has many disadvantages. Diagnosticians are often inconsistent and subject to bias, mood variations, and the pressure of time. In addition, the quantitative and assessment systems employed by raters often lack the sensitivity to allow precision to detect subtle changes in the level of depression. With this as background, we now examine several of the common rating scales employed to measure depression.

Observer-Rated Evaluations

One of the first rating scales primarily designed to assess depression was described in 1960 by Hamilton (12). The rating employs a skilled observer to evaluate a patient during a clinical interview. The test comprises seventeen items that commonly occur in depression (Table 6.1). Most of the items are scored on a continuum of 0 to 4, where 0 represents the absence of a symptom

Table 6.1 Comparison of the Zung and Hamilton Operational Definitions for Depressive Disorders

Zung Scale Item	Hamilton Scale Item	
Pervasive psychic disturbance		
Depressed mood	Depressed mood	
Crying spells		
Physiological disturbance		
Diurnal variation	Diurnal variation	
Sleep disturbance	Insomnia early, middle, late	
Decreased appetite	Somatic symptoms, Gastrointestinal	
Decreased weight	Loss of weight	
Decreased libido	Genital symptoms	
Constipation	Gastrointestinal	
Tachycardia	Somatic anxiety	
Increased fatigue	Work and activities General somatic symptoms	
Psychomotor disturbance		
Psychomotor agitation	Agitation	
Psychomotor retardation	Retardation	
Psychological disturbance		
Confusion		
Emptiness		
Hopelessness		
Indecisiveness	Work and activities	
Irritability		
Dissatisfaction		
Personal devaluation		
Suicidal rumination	Suicide	
	Feelings of guilt	(2)
	Psychic anxiety	(10)
	Hypochondriasis	(15)
	Insight	(17)
	Depersonalization and derealization	(19)
	Paranoid symptoms	(20)
	Obsessional and compulsive symptoms	(21)

and 4 reflects the highest level of severity. The Hamilton scale is the most widely used observer-rated scale for depression. Almost every new antidepressant drug that has been studied for efficacy has depended upon the demonstrated change in improvement over time using this scale. For the busy practitioner, the negative aspect is that it requires a trained observer, favors somatic complaint associated with depression, contains a number of items that measure anxiety as well as neurotic complaints, and is time consuming to perform.

Patient-Rated Evaluations

Beck Depression Inventory.   In 1961, Beck et al. published an interviewer-rated depression inventory consisting of twenty-one categories relating to the symptoms and attitudes of depression (13). During the initial formulation of the inventory, each patient was seen by two psychiatrists who rated the patient on the depth of depression using a four-point scale (none, mild, moderate, and severe, which had values of 0 to 3 respectively). Concurrent validity has been reported through comparisons with other standardized measures of depression. Nussbaum et al. found initial and final correlations between the MMPI D scale and the depression inventory to be 0.75 and 0.69 respectively (14). In a comparison of the depression inventory and Hamilton rating scale for depression, Schwab et al. showed a correlation coefficient of 0.75 (15). In 1972, Beck condensed the scale to thirteen items (16) and used the scale as a self-rating scale.

Of critical importance when testing for depression with the Beck depression inventory is the cutoff score. As a screening device to detect depression among psychiatric patients, a value of 13 is often used. For screening depression among medical patients, Schwab et al. found a cutoff score of 10 to be appropriate, based on the original version of the scale (17).

Zung Self-Rating Depression Scale.   In 1965, Zung published the self-rating depression scale (18) based on a number of commonly agreed upon symptoms most likely to be present in depressed patients and comparable in content to the present diagnostic criteria for a major depressive disorder as specified in the *DSM-III* (Table 6.2).

This scale consists of twenty items, ten of which are worded symptomatically positive, and ten of which are worded symptomatically negative in order to prevent patients from checking a set response of yes or no. In using the test, the patient is asked to rate each item as to how it applies to him or her at the time of testing (or for a given period like during the past week) in the following four quantitative terms: (1) none or a little of the time, (2) some of the time, (3) a good part of the time, and (4) most or all of the time. The self-rating depression scale is constructed so that the less depressed patient will have a lower score on the scale and the more depressed patient will have a higher score. In scoring this depression scale, a value of 1, 2, 3, and 4 is assigned to each response, depending upon whether the item was worded pos-

Table 6.2 Comparison of the Zung and *DSM-III* Operational Definitions for a Depressive Disorder

DSM-III	Zung Self-Rating Depression Scale
Dysphoric mood	
Depressed, sad, blue	Depressed mood
	Crying spells
Hopelessness	Hopelessness
Irritable	Irritability
At least four of the following:	
Poor appetite or	Decreased appetite
significant weight loss	Weight loss
Insomnia	Sleep disturbance
Psychomotor agitation or	Psychomotor agitation
psychomotor retardation	Psychomotor retardation
Loss of interest in usual activities	Emptiness
or decrease in sexual drive	Dissatisfaction
	Decreased libido
Loss of energy, fatigue	Fatigue
Feelings of worthlessness	Personal devaluation
Diminished ability to think	Confusion
or indecisiveness	Indecisiveness
Suicidal thoughts, wish to be dead	Suicidal rumination

itively or negatively. An index for this scale is derived by dividing the sum of the raw scores obtained by 80 and multiplying by 100 to give an index ranging from 25 to 100. The self-rating depression scale index is a measure of how much, in percentage, of the total measurable psychopathology the subject has as defined by the scale. Patients with global ratings of mild to moderate depression have equivalent self-rating depression scale indexes of 50 to 59, patients with moderate to severe depression have indexes of 60 to 69, and those with severe depression have indexes of 70 or above. Subjects who score below 50 on the index have no significant depressive symptomatology.

Correlations between self-rating depression scale indexes obtained from patients and global ratings made by clinicians showed a significantly high correlation ($r = 0.53$) for depressed patients. Likewise, the validity of the Zung scale has been tested and found to have a significant correlation with the Hamilton rating scale for depression (19), the Beck depression inventory (20), and the D scale in the MMPI (21). Additional data demonstrated no correlation between the Zung scale results and age, educational level, annual incomes, or intelligence levels (22). Of added interest were studies showing that this scale has applicability as a screening device for depression across cultural and national boundaries. Collaborative studies performed in Japan,

Australia, Czechoslovakia, the United Kingdom, West Germany, and Switzerland yielded data supporting the correlation between presence and severity of clinical depression and the self-rating depression scale index (20).

In using the self-rating depression scale as a tool for evaluating psychobiological treatments, it is of interest to compare the definition of a depressive disorder as defined by the Food and Drug Administration (FDA) guidelines (23) and the operational definition used in the scale. The FDA guidelines were developed to indicate to investigators of psychotropic drugs the appropriate population of patients to include when specific drugs such as antidepressants or antianxiolytics were to be studied. Table 6.3 shows the basic similarities

Table 6.3 Comparison of the Zung and FDA Guidelines for Psychotropic Drugs Definitions for Depressive Disorders

Zung	FDA Guidelines
Pervasive psychic disturbance	
Depressed mood	Depressed mood
Crying spells	
Physiological disturbance	
Diurnal variation	
Sleep disturbance	Sleep difficulty
Decreased appetite	Poor appetite
Decreased libido	Decrease in libido
Decreased weight	
Constipation	
Tachycardia	
Increased fatigue	Loss of energy
Psychomotor disturbance	
Psychomotor retardation	Retardation
Psychomotor agitation	Agitation
Psychological disturbance	
Confusion	Diminished thinking and concentration
Hopelessness	Helplessness/hopelessness
Irritability	
Indecisiveness	Work and activities
Personal devaluation	Self-reproach or guilt
Emptiness	
Suicidal rumination	Thoughts of death/suicide
Dissatisfaction	Anhedonia
	Anxiety or tension
	Bodily complaints

between them, with the uncommon items being those that measure anxiety and bodily complaints that are in the FDA definition.

The self-rating depression scale has been translated into thirty languages and has been used and cited in over 300 publications (24). Summary results of cross-national studies from North America, South America, Europe, Australia, and Asia of normal subjects and of patients with depression have demonstrated that it is a valid and reliable tool for assessing depression (25) and in assessing change with treatment with antidepressant drugs (26).

In an effort to increase the effectiveness and usefulness of the self-rating depression scale, Zung in 1972 published the depression status inventory (27). This test is a twenty-item, semistructured, interviewer-rated depression instrument that uses the same diagnostic criteria as the self-rating depression scale and whose converted scores have the same range of values. Thus, for researchers and clinicians who want to perform their own ratings of depression and use the identical definition of a depressive disorder as the self-rating scale, this tool is ideally suited. The depression status inventory has a high correlation with the self-rating depression scale ($r = 0.87$). Likewise, its ability to distinguish depressive patients from nondepressed patients was shown by mean indexes of 61 for depressed patients and 48, 51, 52, and 44 respectively for patients diagnosed with schizophrenia, anxiety, personality disorder, and transient situational disturbance.

Significant-Other-Rated Evaluations

Often, the practicing physician would like to be able to find out what the family members or friends of the depressed patient know or think about the patient's illness. Information from such significant-other individuals may at times be the only source of information that is readily and immediately available. A significant-other-rated scale was constructed with the items worded in the third person singular and with the following instructions: "This is a list of 20 sentences, each of which tells us something which we are interested to know about your (relative/friend). Not all of the statements may necessarily apply to him (or her). Other times you may not know which column to check because you do not have the information. In such a case, place a question mark (?) next to that sentence." Results of comparing an interviewer rating and a self-rating with the significant-other rating showed that those items of a more personal and confidential nature were the most difficult for the significant other to rate and that those that were easily observable presented no problem (28).

Rating Scales for Anxiety

Anxiety as a word is used to mean different things such as a mental feeling state, the underlying cause of behavior, a drive, a situational response, and a psychiatric disorder. The focus of measurement of anxiety has been on the use of the word to mean the illness presently called a generalized anxiety disorder. This disorder can be regarded as consisting of fundamental biological changes of a person, whose core manifestations as signs and symptoms can be commonly agreed upon. Based upon such operational criteria, several rating scales for anxiety have been constructed.

Observer-Rated Evaluations

Hamilton Rating Scale for Anxiety.   The Hamilton rating scale was developed as an aid to quantifying the symptoms of patients with diagnoses of a generalized anxiety disorder (29). The fourteen items in the scale measure the psychic and somatic aspects of anxiety using a five-point scale of severity: not present, mild, moderate, severe, and very severe. The scale provides consistent results from rater to rater. As an observer-rated scale, it has been found to be valuable in evaluating treatment intervention including psychobiological treatments. Total scores reflect the severity of the anxiety disorder, while subscores indicate the relative amounts of psychic-affective disturbance and somatic disturbances.

Zung Anxiety Status Inventory.   Zung constructed an instrument to measure the core signs and symptoms of anxiety, using the most commonly agreed upon diagnostic criteria for an anxiety disorder (30). The diagnostic criteria used by Zung are the following:

- Affective symptoms
    - Anxiousness or nervousness
    - Fear
    - Panic
    - Mental disintegration
    - Apprehension
- Somatic symptoms
    - Tremors
    - Body aches and pains
    - Easy fatigability
    - Restlessness
    - Palpitation
    - Dizziness
    - Faintness
    - Dyspnea
    - Paresthesias
    - Nausea and vomiting
    - Urinary frequency

Sweating

Face flushing

Insomnia

Nightmares

These criteria have been compared with those proposed by Hamilton (29) and the FDA guidelines (23), with the results indicating minimal differences among them (31). In using the anxiety status inventory, cues for each of the twenty items are provided for the rater in order to establish consistency in performing the rating. Since the definitions used in this inventory are identical to those used in the self-rated version, comparisons can be made between the observer rating and self-rating for similarities and differences of the patient's clinical condition. The observer rating is performed on the basis of four quantitative terms that are scored from 1 to 4. An index is derived from the sum of the item scores and is converted to a percentage.

Self-Rated Evaluations

The Zung self-rating anxiety scale is based upon the selected diagnostic criteria and operational definition for an anxiety disorder as shown in the preceding list. The items are worded in the everyday language of the patient. In using the scale, the patient is asked to rate each of the twenty items as to how they applied to him or her within a time period in the following four quantitative terms: (1) none or a little of the time, (2) some of the time, (3) a good part of the time, and (4) most or all of the time. The self-rating anxiety scale is constructed so that the less anxious patients will have low scores and the more anxious patients will have high scores. Based upon administering this scale to both normal and anxious subjects, a cutoff index of 45 was established. Subjects who score less than 45 have no significant anxiety, while patients who score between 45 and 59 have minimal to moderate anxiety, between 60 and 74 have marked to severe anxiety, and 75 and over have the most extreme anxiety present. Cross-national studies on normal and anxious subjects have shown the validity and reliability of the self-rating scale in these populations, as well as levels of anxiety for patients in psychiatric as well as nonpsychiatric settings (32). In addition to the observer-rated and self-rated forms of the Zung anxiety scale, a significant-other form is available that can be completed by a family member or friend.

Comparison between Observer-Rated and Self-Rated Scales

Results obtained from evaluating a patient by means of an observer-rated scale like the Hamilton rating scale for depression and a self-rated scale like the Zung self-rating depression scale can be similar, or if dissimilar, one score will be higher than the other. When the scores are concordant, the clinician or researcher feels that a valid estimate of the patient's depressive symptomatology has been made. When the scores disagree, one of the usual interpretations is that one of the scales is not valid or reliable or sensitive to the task. In actuality, both scores are correct, but we have to examine more carefully what each of the scales is measuring.

The usual method of using observer-rated scales allows the inclusion in the scoring procedure of what the observer hears and sees in terms of patient verbal and behavioral manifestations that are related to the disorder. This adds another dimension the patient self-rated scale does not have. In addition, observer bias can enter if patients are seen in certain settings, and if the observer-rater is not careful in excluding this factor as experimental noise. For example, patients examined in inpatient settings may be perceived to be sicker by virtue of being in a hospital, whereas patients examined in an outpatient setting may be perceived to be less sick because they are being rated in an outpatient setting.

Further, differences between observer ratings and self-ratings occur because the contents of the two rating scales may be different. Thus, disagreement between ratings on the same patient using the Hamilton depression and Zung self-rated depression scales can occur because the interviewer-rated Hamilton scale for depression includes items that measure anxiety, as well as neurotic and psychotic variables that are not present in the Zung self-rating depression scale. Other reasons for disconcordance between observer ratings and self-ratings include defense mechanisms that some patients use.

In a study that compared self- versus physician rating, Brown and Zung (19) found that patients who are either sensitizers or repressors tend to show an unreliable correlation between the two scores. Sensitizers are defined as individuals who tend to be oversensitive, to overinterpret, and to ruminate about potential or real threats and conflicts. Their scores on self-ratings will be higher than scores obtained from observer ratings. Repressors are defined as individuals who tend to use avoidance, suppression, repression, and denial of potential threats and conflicts. Their self-rated scores will be lower than observer-rated scores. Such phenomena are usually recognized by the practicing physician and, when present, are accounted for in the final judgment. Last, disagreements between ratings such as self-ratings and nurse's ratings using the NOSIE can occur because each rater perceives a different aspect with regard to what is rated. Patients who improve in their depressive disorder and become more assertive may be perceived by nurses as being uncooperative and scored in a different direction than the patient would. In the final analysis, evaluations of psychobiological treatments performed by different raters (observer, self, significant other, nursing staff) must be put into the context of who is doing the rating, and attempts to reconcile any differences when they occur need to be made in order to understand the patient who is being evaluated.

Although there are disadvantages to the use of self-rating scales, the advantages far exceed them. For example, they provide information that only the patient can provide; they are simple and do not involve the use of trained personnel; they take a short time for the patients to complete; they are easy to score and easily quantifiable; they provide objective data in a standard form; they can be used repeatedly to document change over time and treatment; and they are inexpensive, economical, and cost-effective.

SUMMARY

In order to make quantitative evaluations of psychobiological treatments, the qualitative aspects (the definition of a specific disorder) have to be approached first. Growing out of the context of rating scales and behavior evaluations came a major thrust in the 1970s to make objective psychiatric diagnoses according to standardized and operational criteria. In 1972, Feighner et al. (33) published a set of criteria that represented a compilation of data acquired from years of research on specific psychiatric entities. The criteria pertain to fourteen psychiatric illnesses and helped to provide a standard for evaluating psychiatric diagnosis, prognosis, and treatment.

Still another response to the ambiguity of psychiatric diagnosis came in 1978 when Spitzer et al. published their article on research diagnostic criteria (34). Their goal was to ascribe necessary clinical diagnostic criteria to specific psychiatric illnesses. The criteria included twenty-five major diagnostic categories, many of which were further subdivided into non–mutually exclusive subtypes. For each disorder, the authors present both inclusion and exclusion criteria based on symptoms, signs, duration or course of illness, and severity of impairment. The choice of which diagnostic categories to include in the criteria was a judgment aimed at solving existing problems in psychiatric research. The reliability of the research diagnostic criteria categories to define psychiatric conditions has been tested employing interviewer ratings. When the research diagnostic criteria were employed independently by the raters to make a psychiatric diagnosis, there was good agreement. Thus, the progression of research toward reaching common definitions and constructing rating scales using these definitions has made it possible to begin to evaluate psychobiological treatments quantitatively using the rating scale approach.

REFERENCES

1. Hathaway, S.R., and McKinley, J.C. A multiphasic personality schedule. *J. Psychology* 10:249–254, 1940.
2. Dahlstrom, W.G.; Welsh, G.S.; and Dahlstrom, L.E. *An MMPI Handbook.* Vol. 1: *Clinical Interpretation.* Minneapolis: University of Minnesota Press, 1972.

3. Leverenz, O.W. Minnesota Multiphasic Personality Inventory: Evaluation of its usefulness in a psychiatric service of a station hospital. *War Med.* 4:618–629, 1943.

4. Wise, A.; Jackson, D.; and Rocchio, R. Preoperative psychological testing as a predictor of success in knee surgery. A preliminary report. *Am. J. Sports Med.* 7:287–291, 1979.

5. Pleasant, H.C.; Gilbert, D.; Goldfarb, J.; and Herron, L. The MMPI as a predictor of outcome in low back surgery. *Spine* 4:78–84, 1979.

6. Derogatis, L.R.; Lipman, R.S.; and Covi, L. The SCL-90. An outpatient psychiatric rating scale. *Psychopharm. Bull.* 9:13–28, 1973.

7. Rickels, K.; Lipman, R.S.; Park, L.C.; Covi, L.; Uhlenhuth, E.H.; and Mock, J.E. Doctor warmth and clinic setting in the symptomatic response to minor tranquilizers. *Psychopharmacologia* (Berlin) 20:128–152, 1971.

8. McNair, D.M.; Lorr, M.; and Droppleman, L.F. *Profile of Mood States* (manual). San Diego: Educational and Industrial Testing Service, 1971.

9. Overall, J.E., and Gorham, D.R. The Brief Psychiatric Rating Scale. *Psychol. Rep.* 10:799–812, 1962.

10. Honigfeld, G., and Klett, C.J. The Nurses' Observation Scale for Inpatient Evaluation. A new ward behavior rating scale. *J. Clin. Psychol.* 21:65–71, 1965.

11. American Psychiatric Association. *Diagnostic and Statistical Manual of Mental Disorders*, 3rd ed. Washington, D.C., 1980.

12. Hamilton, M. Development of a rating scale for primary depressive illness. *Br. J. Soc. Clin. Psychol.* 6:278–296, 1967.

13. Beck, A.T.; Ward, C.H.; Mendelson, M.; Mock, J.; and Erbaugh, J. An inventory for measuring depression. *Arch. Gen. Psychiat.* 4:561–571, 1961.

14. Nussbaum, K.; Wittig, B.A.; Hanlon, T.E.; and Kurland, A.A. Intravenous nialamide in the treatment of depressed female patients. *Compr. Psychiat.* 4:105–116, 1963.

15. Schwab, J.J.; Bialow, M.R.; and Holzer, C.E. A comparison of two rating scales for depression. *J. Clin. Psychology* 23:94–96, 1967.

16. Beck, A.T., and Beck, R.W. Screening depressed patients in family practice. A rapid technique. *Postgrad. Med.* 52:81–85, 1972.

17. Schwab, J.J.; Bialow, M.; Brown, J.M.; and Holzer, C.E. Diagnosing depression in medical inpatients. *Ann. Intern. Med.* 67:695–707, 1967.

18. Zung, W.W.K. A self-rating depression scale. *Arch. Gen. Psychiat.* 12:63–70, 1965.

19. Brown, G.L., and Zung, W.W.K. Depression scales. Self- or physician-rating. *Compr. Psychiat.* 13:361–367, 1972.

20. Zung, W.W.K. A cross-cultural survey of symptoms in depression. *Am. J. Psychiat.* 126:116–121, 1969.

21. Zung, W.W.K.; Richards, C.B.; and Short, M.J. Self-rating Depression Scale in an outpatient clinic. *Arch. Gen. Psychiat.* 13:508–515, 1965.

22. Zung, W.W.K. Factors influencing the Self-rating Depression Scale. *Arch. Gen. Psychiat.* 16:543–547, 1967.

23. FDA guidelines for psychotropic drugs. *Psychopharmacol. Bull.* 10:70–91, 1974.

24. Citation Classic, Current Contents 24, June 11, 1979.

25. Zung, W.W.K. How Normal Is Depression? Current Concepts. Scope Publication, 1981.

26. Zung, W.W.K. Evaluating treatment methods for depressive disorders. *Am. J. Psychiat.* 124 (suppl.):40–48, 1968.

27. Zung, W.W.K. The Depression Status Inventory: An adjunct to the Self-rating Depression Scale. *J. Clin. Psychol.* 28:539–543, 1972.
28. Zung, W.W.K.; Coppedge, H.M.; and Green, R.L., Jr. The evaluation of depressive symptomatology: A triadic approach. *Psychotherapy & Psychosom.* 24:170–174, 1974.
29. Hamilton, M. The assessment of anxiety states by rating. *Br. J. Med. Psychol.* 32:50–55, 1959.
30. Zung, W.W.K. A rating instrument for anxiety disorders. *Psychosom.* 12:371–379, 1971.
31. Zung, W.W.K. Assessment of anxiety disorders: Qualitative and quantitative approaches. In *Phenomenology and Treatment of Anxiety*, Fann, W.E., Karacan, I., Pokorny, A., and Williams, R., eds. New York: Spectrum Publications, 1979.
32. Zung, W.W.K. How Normal Is Anxiety? Current Concepts, Scope Publication, 1980.
33. Feighner, J.P.; Robins, E.; Guze, S.B.; Woodruff, R.A.; Winokur, G.; and Munoz, R. Diagnostic criteria for use in psychiatric research. *Arch. Gen. Psychiat.* 26:57–63, 1972.
34. Spitzer, R.L.; Endicott, J.; and Robins, E. Research diagnostic criteria. *Arch. Gen. Psychiat.* 35:773–782, 1978.

PART II

Special Topics

CHAPTER 7

Delirium and Dementia (Organic Brain Syndromes)

C. Edward Coffey
and
E. Wayne Massey

Medical disorders frequently present with neuropsychiatric manifestations. One study found that 43 percent of 2,090 psychiatric outpatients suffered from some medical illness on presentation to a psychiatric clinic (1). The medical disorder alone accounted for all of the psychopathologic findings in 18 percent of the medically ill patients and contributed to or worsened the psychopathology in a further 51 percent of patients. Of 100 new inpatient admissions to a state psychiatric hospital, 46 were discovered to have a medical illness that either caused or aggravated the psychopathologic findings (2).

This chapter focuses on a select group of neuropsychiatric disorders referred to as organic mental disorders. The essential feature of these disorders is a psychological or behavioral abnormality associated with transient or permanent dysfunction of the brain. Organic mental disorders tend to present as one or more organic brain syndromes—i.e., as a particular constellation of psychological or behavioral signs and symptoms that tend to occur together.

The third edition of the American Psychiatric Association's *Diagnostic and Statistical Manual of Mental Disorders (DSM-III)* (3) defines seven purely descriptive organic brain syndromes in three groups:

1. Organic brain syndromes with global cognitive impairment
   Delirium
   Dementia
2. Organic brain syndromes with selective psychological impairment
   Amnestic syndrome
   Organic hallucinosis
3. Organic brain syndromes predominantly manifested by personality disturbance or that closely resemble some of the functional mental disorders
   Organic personality syndrome

Organic affective syndrome
Organic delusional syndrome

The organic brain syndromes are a heterogeneous group of disorders with vastly different clinical presentations. The occurrence, type, severity, course, and outcome of an organic brain syndrome are influenced to a varying degree by several factors (4,5) including:

- Characteristics of the organic causative factor—i.e., its localization, mode of onset, progression, duration, and nature of the underlying pathophysiological process

- Certain psychobiological attributes of the patient—i.e., age, presence of preexisting brain damage, overall medical health, and the patient's basic personality, coping style, intelligence, education, and level of premorbid adjustment

- The patient's social and physical environment—i.e., social isolation, interpersonal conflicts and losses, unfamiliarity with environment, and excessive or deficient sensory input.

Clinically, no behavioral abnormalities may be regarded as characteristic or pathognomonic of the class of organic brain syndromes. Organic brain syndromes display great variability among individuals and in the same individual over time, and more than one organic brain syndrome may be present in individuals simultaneously—e.g., delirium superimposed on a dementia. Nevertheless, certain psychopathological symptoms are more likely than others to be the direct result of cerebral damage or dysfunction. The most common is impairment of cognitive and intellectual functioning including memory, thinking, perception, and attention. A reduced capacity for the control and fine modulation of emotions, drives, and impulses is often impaired in patients with cerebral disease. Another typical feature of an acute or transient and widespread cerebral insult is a disturbance of wakefulness and alertness, often referred to as a "disturbance of consciousness." Patients may also exhibit a variety of compensatory and protective symptoms including concealment, rationalization, minimization, and denial of their cognitive impairment. Finally, such patients may react to their cognitive deficits with a variety of cognitive, emotional, and behavioral symptoms that reflect the patients' understanding of the insult, as modified by the personality, value system, social and economic situation, and other psychosocial variables. These reactive symptoms may include the entire spectrum of neurotic, psychotic, and personality disorders.

The diagnosis of an organic brain syndrome depends upon first the presence of certain behavioral features that define that syndrome and, second, independent or nonpsychological evidence of an antecedent or concurrent cerebral disorder that is judged to be a necessary condition for the syndrome exhibited by the patient. These criteria are discussed in more detail in the following section.

The differential diagnosis of the organic brain syndromes depends upon the predominant clinical features present, as outlined in the decision tree from *DSM-III* (Table 7.1). The focus of treatment of an organic brain syndrome

Table 7.1 Differential Diagnosis of Organic Brain Syndromes

Evidence is gained from either the history, physical examination, or laboratory tests of a specific organic factor that is judged to be etiologically related to the disturbance*

Delirium (also consider underlying dementia)	← Yes	Disturbance of attention, memory, and orientation, developing over a short period of time and fluctuating over time

No
↓

Dementia (also consider superimposed intoxication and withdrawal)	← Yes	Deterioration of previously acquired intellectual abilities of sufficient severity to interfere with social or occupational functioning

No
↓

Amnestic syndrome	← Yes	Short- and long-term memory disturbance is the predominant clinical feature

No
↓

Organic delusional syndrome	← Yes	Delusions are the predominant clinical feature

No
↓

Organic hallucinosis	← Yes	Hallucinations are the predominant clinical feature

No
↓

Organic affective syndrome	← Yes	Disturbance in mood closely resembling those in manic or major depressive episodes

No
↓

Organic personality syndrome	← Yes	Marked change in personality involving either emotional lability, impaired impulse control or social judgment, marked apathy and indifference, or suspiciousness

No
↓

*In the absence of such evidence, an organic factor can be presumed if conditions outside of the organic mental disorders category have been reasonably excluded and if the disturbance meets the symptomatic criteria for dementia.

Source: American Psychiatric Association, *Diagnostic and Statistical Manual of Mental Disorders*, 3rd ed. (Washington, D.C., 1980).

is identification and treatment of the underlying brain disorder. In many cases where this is not possible, all available methods should be employed to restore premorbid psychological functioning if that is feasible, to alleviate suffering, and to ensure optimal compensation for and adjustment to any irreversible losses or deficits of mental abilities. In short, despite the emphasis on etiological treatment, the patient and not just the brain should be the object of therapeutic efforts.

THE MENTAL STATUS EXAMINATION

When an organic brain syndrome is suspected, a mental status examination should be done (6). It is useful to have several simple tests available to screen brain function grossly (7). These tests should be done in an orderly fashion; for example, level of consciousness and attention should be examined first because impairment of these functions will make testing of other functions at best unreliable. A quick screen of the patient's mental status will include (1) describing the patient: include level of consciousness, quality and coherence of spontaneous speech, and spontaneous movements; (2) orientation: define time, place, and person; (3) digit span forward (attention): the numbers are given to the patient once in a slow monotonous voice without cadence, and the patient is required to repeat them back perfectly immediately; (4) short-term memory: go over the names of three unrelated objects repeatedly with the patient until he or she can repeat them perfectly several times; talk about other topics for five minutes and then ask the patient to recall the objects; (5) long-term memory: ask about several famous historical events at a level compatible with the patient's intellectual endowment and education; (6) naming simple objects (dominant hemisphere function): naming objects tests word-finding abilities; (7) drawing objects (nondominant hemisphere function): the patient is asked to copy the examiner's drawing of a square, triangle, Greek cross, and star to test constructional abilities (see Table 7.2).

Social amenities may be well preserved despite a striking loss of intellectual abilities. A patient's statement in response to current-events questions like "I do not keep up with the newspapers" may be a cover-up for time disorientation. A detailed mental status examination will show the organic brain syndrome (8,9). The following section focuses on two of the more common and more interesting organic brain syndromes.

ORGANIC BRAIN SYNDROMES WITH GLOBAL COGNITIVE IMPAIRMENT

Delirium

The term *delirium* derives from the Latin *delirare*, which literally means "off the track." As used here, delirium denotes a transient organic mental dis-

Table 7.2 Mental Status Examination

Item	Assessment
Appearance	Personal grooming, attention to garments and posture
Behavior	Gestures, movements; ability to sit or wait in conversation
Orientation	Time orientation usually the first to crumble (never fail to know one's own name or identity unless in coma)
Speech	Volume and rate, clarity and coherence; ratio of substance words (verbs, nouns) to adjectives, articles, and conjunctions
Mood	Responsiveness, flexibility; normal, happy, sad, apathetic
Memory	Remembering three objects after five minutes, a short story, meals yesterday or from today's breakfast; digit span is test of alertness more than memory; old memories may last despite bad disease; recent memory most important
Intelligence	Current events, math (serial 7s), spelling, presidents backward
Thought content	Hallucinations, illusions, delusions, suicidal or homicidal ideation, paranoia
Unique interests	These may need to be asked: i.e., a gourmet cook should be able to describe favorite dish
Understanding	Simple conversation may be sufficient; ask meaning of a short story; complex commands
Judgment and insight	Proverbs; social-behavior tests: e.g., "What do you do if you see a fire in a theatre?" or simply ask "Why am I asking you all of these questions?"

order of relatively acute onset, characterized by global impairment of cognitive functions and widespread disturbance of cerebral metabolism (5,10). This syndrome has many synonyms—e.g., metabolic encephalopathy (11), exogenous metabolic brain disease (11), acute brain syndrome (10), toxic psychosis (5), and syndrome of cerebral insufficiency (12). The common denominator in these variations is a distortion of cerebral cellular metabolism resulting from an insult to the brain (5,10).

Epidemiology

Relatively few data exist with regard to the epidemiology of delirium, but according to the best estimates, delirium of some degree of severity may be manifest in 5 to 15 percent of all patients on general medical and surgical wards (10,13). The incidence may be higher on intensive care units (2 to 40 percent) (14,15,16), following open heart and coronary bypass surgery (30 to 60 percent) (17), and in patients with severe burns (20 to 30 percent) (18,19). The incidence and prevalence of delirium are especially high in patients sixty years of age and older (46 to 80 percent) (17,20,21). Delirium is the most common disorder diagnosed by consultation-liaison psychiatrists in general hospitals (10) and may be the most common mental disorder to which humans are subject.

Etiology

Delirium may result from a number of factors, acting singly or in combination, that result in widespread derangement of cerebral metabolism. A necessary condition for delirium to occur is the presence of one or more organic factors, the most common of which are listed in the following:

- Intoxication by Drugs and Poisons

    Drugs: anticholinergic agents, sedative-hypnotics, digitalis derivatives, opiates, corticosteroids, salicylates, antibiotics, anticonvulsants, antiarrhythmic and antihypertensive drugs, antineoplastic agents, cimetidine, lithium, antiparkinson agents, disulfiram, indomethacin, bismuth salts, phencyclidine

    Alcohol: ethyl and methyl

    Addictive inhalants: gasoline, glue, ether, nitrous oxide, nitrites

    Industrial poisons: carbon disulphide, organic solvents, methyl chloride and bromide, heavy metals, organophosphorus insecticides, carbon monoxide

    Snakebite

    Poisonous plants and mushrooms

- Withdrawal Syndromes

    Alcohol: delirium tremens

    Sedatives and hypnotics: barbiturates, chloral hydrate, chlordiazepoxide, diazepam, ethchlorvynol, glutethimide, meprobamate, methyprylon, paraldehyde

    Amphetamines

    Nutritional, Hormonal, and Metabolic Disorders

    Hypoxia

    Hypoglycemia

    Hepatic, renal, pancreatic, pulmonary insufficiency (encephalopathy)

    Avitaminosis: nicotinic acid, thiamine, cyanocobalamine (vitamin 7_{12}), folate, pyridoxine

    Hypervitaminosis: intoxication by vitamins A and D

    Hormonal disorders: hyperinsulinism, hyperthyroidism, hypothyroidism, hypopituitarism, Addison's disease, Cushing's syndrome, hypoparathyroidism, hyperparathyroidism

Disorders of fluid and electrolyte metabolism:

Dehydration, water intoxication

Alkalosis, acidosis

Hypernatremia, hyponatremia, hyperkalemia, hypokalemia, hypercalcemia, hypocalcemia, hypermagnesemia, hypomagnesemia

- Errors of metabolism:

Porphyria

Carcinoid syndrome

Hepatolenticular degeneration (Wilson's disease)

- Infections

Systemic: pneumonia, typhoid, typhus, acute rheumatic fever, malaria, influenza, mumps, diphtheria, brucellosis, infectious mononucleosis, infectious hepatitis, malaria, subacute bacterial endocarditis, bacteremia, septicemia, Rocky Mountain spotted fever, legionnaires' disease

Intracranial: acute, subacute, and chronic:

Viral encephalitis, aseptic meningitis, rabies

Bacterial meningitis: meningococcal, pneumococcal, hemophilus influenza, etc. (22)

A variety of factors may predispose a person to delirium, including age of sixty years and older (20,23), drug addiction, and brain damage (10). Psychological stress, sleep and sensory deprivation, severe fatigue, and prolonged immobilization may facilitate the onset and/or increase the severity of delirium (10). Psychological predisposing factors have been postulated, but supporting data are lacking (10).

Pathophysiology

Data suggest that delirium is mediated by a widespread disturbance of cerebral metabolism coupled with an alteration in central nervous system neurotransmitter activity. Evidence for altered brain metabolism is provided by studies that consistently describe a bilateral, diffuse abnormality of EEG background activity in delirium (12,24). Most often there is slowing of the dominant EEG rhythm, but low-voltage fast activity may predominate in agitated deliria—e.g., delirium tremens (24). Changes in cerebral metabolism may be accompanied by altered central nervous system neurotransmitter synthesis, activity, and receptor sensitivity (25). These changes have been postulated to underlie delirium associated with anticholinergic drugs, cimetidine and alcohol (decreased cholinergic activity) (25), with prolonged levodopa therapy (serotonergic supersensitivity) (26), and with delirium tremens (increased central noradrenergic activity) (27).

Since disordered cognition and wakefulness are prominent features of delirium, both cortical and subcortical structures likely are involved. Neuropathologic changes are relatively nonspecific and usually reversible and include diffuse cerebral swelling and pallor, swelling of cortical and hippocampal neurons, and dissolution of Nissl granules (10).

Clinical Features

Delirium is characterized by concurrent disturbances of wakefulness and sensorium, cognition, and psychomotor activity. Some level of disordered wakefulness and sensorium is a sine qua non for the diagnosis of delirium. This may be manifested by disturbed attention to and/or reduced awareness of self and the environment. In delirium, the state of the patient's level of awareness may range from minimum neglect of details to coma, but it is always reduced. The patient's level of arousal and alertness (readiness to respond) may be increased or decreased, but vigilance (sustained attention) is invariably reduced. These features suggest that delirium may be at least in part a disorder of wakefulness (10).

A second core feature of delirium is relatively global impairment of cognition—i.e., those functions essential to the processing of information. Some degree of impaired perception is invariably present, with resultant spatiotemporal disorientation, illusions (erroneous or misunderstood perceptions), and hallucinations (false perceptions). All of these phenomena are more common when sensory discrimination is made difficult. Thinking is invariably disorganized to some degree. Whether thoughts are slowed and impoverished or pressured, purposive problem solving, reasoning, and abstraction are reduced. Delusions (false beliefs) may result and are often elaborated from illusions (misperceptions). Finally, memory is invariably impaired, including retrograde and antegrade recall, resulting in partial amnesia for the course of the delirium.

The third essential feature of delirium involves disturbances of psychomotor activity. This feature may be manifested by catatonic stupor, lethargy, or purposeless hyperactivity, often with rapid unpredictable shifts from one to another. Purposeful modulations of behavior are almost always impossible in delirium. A variety of involuntary or semipurposeful movements may be present, including tremor, automatisms, and dysgraphia. Two movement disturbances—bilateral asterixis and multifocal myoclonus—have been considered virtually pathognomonic for delirium (11). The symptoms and signs of delirium characteristically fluctuate but usually are worse at night than during the day.

Delirium most commonly develops acutely but may begin insidiously in a setting of slowly evolving disturbances—e.g., endocrinopathies. Prodromata, including insomnia, restlessness, vivid dreams, nightmares, and oneiric mentation, may precede delirium by hours or even days. A wide range of emotional disturbances may be present, with fear or anxiety, depression, and apathy the most common. Autonomic arousal may be manifested by tachycardia, facial flushing, mydriasis, diaphoresis, and hypertension. These symptoms only serve to highlight the clinical variability that is the hallmark of delirium (28).

The outcome of the delirium depends upon the underlying cause. An episode of delirium usually lasts about one week and rarely longer than one month. Although full recovery of premorbid functioning is most common, transition to another organic brain syndrome (e.g., dementia) or death may eventuate. Commonly, delirium is complicated by an injury sustained in falling out of bed or in an attempted fight.

Diagnosis

The diagnosis of delirium is made at the bedside by recognizing the clinical syndrome. Diagnostic criteria for delirium include (3):

- Clouding of consciousness (reduced clarity and awareness of environment) and disturbances of attention

  At least two of the following:

  Perceptual disturbance: misinterpretations, illusions, or hallucinations; speech that is at times incoherent; disturbances of sleep-wakefulness cycle with insomnia or daytime drowsiness; increased or decreased psychomotor activity

- Disorientation and memory impairment
- Clinical features that develop over a short period of time (usually hours to days) and that tend to fluctuate over the course of a day
- Evidence, from the history, physical examination, or laboratory tests, of a specific organic factor judged to be etiologically related to the disturbance

Once the diagnosis of delirium has been made, a thorough search for its cause or causes is required. In many cases the cause may be obvious, but in others, the following appropriate laboratory procedures may aid the investigation:

- Blood chemistries: glucose, electrolytes, blood urea nitrogen, liver enzymes, arterial blood gases
- Hemogram
- Urinalysis
- Drug screen
- Serum protein electrophoresis

- LE cell preparation, antinuclear antibody, Westergren erythrocyte sedimentation rate

- ECG (consider Holter monitoring)

- Chest X-ray

- EEG

- Cerebrospinal fluid examination including protein, glucose, cell count, gram stain, serology, cryptococcal antigen, and protein electrophoresis

- Vitamin B_{12}, folate levels

- Computerized axial tomography of the brain

- Serological test for syphilis

- Serum thyroxine and cortisol

- Heavy metal screen

- Urinary porphobilinogen and 5-hydroxyindoleacetic acid

The differential diagnosis of delirium includes dementia; certain psychotic disorders marked by hallucinations, delusions, and disordered thinking; and speech and factitious disorders with psychological symptoms. Both delirium and dementia are characterized by impaired cognition, but dementia is a relatively stable global cognitive disorder that is not accompanied by the fluctuating disturbances of wakefulness and sensorium pathognomonic of delirium. Similarly, in schizophrenia and hysteria, there is usually neither alteration in wakefulness and sensorium nor the cognitive impairment and memory loss seen in delirium (see Table 7.1). Asterixis and multifocal myoclonus are not features of schizophrenia or hysteria. Nevertheless, distinguishing between schizophrenia and delirium may be difficult, in which case the EEG and sodium amytal interview are useful aids in the differential diagnosis (5,29).

Treatment

The management of delirium requires a dual approach: etiologic and symptomatic. Correct diagnosis of the causative agent or agents and appropriate therapy directed at the underlying pathology are essential. In many cases, more than one putative pathogen may be identified (e.g., drug toxicity with anemia, hypoxia, and fluid and electrolyte imbalance), and all must be corrected. A history of current alcohol and all other drug use is essential since virtually any drug may result in delirium through overdose, withdrawal, idiosyncratic sensitivity, and so on. In such cases, all nonessential medications should be gradually tapered and eventually discontinued. Too often, the cause of the delirium is never found.

Symptomatic and supportive measures designed to relieve distress and prevent complications constitute the second arm of the overall approach to managing delirium. Adequate nutrition, fluid intake, electrolyte balance, and vitamin supply must be maintained. The environment of the patient is very important and should be structured to avoid sensory overload, monotony, and deprivation; to decrease unfamiliarity; and to provide appropriate social support and sensory stimulation. Optimally, the patient is placed in a single, quiet but not silent, well-lighted room with a dimmed light at night. Extraneous confusing noises including hospital intercom messages should be kept to an absolute minimum. The patient should be provided with sensory cues to support reality, spatial-temporal orientation, and a sense of familiarity. The nursing staff and family can be especially helpful by providing encouragement, reorientation, and a sense of familiarity (30). Close monitoring of the patient's mental status and behavior are mandatory.

The specific treatment of each of the numerous disorders that may cause delirium is beyond the scope of this chapter. However, delirium is often a neuropsychiatric emergency in that certain conditions immediately threaten permanent brain damage or life. These include hypoglycemia, diabetic ketosis, hyperosmolar state, hypoxia and anoxia, hyperthermia, and Wernicke's encephalopathy. Consequently, we recommend the following approach to every patient initially presenting with delirium, without exception:

- Establish an adequate airway and ensure that the patient is breathing.

- Ensure adequate blood perfusion to the brain.

- Obtain blood studies immediately (hemogram, serum glucose, electrolytes, blood urea nitrogen, arterial blood gas) while establishing an IV line.

- Administer 100 ml of 50 percent dextrose and 100 mg of thiamine IV.

These procedures may not bring about immediate improvement but will at least prevent further cerebral damage pending definitive diagnostic studies.

Because medications may complicate the clinical picture and further confound the disorder, their use in delirium is limited to certain specific indications. A restless, agitated, or fearful patient needs sedation to prevent accidents and complications like insomnia. No drug is entirely without potential risks, but haloperidol has proved effective, potent, and relatively nontoxic and is the drug of choice in most cases of delirium (31). Initially, the patient receives from 2 to 10 mg IM, to be repeated hourly until agitation subsides. For most patients, the effective total daily dose ranges from 10 to 60 mg. Once stable, oral medication may be substituted at a total daily dose roughly two times the parenteral dose for equivalent therapeutic efficacy. The serum half-life allows for twice daily dosing, with the majority (roughly two-thirds) given at bedtime. It is important to note that antipsychotic medications can precipitate hypothermia in myxedematous patients or hepatic coma in patients with cirrhosis. Thus, hepatic encephalopathy is best managed with a benzodiazepine such as oxazepam or diazepam (32). Physostigmine is the drug of choice for patients with anticholinergic delirium (33). In alcohol and drug withdrawal deliria, the benzodiazepines are preferred (34). Close monitoring of the patient's mental status and behavior are mandatory for the duration of delirium. Early psychiatric referral can aid in the diagnosis and therapy, and skillful liaison may help prevent progression of symptoms (10).

Dementia

Dementia refers to a global decline in higher intellectual functions in an otherwise alert patient (35,36). Approximately one million Americans over sixty-five years old, and many younger than sixty-five, meet the criteria for dementia (37). It is one of the most feared and disabling aspects of aging.

Although many individuals maintain full cognitive function as they age, normal aging may be associated with mild cognitive impairment. A slight slowing of intellectual processes and some degree of mild forgetfulness characterize this "benign senescent forgetfulness" (23,38,39). It is a normal concomitant of aging and is not, by itself, prognostic of a progressive deterioration (38). Dementia, however, is *not* a normal or inevitable consequence of aging, and any patient who develops dementia must receive a thorough neuropsychiatric evaluation.

Diagnosis

Impairment of recent memory typically heralds the onset of dementia. Patients are unable to recall events occurring only minutes earlier, although they remember events from the distant past in detail. Eventually, higher cognitive functions such as reading, writing, calculation, visuospatial construction, and even speech (40) are lost. Psychiatric symptoms including personality change, irritability, emotional lability and frank psychoses with delusions, hallucinations, and paranoia may eventually accompany the cognitive deterioration.

The diagnostic criteria for dementia listed in *DSM-III* (3) include the following:

- A loss of intellectual abilities of sufficient severity to interfere with social or occupational functioning

- Memory impairment

- At least one of the following:

    Impairment of abstract thinking as manifested by concrete interpretation of proverbs, inability to find similarities and differences between related words, difficulty in defining words and concepts, and other similar tasks

    Impaired judgment

Other disturbances of higher cortical function, such as aphasia (disorder of language due to brain dysfunction), apraxia (inability to carry out motor activities despite intact comprehension and motor function), agnosia (failure to recognize or identify objects despite intact sensory function), constructional difficulty (e.g., inability to copy three-dimensional figures, assemble blocks, or arrange sticks in specific designs)

Personality change (i.e., alteration or accentuation of premorbid traits)

- State of consciousness not clouded (i.e., does not meet the criteria for delirium or intoxication although these may be superimposed)

- Either the first or both of the following:

Evidence from the history, physical examination, or laboratory tests of a specific organic factor that is judged to be etiologically related to the disturbance

In the absence of such evidence, an organic factor necessary for the syndrome can be presumed if conditions other than organic mental disorders have been reasonably excluded and if the behavior change represents cognitive impairment in a variety of areas

Etiology and Differential Diagnosis

Initially, the physician must determine if the patient has dementia or minor memory lapses of normal aging. As is recognized in *DSM-III*, dementia is a chronic, progressive deterioration of intellectual and cognitive functions that must be of sufficient severity to interfere with a person's ability to function normally.

The following list shows the many possible causes of dementia, but the majority of cases is associated with degenerative diseases of the central nervous system (41,42,43,44,45):

- Diffuse Parenchymatous Disease

Alzheimer's, Parkinson's syndrome, Parkinson/dementia complex, Pick's, Jakob-Creutzfeldt, Huntington's disease, Kraepelin's disease, Hallervorden-Spatz, spinocerebellar degeneration, progressive myoclonic epilepsy, Steel-Richardson-Olchefsky (progressive supranuclear palsy)

- Metabolic Disorders

Myxedema, Wilson's disease, liver failure, Cushing's syndrome, uremia, hypoparathyroidism, hyperparathyroidism

- Cardiovascular Disorders

Atherosclerosis, inflammatory vasculitis, subcortical arteriosclerotic encephalopathy, arterio-venous malformation, atrial myxoma

    Hypoxia

- Normal Pressure Hydrocephalus
- Nutritional Deficiencies

    Wernicke-Korsakoff, B_{12} deficiency, Marchiafava-Bignami, pellagra, Strachen's syndrome

- Toxins

    Metals (Pb, Hg), organic compounds, carbon monoxide

- Drugs

    Therapeutic and abuse

- Tumors

    Meningioma, glioma, metastatic

- Infections

    Brain abscess, meningitis (bacterial, fungal), viral encephalitis, Behçet's, kuru, lues

- Trauma

    Punch drunk, heat stroke, subdural hematomas, open and closed head injury

- Demyelinating

    Multiple sclerosis

- Degenerative

    Myotonic dystrophy

- Inflammatory

    Sarcoidosis, granulomatous arteritis, Whipple's disease (cerebral)

Post mortem studies in geriatric inpatients with dementia have demonstrated that 70 percent of cases are due to Alzheimer's disease, either alone or in combination with vascular disease (46). Alzheimer's disease accounts for at least 55 percent of cases of senile dementia (42,47) and is probably the most common cause of dementia.

    Fifteen percent of patients who meet criteria for dementia have potentially reversible disorders. Another 20 to 25 percent of patients have disorders that may be arrested with proper diagnosis and treatment (43,44,45,48). The diagnostic workup is directed toward identifying these treatable conditions (see Table 7.3).

    Depression must be a serious consideration in all cases. A primary depression and pseudodementia can be difficult to distinguish from depression secondary to dementia. A mental status examination and appropriate studies are required to rule out dementia reliably (41,49,50,51,52,53).

Table 7.3 Laboratory Evaluation of Dementia

Laboratory Test	Result
Chest X-ray	Tumor, chronic lung disease
EEG	Diffuse cerebral dysfunction, focal abnormality, temporal lobe foci
Brain CT scan, NMR, PET	Atrophy, subdural hematoma, mass lesion, normal pressure hydrocephalus, lacunae
Skull X-ray	Pineal shift, increased intracranial pressure
ECG	Arrhythmia, remote infarction
Urinalysis	Renal or hepatic disease
Tuberculosis skin test	Tuberculosis
Blood evaluation	
Complete blood count	Anemia (megaloblastic or hypochromic)
Serologic test for syphilis	Tertiary central nervous system syphilis
Drug levels	Barbiturates, bromides, phenothiazines, other
Electrolytes	Pulmonary, renal, or endocrine dysfunction
Whole blood urea nitrogen/ Creatinine	Kidney disease
Liver functions	Hepatic encephalopathy
Thyroid panel	Graves disease, myxedema
B_{12} level/Schilling test	Impaired B_{12} absorption
Cerebrospinal fluid	Chronic infection (cryptococcus, tuberculosis, syphilis), degenerative central nervous system disease, granulomatosis arteritis

Multi-infarct dementia (54) may be distinguished from Alzheimer's disease by the abruptness in onset and fluctuating course. Of course, these problems may coexist (46).

Dementia secondary to normal pressure hydrocephalus is characterized by gait disturbance, usually preceding mental impairment, and urinary incontinence. Memory loss may be mild without language or constructional problems.

Korsakoff's psychosis is a disorder of short-term memory that occurs in patients with prolonged alcohol intake. Often it is accompanied by an ataxic gait and neuropathy.

Tumors, particularly in the frontal lobe, and subdural hematoma may present with dementia. Usually focal neurologic signs, headache, and papilledema are present. Brainstem tumors are reported to cause dementia (55).

Metabolic causes of dementia include thyroid and parathyroid disease (56), hepatic failure, and pernicious anemia. All may have a sensorimotor neuropathy or other neurologic signs to suggest the diagnosis (43,48).

Degenerative processes other than Alzheimer's disease may cause dementia. Accompanying clinical signs such as tremor, rigidity, and bradykinesia in parkinsonism, chorea in Huntington's disease, myoclonus in

Jakob-Creutzfeldt disease, or absence of vertical gaze in progressive supra-nuclear palsy will aid in diagnosis.

Neurosyphilis, although now rare, must be remembered as an infectious cause of dementia. Herpes simplex encephalitis and herpes zoster ophthalmicus with central nervous system involvement are other considerations. Dementia with pulmonary infiltrates may suggest a vasculitis or sarcoidosis (57).

Table 7.3 illustrates the laboratory studies useful in evaluation of the patient with dementia. The EEG may show focal slowing in structural brain disease or diffuse slowing in primary degenerative and metabolic diseases (52,58,59,60,61,62,63,64,65,66). Computerized brain tomography may reveal focal structural disease (tumor, infarct, subdural hematoma, hydrocephalus) or cortical atrophy (8,49,67,68,69,70,71,72,73,74). Regional blood flow (75,76,77), evoked potentials (78,79), positron emission tomography (PET), and nuclear magnetic resonance (NMR) studies may also be of help.

Pathophysiology of Alzheimer's Disease

The morphologic abnormalities found in Alzheimer's form of dementia may be seen, although to a lesser degree, in the brain tissue of normal elderly people. It has been suggested that the disease represents a situation where clinical signs and symptoms do not appear until after a certain number of tissue alterations exist (47). This threshold for the emergence of symptoms undoubtedly differs across individuals.

Grossly, the brain is atrophic; brain weight varies considerably but is commonly between 950 and 1,100 gm (47). This weight loss corresponds principally to shrinkage of cerebral white matter. Although the atrophy is diffuse, it is often most prominent in the frontal and temporal (hippocampal gyrus) regions. The deep structures of the diencephalon and brainstem are usually normal.

Changes in cortical cellularity are common. Small neurons (40 to 90 microns) from the mid-frontal region and large neurons (greater than 90 microns) from the frontal and temporal areas are reduced in number (47). Fibrous astrocytes are increased in the glial layers (II–VI) of the cerebral cortex.

The diagnosis of Alzheimer's disease rests ultimately on demonstration of the classic histological changes—neuritic (senile) plaques and neurofibrillary tangles. Senile plaques and neurofibrillary tangles are seen in intellectually normal old people but are largely confined to the hippocampus. In Alzheimer's disease, these histological changes are found throughout the cerebral cortex and in certain deeper gray areas (substantia inominata, claustrum, hypothalamus, pontine tegmentum, and floor of the fourth ventricle). The quantity of senile plaques and neurofibrillary tangles correlates highly with the degree of dementia (80).

The senile plaques have a central core of extracellular amyloid fibers surrounded by abnormal neurites and sometimes tangles. Glial fibers and microglial cells are also present. Amyloid may infiltrate the vascular walls.

Neurofibrillary tangles usually occupy the cell body of medium and large neurons. These tangles are composed of a pair of twisted filaments, called paired helical filaments, located in the cytoplasm of neurons. In animal preparations, aluminum may lead to formation of neurofibrillary tangles. Some authors (81) have reported elevated brain aluminum content in patients with Alzheimer's disease, but brain aluminum does increase with age (82,83). Since aluminum is located in the nuclei of neurons with tangles rather than in the adjacent normal neurons, a relationship between tangles and aluminum may exist.

Other microscopic changes found in the hippocampus of patients with dementia include the granulovacuolar change of Simchowicz (84) and the Hirano body (85)—both lesions are also found in the normal elderly but only in small numbers.

Evidence indicates that neurotransmitter systems may be altered in Alzheimer's disease (86,87,88,89). Perhaps the most important of these changes involves the cholinergic system. The activity of choline acetyltransferase (ChAT), the biosynthetic enzyme for acetylcholine, is significantly reduced in post mortem cerebral cortex from Alzheimer's patients (87,88,90,91). The ChAT deficit has been confirmed in temporal cortical biopsy material (92,93) where a reduced capacity for acetylcholine synthesis has been directly demonstrated (94). On the basis of animal studies, the major contribution to ChAT activity appears to derive from subcortical cholinergic cells of the nucleus basalis of Meynert (95,96), located in the basal forebrain. It has been suggested that the cholinergic lesion in Alzheimer's disease lies in the subcortical afferent neuronal processes rather than in the cholinergic neurons intrinsic to the neocortex (89).

Acetylcholinesterase has also been found to be reduced in Alzheimer's disease (97,98). Muscarinic cholinergic receptors are apparently normal (91,92,99); nicotinic receptors have not been adequately studied.

The cholinergic deficit in Alzheimer's disease has generated several possible therapeutic concepts, to be discussed later. The deficiency in ChAT is not unique to Alzheimer's disease, however. Reduced ChAT activity has been reported in adults with Down's syndrome (100), in Jakob-Creutzfeldt disease (100), and in alcoholic dementia (101,102).

A loss of noradrenergic cell bodies from the locus coeruleus (103,104) and reduced activity of the noradrenergic synthetic enzyme dopamine-β-hydroxylase (105) has been demonstrated in Alzheimer's disease. This noradrenergic deficit does not appear to be as widespread as the cholinergic deficit. Other systems that project to the neocortex and that may be altered in Alzheimer's disease include dopamine (106), serotonin (106), substance P (107), and somatostatin (107,108); abnormalities of these systems await further definition.

The existence of a genetic factor in Alzheimer's disease is well established. A number of families with apparent autosomal dominant transmission have been reported (47). Larsson and associates (110) suggested the existence of a predisposing autosomal dominant gene with age-related penetrance reaching 40 percent at age ninety. They estimated the gene frequency at 12 percent. Twin studies strongly implicate a genetic factor. Jarvik et al. (73) reported a concordance of 61 percent for organic brain syndrome in elderly monozygotic twin pairs. Kallmann (111) found the concordance of Alzheimer's disease or senile dementia in monozygotic twins to be 42.8 percent; in dizygotic twins, 8.9 percent; in other siblings, 6.5 percent; and in parents, 3.4 percent. Environmental factors may also be important in these data. A genetic marker, haptoglobin-1, has been reported to be highly correlated in patients from the Netherlands with dementia (112).

Chromosomal abnormalities may predispose to Alzheimer's disease. Individuals with Down's syndrome who live more than thirty to forty years almost invariably develop the morphologic and biochemical changes of Alzheimer's disease, including neuritic plaques, neurofibrillary tangles, and loss of ChAT (113). These are usually accompanied by clinical changes, suggesting further cognitive impairment. Also, an increase in Down's syndrome in relatives of Alzheimer's probands has been reported (113).

Autoimmune disease has also been suggested as an etiology for Alzheimer's disease (114). Elderly humans with autoantibodies (115), with low suppressor T cell activity (116), or with impaired cutaneous hypersensitivity (117) are at increased risk of death. A decrease in specific immunoglobulins in Alzheimer's disease has been reported, but this is likely a secondary phenomenon (118). Increases in specific major histocompatibility haplotypes have been reported but not confirmed (119,120,121,122,123).

Evidence suggesting a viral etiology for dementia is indirect. Inoculation of the scrapie agent into certain strains of mice causes an encephalopathy and neuritic plaques made of amyloid core and abnormal neurites (124) that are remarkably similar to the plaques in human Alzheimer's disease.

Treatment

Etiologic. In those cases in which dementia develops secondary to other medical disorders (see list of causes of dementia), treatment should be directed at the underlying causative agent or agents. Metabolic and nutritional derangements should be corrected, vascular risk factors controlled, infections treated, structural lesions repaired, and unnecessary drugs and toxins removed. Obviously, attention to diagnostic detail (see Table 7.3) is essential if potentially treatable causes of dementia are to be identified and corrected prior to the development of irreversible brain damage (43,44,125,126).

Successful pharmacologic treatment that reverses the cognitive deficits of Alzheimer's disease is lacking at present. Numerous agents have been variously tested, including vasodilators, anticoagulants, Gerovital #3, psychostimulants, nootropics, neuropeptides, and neurotransmitters (127). Consistent improvement with these therapies has not been demonstrated.

The evidence (discussed earlier) for a cholinergic deficiency in Alzheimer's disease may provide a rational basis for attempts at treatment. It has been suggested that replenishing the cholinergic deficit might improve or reverse cognitive deterioration. Inhibiting the hydrolysis of acetylcholine with physostigmine is one such approach, and memory improvement has been observed in a small number of patients (128,129,130) despite side effects.

In animals, administration of the acetylcholine precursors choline and lecithin (a choline-containing phospholipid) results in an increase in both the synthesis and release of acetylcholine (131,132). Unfortunately, clinical trials with choline and lecithin in humans have been disappointing (133,134,135). One possible explanation for these negative findings might be that a precursor-loading strategy depends upon a minimum number of intact cholinergic neurons that can continue synthesizing acetylcholine from the precursors. In Alzheimer's disease, the residual population of cholinergic neurons may be inadequate.

An alternative approach would be the use of direct cholinergic agonists such as oxotremine and arecholine, especially given that the concentration of muscarinic receptors remains normal even in advanced Alzheimer's disease (91,99). These agents are limited by their side effects. Attempts to develop selective agonists for receptor subtypes (136) and to increase the sensitivity of cholinergic receptors may prove useful. A combination of these approaches might be indicated (129,130). Efforts at correcting noradrenergic or dopaminergic deficits with L-dopa have been unsuccessful (137).

Symptomatic.   Although the majority of patients with dementia cannot be cured, much can be done to maximize remaining intellectual function, to relieve distress, and to prevent complications.

The patient's visual and auditory acuity should be maximized. Visual and auditory environmental clues are the most basic sources of orientation, and when they are lost or obscured, confusion may ensue. The person with slight memory loss and compromised orientation who loses continuity of the environment may become rapidly confused, frightened, and even psychotic because of isolation and misperceptions of the environment. A familiar example is the so-called sundown syndrome in which an apparently stable elderly person admitted to the hospital for a minor problem becomes paranoid and combative at night but seems well during daylight hours the next day. A lamp lit in the room to maintain visual environmental clues or a radio on low volume for auditory stimulus may be sufficient to avert the sundown syndrome.

Any superimposed medical illness may precipitate a deterioration in cognitive functioning in the demented patient. Anxiety and depression are common in the elderly (50,51,53,138) and also may be accompanied by significant cognitive impairment. Prompt diagnosis and appropriate therapy of these conditions can result in marked improvement in intellectual functioning (139). Adequate fluid and nutrition are obviously mandatory but are frequently neglected.

Drug pharmacokinetics are altered significantly in the elderly (140,141) and dictate a need for conservative drug administration. The absorption, distribution, metabolism, and excretion of drugs by the elderly make them especially sensitive to toxic side effects. Sleep and pain medications and anticholinergic agents are common causes of intellectual deterioration and frank delirium in the elderly. Unfortunately, many elderly patients are on numerous medications, placing them at great risk for side effects resulting from drug interactions (140).

Proper physical and intellectual activity are important. Depriving elderly people of work or activity because of their age rather than their ability invariably results in loss of self-worth and may worsen the cognitive deficits. The elderly are often patronized and arbitrarily excluded from social roles. Such discrimination may exaggerate the effects of physical and psychological aging. Giving the elderly responsibilities to match their abilities will enhance self-respect and help them to maintain a functioning level.

Sleep patterns change with aging, including a diminished need for sleep, frequent awakenings from sleep, a reduction of stage III sleep, and disappearance of stage IV sleep (64,65). For this reason, elderly people may complain of not sleeping deeply or of awakening often during the night. Concern about lack of sleep may be more disturbing than insomnia. Reassuring the patient that these changes are a natural accompaniment of aging may relieve much of the distress. The elderly and patients with dementia often have a reversal in their sleep cycle. This is best managed without medications by gradually readjusting the sleep cycle so that patients spend more daytime hours awake and more nighttime hours asleep. Sedatives should be avoided whenever possible because of the increased risk of toxic side effects (141,142).

Essential to the care of the elderly and demented is family counseling about the disease process and progression. The family's perception of the demented patient's disability should be determined. The family's interpretation may not agree with the patient's view or that of the physician. The capabilities and limitations of the patient must be clearly explained. Studies indicate that normal aging people show no loss of acquired knowledge but a decline in their ability to obtain new knowledge (47). Thus, older people need more time to incorporate new information and may be more careful and discriminating with new information (47). Specific training for the family will enable them to be more effective caretakers. In addition, a number of community resources are available to assist the family, including Homemaker Home-Health Aide Services, Visiting Nurse Association, Meals-on-Wheels, telephone services, Alzheimer's support groups, social services, and local churches.

Attention should be paid to the effects of the patient's illness on the spouse and family. The spouse must now assume the roles and previous responsibilities of the patient. This will be especially difficult when the spouse is facing his or her own declining physical and intellectual capabilities. Financial hardship may ensue. Professional legal advice should be obtained early to ensure proper management of the estate. It is not surprising that these problems may eventually overwhelm the spouse, resulting in severe anxiety and depression. Social isolation aggravates the situation because friends no longer invite the couple out. The physician must be alert to these problems.

Unfortunately, the dementing illness may eventually progress to the point at which the patient can no longer be cared for at home. The physician may be extremely valuable here by helping the family to determine when nursing home placement is indicated, making the appropriate arrangements for transfer, and perhaps most important, assuaging the family's guilt over abandoning one of their members.

In summary, treatment of dementia is far from hopeless. Management depends upon prompt diagnosis and treatment, including treatment of superimposed medical disorders and attention to the psychological and social aspects of the patient's illness.

REFERENCES

1. Koranyi, E.K. Morbidity and rate of undiagnosed physical illness in a psychiatric clinic population. *Arch. Gen. Psychiatry* 36:414–419, 1979.
2. Hall, R.C.W.; Gardner, E.R.; and Stickney, S.K. Physical illness manifesting as psychiatric disease: II. Analysis of a state hospital inpatient population. *Arch. Gen. Psychiatry* 37:989–995, 1980.
3. American Psychiatric Association. *Diagnostic and Statistical Manual of Mental Disorders*, 3rd ed. Washington, D.C., 1980.
4. Kahana, R.J., and Bibring, G.L. Personality types in medical management. In *Psychiatry and Medical Practice in a General Hospital*, Zinberg, N.E., ed. New York: International University Press, 1964; 108–123.
5. Lipowski, Z.J. *Delirium: Acute Brain Failure in Man*. Springfield, Ill.: Charles C Thomas, 1980.
6. Strub, R.L., and Black, F.W. *The Mental Status Examination in Neurology*. Philadelphia: F.A. Davis Co., 1977.
7. Folstein, M.F.; Folstein, S.E.; and McHugh, P.R. "Mini-mental state": A practical method for grading the cognitive state of patients for the clinician. *J. Psychiatr. Res.* 12:189–198, 1975.
8. Jacobs, J.W.; Bernhard, M.R.; Dalgado, A.; and Strain, J.J. Screening for organic mental syndromes in the medically ill. *Ann. Intern. Med.* 86:40–46, 1977.
9. Parozzolo, F., and Kerr, K. Neuropsychological assessment of dementia. In *The Aging Nervous System*, vol. 1, Pirozzolo, F., and Maletta, G., eds. New York: Praeger, 1980.
10. Lipowski, Z.J. Organic mental disorder: Introduction and review of syndromes. In *Comprehensive Textbook of Psychiatry*, vol. 1, Kaplan, H.I., Freedman, A.M., and Sadock, B.J., eds. Baltimore: Williams and Wilkins, 1980, pp. 1359–1391.
11. Plum, F., and Posner, J.B. *The Diagnosis of Stupor and Coma*, 3rd ed. Philadelphia: F.A. Davis, 1980.
12. Romano, J., and Engel, G.L. Delirium. I. Electroencephalographic data. *Arch. Neurol. Psychiat.* 51:356–377, 1944.
13. Turner, G.O. *The Cardiovascular Care Unit*. New York: John Wiley and Sons, 1978.
14. Hale, M.; Koss, N.; and Kerstein, M. Psychiatric complications in a surgical ICU. *Crit. Care Med.* 5:199–203, 1977.

15. Katz, N.M.; Agle, D.P.; DePalma, R.G.; and DeCosse, J.J. Delirium in surgical patients under intensive care. *Arch. Surg.* 104:310–313, 1972.
16. Wilson, L.M. Intensive care delirium. *Arch. Intern. Med.* 130:225–226, 1972.
17. Titchener, J.L.; Zwerling, I.; and Gottschalk, L. Psychosis in surgical patients. *Surg. Gynecol. Obstet.* 102:59–65, 1956.
18. Andreasen, N.J.C.; Noyes, R.; and Hartford, C.E. Management of emotional reactions in seriously burned adults. *N. Engl. J. Med.* 286:65–69, 1972.
19. Antoon, A.Y.; Volpe, J.J.; and Crawford, J.D. Burn encephalopathy in children. *Pediatrics* 50:609–616, 1972.
20. Bedford, P.D. General medical aspects of confusional states in elderly people. *Br. Med. J.* 2:185–188, 1959.
21. Simon, A., and Cahan, R.B. The acute brain syndrome in geriatric patients. *Psychiatr. Res. Rep.* 16:8–21, 1963.
22. Lipowski, Z.J. *Delirium, Acute Brain Failure in Man.* Springfield, Illinois: Charles C Thomas, 1980.
23. Blazer, D.G., and Friedman, S.W. Depression in late life. *Family Physician* 3:72–89, 1979.
24. Pro, J.D., and Wells, C.E. The use of the electroencephalogram in the diagnosis of delirium. *Dis. Nerv. Syst.* 38:804–808, 1977.
25. Blass, J.D., and Gibson, G.E. Carbohydrate and acetylcholine synthesis: Implications for cognitive disorders. In *Brain Acetylcholine and Neuropsychiatric Disease,* Davis, K.L., and Berger, P.A., eds. New York: Plenum, 1979, pp 215–236.
26. Nausieda, P.A.; Kaplan, L.R.; and Weber, S. Sleep disruption and psychosis induced by chronic levodopa therapy. *Neurology* 29:553, 1979.
27. Athen, D.; Beckman, H.; and Ackenheil, M. Biochemical investigations into the alcoholic delirium: Alteration of biogenic amines. *Arch. Psychiat. Nervenkr.* 224:129–140, 1977.
28. Wolff, H.G., and Curran, D. Nature of delirium and allied states. *Arch. Neurol. Psychiatry* 33:1175–1215, 1935.
29. Ward, N.G.; Rowlett, D.B.; and Burke, P. Sodium amylbarbitone in the differential diagnosis of confusion. *Am. J. Psychiatry* 135:75–78, 1978.
30. Gerdes, L. The confused or delirious patient. *Am. J. Nursing* 68:1228–1233, 1968.
31. Ayd, F.J. Haloperidol: Twenty years' clinical experience. *J. Clin. Psychiatry* 39:807–814, 1978.
32. Editorial: Sedation in liver disease. *Br. Med. J.* 1:1241–1242, 1977.
33. Granacher, R.P., and Baldessarini, R.J. Physostigmine. *Arch. Gen. Psychiatry* 32:375–380, 1975.
34. Holzbach, E., and Buhler, K.E. Behandlung der delirium tremens mit haldo. *Nervenarzt* 49:405–409, 1978.
35. Terry, R.D. Dementia. *Arch. Neurol.* 33:1–7, 1976.
36. Terry, R.D., and Davies, P. Dementia of the Alzheimer type. *Ann. Rev. Neurosci.* 3:77, 1980.
37. Katzman, R. The prevalence and malignancy of Alzheimer's disease. *Arch. Neurol.* 33:127–132, 1976.
38. Kral, V.A. Senescent forgetfulness: Benign and malignant. *Can. Med. Assoc. J.* 86:257, 1962.
39. Pfeiffer, E. Handling the distressed older patient. *Geriatrics* 34(2):23–29, 1979.
40. Rochford, G. A study of naming errors in dysphasic and in demented patients. *Neuropsychologia* 9:437, 1971.

41. Katzman, R., Karasu, T. Differential diagnosis of dementia. In *Neurological and Sensory Disorders in the Elderly*, Fields, W., ed. New York: Stratton Intercontinental Book Corporation, 1978, pp. 103–134.
42. Katzman, R.; Terry, R.D.; and Bick, K.L., eds. *Alzheimer's Disease: Senile Dementia and Related Disorders*. New York: Raven Press, 1978, p. 595.
43. Wells, C.E., ed. *Dementia*. Philadelphia: F.A. Davis Company, 1971.
44. Wells, C.E. Chronic brain disease: An overview. *Am. J. Psychiatry* 135:1–12, 1978.
45. Wells, C.E. Editorial: Role of stroke in dementia. *Stroke* 9:1–3, 1978.
46. Tomlinson, B.E.; Blessed, G.; and Roth, M. Observations on the brains of demented old people. *J. Neurol. Sci.* 11:205, 1970.
47. Katzman, R., and Terry, R.D. *The Neurology of Aging*. Philadelphia: F.A. Davis Company, 1983.
48. Wells, C.E. Treatable form of dementia. In *Update II: Harrison's Principles of Internal Medicine*, Isselbacher, K.J., Adams, R.D., Braunwald, E., Martin, J.B., Petersdorf, R.J., and Wilson, J.D., eds. New York: McGraw-Hill, 1981.
49. Brinkman, S.D.; Sarwar, M.; Levin, H.S.; and Morris, H.H. Quantitative indexes of computed tomography in dementia and normal aging. *Radiology* 138:89–92, 1981.
50. Kiloh, L.G. Pseudo-dementia. *Acta Psychiat. Scand.* 37:336, 1961.
51. Libow, L.S. Pseudo-senility: Acute and reversible organic brain syndromes. *J. Am. Geriat. Soc.* 21:112, 1973.
52. McAdam, W., and Robinson, R.A. Senile intellectual deterioration and the electroencephalogram: A quantitative correlation. *J. Ment. Sci.* 102:819, 1956.
53. Post, F. Dementia, depression and pseudodementia. In *Psychiatric Aspects of Neurologic Disease*, Benson, D.F., and Blumer, D., eds. New York: Grune and Stratton, 1975, pp. 99–120.
54. Souranden, P., and Walinder, J. Hereditary multi-infarct dementia. *Acta Neuropathologica* 39:247–254, 1977.
55. Wallack, E.M.; Reaves, W.M.; and Hall, C.D. Primary brain stem reticulum cell sarcoma causing dementia. *Dis. Nerv. Sys.* 6:744–747, 1979.
56. Slyter, H. Idiopathic hypoparathyroidism presenting as dementia. *Neurology* 29:393–394, 1979.
57. Cordingley, G.; Navarro, C.; Breist, J.C.M.; and Healton, E.B. Sarcoidosis presenting as senile dementia. *Neurology* 31:1148–1151, 1981.
58. Ehle, A.L., and Johnson, P.C. Rapidly evolving EEG changes in a case of Alzheimer's disease. *Ann. Neurol.* 1:593, 1977.
59. Gordon, E.B., and Sim, M. The EEG in presenile dementia. *J. Neurol. Neurosurg. and Psychiatry* 30:285, 1967.
60. Johannesson, G.; Brun, A.; Gustafson, I.; and Ingvar, D.H. EEG in presenile dementia related to cerebral blood flow and autopsy findings. *Acta Neurol. Scand.* 56:89, 1977.
61. Letemendia, F., and Pampiglione, G. Clinical and electroencephalographic observations in Alzheimer's disease. *J. Neurol. Neurosurg. and Psychiatry* 21:167, 1958.
62. Liddell, D.W. Investigations of EEG findings in presenile dementia. *J. Neurol. Neurosurg. and Psychiatry* 21:173, 1958.
63. Muller, H.F., and Kral, V.A. The electroencephalogram in advanced senile dementia. *J. Am. Geront. Soc.* 15:5, 415, 1967.

64. Obrist, W.D. Electroencephalography in aging and dementia. In *Alzheimer's Disease: Senile Dementia and Related Disorders*, Katzman, R., Terry, R.D., and Brick, K.L. eds. New York: Raven Press, 1978, p. 227.

65. Roberts, M.A.; McGeorge, A.P.; and Caird, F.I. Electroencephalography and computerized tomography in vascular and non-vascular dementia in old age. *J. Neurol. Neurosurg. and Psychiatry* 41:903, 1978.

66. Swain, J. M. Electroencephalographic abnormalities in presenile atrophy. *Neurology* 9:722, 1959.

67. Earnest, M.P.; Heaton, R.K.; Wilkinson, W.E.; and Manke, W.F. Cortical atrophy, ventricular enlargement and intellectual impairment in the aged. *Neurology* 29:1138–1143, 1979.

68. George, A.E.; deLeon, M.J.; Ferris, S.H.; and Kricheff, I.I. Parenchymal CT correlates of senile dementia (Alzheimer disease): Loss of gray-white matter discriminability. *Am. J. Neuroradiology* 2:205–213, 1981.

69. Huckman, M.S.; Fox, J.; and Topel, J. The validity of criteria for the evaluation of cerebral atrophy by computed tomography. *Radiology* 116:85–92, 1975.

70. Jacoby, R., and Levy, R. CT scanning and the investigation of dementia: A review. *J. Royal Society* 73:366–369, 1980.

71. Jacoby, R.; Levy, R.; and Dawson, J.M. Computed tomography in the elderly: I. The normal population. *Br. J. Psychiatry* 136:249–255, 1980.

72. Jacoby, R., and Levy, R. Computed tomography in the elderly: II. Senile dementia: Diagnosis and functional impairment. *Br. J. Psychiatry* 136:256–269, 1980.

73. Jarvik, L.F.; Ruth, V.; and Matsuyama, S.S. Organic brain syndrome and aging. A six year follow-up of surviving twins. *Arch. Gen. Psychiatry* 37:280, 1980.

74. Naeser, M.A.; Gebhardt, C.; and Levine, H.L. Decreased computerized tomography numbers in patients with presenile dementia. *Arch. Neurol.* 37:401–409, 1980.

75. Naritomi, H.; Meyer, J.S.; Sakai, F.; Yamaguchi, F.; and Shaw, T. Effects of advancing age on regional cerebral blood flow. *Arch. Neurol.* 36:410–416, 1979.

76. Obrist, W.D. Cerebral circulatory changes in normal aging and dementia. Bayer-Symposium VII. Brain functions in old age. Hoffmeister, F. and Muller, C., eds. Berlin: Springer-Verlag, 1979, pp. 278-287.

77. Smith, C.B.; Goochee, C.; Rapoport, S.I.; and Sokoloff, L. Effects of aging on local rates of cerebral glucose utilization in the rat. *Brain* 103:351–365, 1980.

78. Bodis-Woolner, T., and Yahr, M. Measurements of visual evoked potentials in Parkinson's disease. *Brain* 101:661, 1978.

79. Celesia, C.G., and Daly, R.F. Effects of aging on visual evoked responses. *Arch. Neurol.* 34:403, 1977.

80. Blessed, G.; Tomlinson, B.E.; and Roth, M. The association between quantitative measurements of dementia and of senile changes in the cerebral gray matter of elderly subjects. *Br. J. Psychiatry* 114:797, 1968.

81. Crapper, D.R.; Krishnan, S.S.; and Dalton, A.J. Brain aluminum distribution in Alzheimer's disease and experimental neurofibrillary degeneration. *Science* 180:511, 1973.

82. McDermott, J.R.; Smith, I.A.; Iqbal, K.; and Wisnicwski, H.M. Brain aluminum in aging and Alzheimer's disease. *Neurology* 29:809–814, 1979.

83. Markesbery, W.R.; Ehmann, W.D.; and Houssain, T.I.M. Brain trace element levels in Alzheimer's disease by instrumental neutron activation analysis. *J. Neuropathol. Exp. Neurol.* 40:359, 1981.

84. Simchowicz, T. Histopathologische Studien über die senile demenz. In *Histologie und histopathologische Arbeiten über die Grosshirnrinde*, vol. 4, Nissl, F., and Alzheimer, A., eds. Jena, Germany: Fisher, 1911, p. 267.
85. Hirano, A.; Dembitzer, H.M.; and Kurland, L.T. The fine structure of some intraganglionic alterations. Neurofibrillary tangles, ganulo-vascular bodies and "rod-like" structures as seen in Guam amyotrophic lateral sclerosis and Parkinsonism-dementia complex. *J. Neuropathol. Exp. Neurol.* 27:167, 1968.
86. Coyle, J.T.; Price, D.T.; and DeLong, M.R. Alzheimer's disease: A disorder of cortical cholinergic innervation. *Science* 219:1184–1189, 1983.
87. Bowen, D.M., and Davison, A.N. Biochemical changes in the normal aging brain and in dementia. *Psych Med* 10:315–321, 1980.
88. Davies, P. Neurotransmitter-related enzymes in senile dementia of the Alzheimer type. *Brain Res.* 171:319, 1979.
89. Rossor, M.N. Neurotransmitters and CNS disease. *Lancet* 2:1200–1204, 1982.
90. Bowen, D.M.; Smith, C.B.; White, P.; and Davison, A.N. Neurotransmitter-related enzymes and indices of hypoxia in senile dementia and other abiotrophies. *Brain* 99:459–496, 1976.
91. Perry, E.K.; Perry, R.H.; Blessed, G.; and Tomlinson, B.E. Necropsy evidence of central cholinergic deficits in senile dementia. *Lancet* 1:189, 1977.
92. Bowen, D.M.; Spillane, J.A.; and Curzon, G. Accelerated aging or selective neuronal loss as an important cause of dementia. *Lancet* 1:11–14, 1979.
93. Spillane, J.A.; White, P.; and Goodhardt, M.J. Selective vulnerability of neurones in organic dementia. *Nature* 266:558–559, 1977.
94. Sims, N.R.; Bowen, D.M.; and Smith, C.C.T. Glucose metabolism and acetylcholine synthesis in relation to neuronal activity in Alzheimer's disease. *Lancet* 1:333–335, 1980.
95. Mesulam, M.M., and Van Hoesen, G.W. Acetylcholinesterase-rich projections from the basal forebrain of the rhesus monkey to neocortex. *Brain Res.* 109:152–157, 1976.
96. Johnston, M.V.; McKinney, M.; and Coyle, J.T. Neocortical cholinergic innervation: A description of extrinsic and intrinsic components in the rat. *Exp. Brain Res.* 43:159–172, 1981.
97. Davies, P., and Maloney, A.J. Selective loss of central cholinergic neurones in Alzheimer's disease. *Lancet* 2:1403, 1976.
98. Pope, A.; Hess, H.H.; and Lewin, E. Microchemical pathology of the cerebral cortex in presenile dementias. *Trans. Am. Neurol. Assoc.* 89:15, 1965.
99. Davies, P., and Verth, A.H. Regional distribution of muscarinic acetylcholine receptor in normal and Alzheimer's-type dementia brains. *Brain Res.* 138:385–392, 1978.
100. Yates, C.M.; Simpson, J.; and Maloney, A.F.J. Alzheimer's-like cholinergic deficiency in Down's syndrome. *Lancet* 2:979, 1980.
101. Antuono, P.; Sorbi, S.; and Bracco, L. A discrete sampling technique in senile dementia of the Alzheimer type and alcoholic dementia: Study of the cholinergic system. In *Aging of the Brain and Dementia*. Aging series, vol. 13, Amaducci, L., Davison, A.N., and Antuono, P., eds. New York: Raven Press, 1980, p. 151.
102. Nordberg, A.; Adolfsson, R.; and Aquilonius, S.M. Brain enzymes and acetylcholine receptors in dementia of Alzheimer type and chronic alcohol abuse. In *Aging of the Brain and Dementia*. Aging series, vol. 13, Amaducci, L.,

Davison, A.N., and Antuono, P., eds. New York: Raven Press, 1980, p. 169.

103. Mann, D.M.A.; Lincoln, J.; and Yates, P.O. Changes in the monoamine containing neurones of the human CNS in senile dementia. *Br. J. Psychiatry* 136:533, 1980.

104. Tomlinson, B.E.; Irvin, D.; and Blessed, G. Cell loss in the locus coeruleus in senile dementia of the Alzheimer type. *J. Neurol. Sci.* 49:419, 1975.

105. Cross, A.J.; Crow, T.J.; and Perry, E.K. Reduced dopamine-beta-hydroxylase activity in Alzheimer's disease. *Br. Med. J.* 282:93, 1981.

106. Gottfries, C.G. Amine metabolism in normal ageing and in dementia disorders. In *Biochemistry of Dementia*, Roberts, P.J., ed. Chichester: John Wiley & Sons, 1980, p. 213.

107. Crystal, H.A., and Davies, P. Cortical substance P-like immunoreactivity in cases of Alzheimer's disease and senile dementia of the Alzheimer's type. *J. Neurochem.* 38:1781–1784, 1983.

108. Davies, P.; Katzman, R.; and Terry, R.D. Reduced somatostatin-like immunoreactivity in cerebral cortex from cases of Alzheimer disease and Alzheimer senile dementia. *Nature* (London) 288:279, 1980.

109. Davies, P., and Terry, R.D. Cortical somatostatin-like immunoreactivity in cases of Alzheimer's disease and senile dementia of the Alzheimer type. *Neurobiology of Aging* 2:9, 1981.

110. Larsson, T.; Sjogren, T.; and Jacobson, G. Senile dementia. *Acta Psychiatr. Scand.* 39 (suppl. 167):3, 1963.

111. Kallmann, F.J. Genetic aspects of mental disorders in later life. In *Mental Disorders in Later Life*, 2nd ed., Kaplan, O.J., ed. Stanford: Stanford University Press, 1956, p. 26.

112. Stam, F.C., and Op Den Velde, W. Haptoglobin types in Alzheimer's disease and senile dementia. In *Alzheimer's Disease: Senile Dementia and Related Disorders*. Aging series, vol. 7, Katzman, R., Terry, R.D., Bick, K.L., eds. New York: Raven Press, 1978, p. 279.

113. Heston, L.L., and White, J. A family study of Alzheimer's disease and senile dementia: An interim report. *Proceedings of the American Psychopathology Association* 69:63, 1980.

114. Weksler, M.E., and Hutteroth, T.H. Impaired lymphocyte function in aged humans. *J. Clin. Invest.* 53:99–104, 1974.

115. MacKay, I. Aging and immunological function in man. *Gerontologia* 18:285–304, 1972.

116. Hallgren, H.M., and Unis, E.J. Suppressor lymphocytes in young and aged humans. *J. Immunol.* 1118:2004–2008, 1977.

117. Roberts-Thompson,I.C.; Whittingham, S.; Youngchaiyud, U.; and MacKay, T. Aging immune response and mortality. *Lancet* 2:368–370, 1974.

118. Sulkava, R.; Koshimies, S.; and Wikstrom, J. HLA antigens in Alzheimer's disease. *Tissue Antigens* 16:191, 1980.

119. Henschke, P.J.; Bell, D.A.; and Cape, R.D.T. Alzheimer's disease and HLA. *Tissue Antigens* 12:132, 1978.

120. Hodge, S.E., and Walford, R.L. HLA distribution in aged normals. In *Histocompatibility Testing*, 1980, p. 722.

121. Mucuruvo, H.; Ivanyi, P.; Sajdlova, H.; and Trojan, J. HLA antigens in aged persons. *Tissue Antigens* 6:269, 1975.

122. Walford, R.L., and Hodge, S.E. HLA distribution in Alzheimer's disease. In *Histocompatibility Testing*, 1980, p. 727.

123. Wilcox, C.B.; Caspary, E.A.; and Behen, P.O. Histocompatibility antigens in Alzheimer's disease. *Eur. Neurol.* 19:262, 1980.
124. Wisniewski, H.M.; Moretz, R.C.; and Lossinsky, A.S. Evidence for induction of localized amyloid deposits and neuritic plaques by an infectious agent. *Ann. Neurol.* 10:517–522, 1981.
125. Katzman, R. Early detection of senile dementia. *Hospital Practice*, pp. 61–76, June 1981.
126. Liston, E.H. Diagnostic delay in presenile dementia. *J. Clin. Psychiatry* 39:599, 1978.
127. Reisberg, B.; Ferris, S.H.; and Gershon, S. An overview of pharmacologic treatment of cognitive decline in the aged. *Am. J. Psychiatry* 138:593–600, 1981.
128. Muromoto, O.; Sugishita, M.; Sugita, H.; and Toyokura, Y. Effect of physostigmine on constructional and memory tasks in Alzheimer's disease. *Arch. Neurol.* 36:501, 1979.
129. Peters, B.H., and Levin, H.S. Effects of physostigmine and lecithin on memory in Alzheimer's disease. *Ann. Neurol.* 6:219–221, 1979.
130. Thal, L.J.; Fuld, P.A.; Mashv, D.M.; and Sharpless, N.S. Oral physostigmine and lecithin improve memory in Alzheimer's disease. *Ann. Neurol.* 13:491–496, 1983.
131. Cohen, E.L., and Wartman, R.J. Brain acetylcholine: Control by dietary choline. *Science* 191:561–562, 1976.
132. Hirsch, M.J., and Wurtman, R.J. Lecithin consumption elevates acetylcholine concentrations in rat brain and adrenal gland. *Science* 202:223–225, 1978.
133. Corkin, S.; Davis, K.L.; Growdon, J.H.; Usdin, E.; and Wurtman, R. J., eds. *Alzheimer's Disease: A Report of Progress in Research.* Aging, vol. 19. New York: Raven Press, 1982.
134. Davis, K.L.; Mohs, R.C.; and Tinklenberg, J.R. Cholinomimetics and memory: The effect of choline chloride. *Arch. Neurol.* 37:49, 1980.
135. Drachman, D.A., and Leavitt, J. Human memory and the cholinergic system: A relationship to aging. *Arch. Neurol.* 30:113, 1974.
136. Hammer, R.; Berrie, C.P.; Girdsell, N.J.M.; Burgen, A.S.V.; and Hulme, E.C. Pirenzepine distinguishes between different subclasses of muscarinic receptor. *Nature* 283:90–92, 1980.
137. Bartus, R.T.; Dean, R.L.; Beer, B.; and Lippa, A.S. The cholinergic hypothesis of geriatric memory dysfunction. *Science* 217:408–417, 1982.
138. Folstein, M.F., and McHugh, P.R. Dementia syndrome of depression. In *Alzheimer's Disease: Senile Dementia and Related Disorders*, Katzman, R., Terry, R.D., and Bick, K.L., eds. New York: Raven Press, 1978, p. 87.
139. Sternberg, D.E., and Jarvick, M.E. Memory functions in depression. Improvement with antidepressant medication. *Arch. Gen. Psychiatry* 33:219, 1976.
140. Salzman, C. A primer on geriatric psychopharmacology. *Am. J. Psychiatry* 139:67–74, 1982.
141. Thompson, T.L.; Moran, M.G.; and Nies, A.S. Psychotropic drug use in the elderly. *N. Engl. J. Med.* 308:134–138, 194–199, 1983.
142. Barnes, R.; Veith, R.; and Okimoto, J. Efficacy of antipsychotic medications in behaviorally disturbed dementia patients. *Am. J. Psychiatry* 139:1170–1174, 1982.

CHAPTER 8

Chronic Pain

Allan A. Maltbie

Pain is perhaps the most dreaded human life experience. It is the preeminent sensory experience through which the individual judges a disease process to be present. Acute pain serves as a warning and is a characteristic experience of active illness or injury that disappears with recovery of health. Biologically, acute pain provides an alerting mechanism to enhance survival (1). In addition, the sudden onset of acute pain in one person generates an enormous empathic response from others (2). How much does it hurt? is the question often equated with How bad is it? or How serious is the condition? Pain is synonymous with a threat to life.

The situation is quite different with chronic pain where the pain no longer serves a warning function (1). Chronic pain, regardless of etiology, becomes a burden to be borne by the sufferer. Individuals with chronic pain commonly seek out medical assistance with the expectation of relieving their suffering. This chapter considers the problem of chronic pain from a psychiatric perspective. This includes a consideration of the diagnostic approach to the chronic pain patient where the phenomenon of chronic pain is considered from a psychodynamic as well as psychobiologic viewpoint. In addition, a consideration of psychiatric approaches to treatment with an emphasis on the pharmacologic approaches to chronic pain management is discussed.

FORMS OF CHRONIC PAIN

Chronic pain is often divided into two forms. In the first, medical evaluation reveals the presence of a pathological process believed by the physician to be a likely physical source of distress to explain the pain complaints. Since a mechanical nociceptive noxious stimulus can be postulated to account for the perceived discomfort, organic pain is diagnosed. In the second form, medical examination fails to define a pathologic process whereby the painful experiences can be medically explained. Here, functional pain is the diagnosis. Thus, the chronic pain of patients has traditionally been viewed as either organic or functional. Often, after multiple therapeutic interventions have failed to alter apparent chronic organic pain complaints, the diagnostic impression is altered to one of a chronic functional pain syndrome.

This dualistic view of pain as being either real or imagined represents a persistence in modern medical thought of the archaic belief that mind and body are separate and unrelated. In this view, body function is in the purview of medical science, and mind represents a more philosophic concept. While organic pain complaints are seen as entirely physical and hence medically understandable, the functional, or supratentorial pain is not viewed as a real medical disorder but as a disturbance of mind.

The fallacy of this dualistic mind/body separation becomes eminently apparent when one looks at the patient population being considered. The degree of suffering and impaired function often is weakly correlated at best with severity of organic pathology as observed in those patients having clearcut organic findings. Clearly, the complaint of pain involves far more than the simple presence or absence of an external noxious stimulus.

PSYCHOLOGICAL ASPECTS OF CHRONIC PAIN

Freud described pain as being an affective response to injury (4). He considered chronic pain as representing an emotional investment or preoccupation with the pain experience that may be so all consuming that it renders the sufferer incapable of functioning. He hypothesized a similarity between the processes of chronic pain and mourning where for each situation an adjustment to reality is necessitated. With mourning, there is a loss while with pain, there is an injury. In both situations, the reality of these life disruptions may be denied. With time, the reality of loss typically forces the breakdown of denial and subsequent adaptation through the mourning process. However, denial is less threatened with pain as long as treatable active disease is suspected. Consequently, the perpetual search for cure encountered in many chronic pain patients may be understood as an avoidance of the reality of this injured state that is now a part of their lives. This denial interferes with adaptive life adjustments that include acceptance of the painful state and productive coping despite it.

In a classic paper, Rangell (5) observed that the adaptation to chronic pain may be understood as a product of the past psychological development of the individual and the total personality structure. The experience of pain or illness may activate unconscious longings or provoke latent neurotic conflicts. In addition, pain as a perceived experience may become incorporated into a preexisting neurotic or psychotic process. Rangell defined the normal response of a person with pain as the taking of appropriate measures to avoid pain, which includes the ability to tolerate and utilize as warnings small amounts of pain and, second, the capacity to react appropriately in kind and degree to pain that is unavoidable. He discussed patients with psychogenic pain as being those who seem to seek rather than avoid pain as an experience.

He describes possible unconscious motivations for pain-seeking behavior, like masochism where the pain may serve some erotic function or gratify a sense of guilt or a need for punishment.

In another classic article, Engel (6) further elaborated the problem of psychogenic pain through a consideration of the "pain prone patient." He believed that some individuals were inherently vulnerable to chronic pain and listed the following six specific premorbid characteristics he had observed clinically to be frequently present: (1) a prominence of guilt in the personality structure and use of pain to expiate guilt; (2) a childhood history of harsh disciplinary actions regularly used against the patient; (3) problems with the direct expression of anger where a pattern of turning the anger onto the self is observable; (4) the presence of a history of chronic suffering, recurrent defeats, and problems accepting success; (5) the presence of strong conflicts over sexual impulses that, combined with aggressive and guilt feelings, are symbolically expressed through pain; and (6) the presence of conflicts over the loss or potential loss of an individual with whom the patient is close.

PSYCHOGENIC PAIN DISORDER

With the publication of the *DSM-III* (7), the classification "psychogenic pain disorder" was introduced as a separate category under the category of "somatoform disorders." A characteristic common to all of the somatoform disorders is the presence of physical symptomatology suggesting physical disorder but where no organic findings or known pathophysiologic mechanisms are available to account for the perceived symptoms. In addition, the symptoms must not be under voluntary control, and psychological mechanisms are believed to play a prominent role in the development of the symptoms.

Prior to the publication of the *DSM-III*, conversion disorder and psychogenic pain disorder had not been separated as different diagnostic entities. In fact, chronic pain in the absence of demonstrable physical pathology that seemed to serve a psychological defensive function was diagnosed as conversion. Consequently, much of the literature regarding conversion phenomena includes this population of patients, making no distinction between psychogenic pain and conversion.

Bishop and Torch (8) reported a retrospective study in 1979 designed to contrast the categories of conversion disorder versus psychogenic pain disorder (psychalgia). The authors reviewed 285 charts where diagnoses of hysterical conversion had been made and where organic factors had been reasonably ruled out. For comparison, they identified a control group of 94 random cases having *DSM-III* neurotic diagnoses other than conversion or psychogenic pain. They attempted to rediagnose the 285 patients by *DSM-III* standards. They classified patients as definite conversion or psychogenic pain when they met all the standards of *DSM-III* and as probable cases where three or more of the *DSM-III* criteria were met. From the 285, 63 definite and 28 probable conversion disorders were identified, while 9 definite and 71 probable psychogenic pain disorders were found. Cases meeting criteria for both disorders were excluded. Each of the subgroups plus the controls was then compared by a variety of demographic and clinical variables.

No significant differences between the definite and probable groups of each category were identified, and no significant differences were found to discriminate patients with psychogenic pain disorder from those with conversion disorder. This finding was in contrast to the control group that varied significantly from both the conversion and pain groups on five specific variables: (1) symptoms possessing a psychological defensive function, (2) symptoms possessing conflictual content, (3) evident secondary gains, (4) positive history of trauma preceding the symptom onset, and (5) past history of conversion phenomenon. These findings would suggest that the division of conversion disorder and psychogenic pain disorder into two separate diagnostic entities as defined in *DSM-III* may be artificial.

DSM-III criteria needed to make the diagnosis of psychogenic pain disorder differ essentially in the predominant complaint: pain versus a wide variety of alteration or loss in physical function. Table 8.1 contrasts the diagnostic criteria by *DSM-III* for these two conditions.

CONVERSION AND PSYCHOGENIC PAIN

Conversion, a term originally introduced by Freud, defines a psychic mechanism whereby an unconscious impulse or wish is kept from consciousness through the development of a physical symptom suggesting illness. Through this mechanism, a forbidden unconscious impulse is prevented from expression by the process of being converted to a relatively less threatening physical complaint. Thus, the sudden appearance of a physical symptom avoids the conscious realization or expression of an aggressive or sexual impulse. Often the symptom may have symbolic significance to the underlying conflict—e.g., a pain in the neck suddenly appearing during a visit from a demanding mother-in-law. Such a defensive function is usually referred to as "primary gain" where, through the conversion symptom, the unconscious conflict is kept from conscious awareness.

Conversional symptoms including psychogenic pain often appear suddenly in affectively charged situations. Here, the primary gain is usually apparent, with the disabling effects of the symptom preventing the recognition or expression of the conflicted impulses. Often with an apparent serious and sudden state of physical distress, the person suffering the disorder seems strikingly unconcerned. This lack of concern has been referred to as "la belle indifférence." Such an indifferent attitude is clearly in marked contrast with the apparent catastrophic medical situation, but from a psychodynamic perspective it is easily understandable in terms of the defensive relief provided

Table 8.1 *DSM-III* Diagnostic Criteria for Conversion and Psychogenic Pain Disorders

Criterion	Psychogenic Pain Disorder	Conversion Disorder
Predominant disturbance	Pain as symptom complaint	Loss or alteration in physical function
Organic medical findings	Pain not medically explained either by physical disorder or pathophysiologic mechanism. When organic findings present, severity of pain complaint far in excess of observed pathology	Symptom not medically explained either by physical disorder or pathophysiologic mechanism. No organic findings present.
Judged voluntary or involuntary	Involuntary (unconscious)	Involuntary (unconscious)
Qualifiers	At least one of the following judged to be etiologically involved: Presence of a temporal relationship between an affectively charged conflictual event and the onset or exacerbation of the pain; Pain enables individual to avoid some noxious activity; Pain enables individual to get support from the environment	At least one of the following judged to be etiologically involved: Presence of a temporal relationship between an affectively charged conflictual event and the onset or exacerbation of the symptom; Symptom enables individual to avoid some noxious activity; Symptom enables individual to get support from the environment
Exclusions	Not due to somatization disorder or other mental disorder.	Not due to somatization disorder or other mental disorder; Not limited to pain or disturbance in sexual function.

by the conversion phenomenon, the primary gain. Many conversion symptoms are relatively transient in nature, serving a defensive primary gain and remitting once the stressful situation has passed.

In contrast to the acute conversional symptoms, chronic conversion may persist for months, years, or even a lifetime. Chronic conversional symptoms would be more commonly encountered by practicing physicians in the pain clinic and are understood somewhat differently than those mentioned earlier. With chronic conversion, the afflicted individual may seem severely disabled and distressed by the symptom. In this situation, the primary gain is of much less significance in comparison to the alterations in life-style and interpersonal relationships that have resulted from the continued physical disability. The special status of the sick role provides the secondary gain where the perpetuation of the symptom may be rewarded by financial aid, as well as through enhanced attention and special treatment from others. As a result, chronic conversional or psychogenic pain symptoms are predominantly centered around secondary gain factors. The resultant psychological regression with increased dependence is justified by the physical complaint. Consequently, the chronic pain or conversion symptom becomes a necessary condition for the maintenance of the secondary gain and, as such, is incorporated in the personality structure essentially as a maladaptive life-style.

Since the 1960s, numerous investigators have attempted to define and characterize the conversion phenomenon better through various retrospective and follow-up study designs. These studies have helped define the nature of patients presenting with conversion symptomatology, as well as to characterize the differential diagnostic problems and diagnostic mistakes often made with this difficult and complex population.

Organic Disease

Perhaps the single most disturbing finding in the literature is the high incidence observed of organic disease initially misdiagnosed as hysterical (11,12,13,14,15,16,17,18). Reports of incidence range from a low of 14 percent to a high of 56 percent of patients initially misdiagnosed as suffering from conversion disorders where organic diseases later were correctly diagnosed. These data are particularly worrisome since the diagnosis of conversion or psychogenic pain may be associated with a later presumption that physical complaints in such a patient are most likely hysterical and deserve only cursory assessment. Thus, there may be a hazard of a cry-wolf reaction on the part of the physician caring for the patient who is presumed to have psychogenic symptomatology.

Another related and common clinical observation is that of psychogenic or conversional overlay complicating the presentation of organic medical disorders. Slater and Glighero (16), in a ten-year follow-up of seventy-three patients initially diagnosed as having hysterical conversion, reported that 26 percent of the original number had demonstrable hysterical overlay superimposed upon clear organic pathology. An additional 30 percent were found to be truly organic. The phenomenon of overlay often serves to confuse the medical data base. One must always consider the possibility that a combination of organic pathology with psychogenic symptomatology may be present. The positive demonstration of an organic disease or a psychogenic symptom does not rule out the possible coexistence of the other. The physician is often confronted by patients with known organic disease whose complaints are exaggerated far out of proportion to the observed pathology or are not in keeping with known pathophysiologic mechanisms. For such patients, a reasonable suspicion would be that a superimposed conversional process is serving a psychological defensive function, utilizing the existing organic disorder as a symptom model.

Depression

Another frequent observation in this series of studies is the occurrence of clinical depression among patients diagnosed as having psychogenic pain or conversional disorders (10,11,12,16). The reported incidence of overt depressive disorder in this population ranged from a low of 12 percent to a high of 30 percent. Two studies (11,12) described additional covert depression, resulting in a combined incidence of depressive illness of 50 percent in one study and 57 percent in the other. This interesting correlation between depressive disorder and chronic conversion or psychogenic pain disorder is particularly noteworthy and is addressed later in the chapter.

Schizophrenia

While far less common than depression, diagnoses of schizophrenia presenting initially with conversional or psychogenic symptomatology were also observed (10,12,16). In these reports, 3 to 14 percent of patients initially diagnosed as conversional were later found to be schizophrenic. Here, the psychogenic symptom is thought to provide a last desperate defensive effort to ward off the psychotic process. Clinically, additional diagnostic evidence and support of a primary diagnosis of schizophrenia should be present. Various pain complaints or hypochondriacal preoccupations are often observed early in the course of schizophrenia, and at times, somatic delusions may be the primary presenting symptom (19). Typically, the complaints are sufficiently bizarre to be clearly a product of psychosis, but occasionally only after careful questioning will the delusional quality of the complaint emerge. The sodium amytal interview has been reported as a helpful diagnostic tool when underlying schizophrenic pathology is suspected (20).

Acute versus Chronic Forms of Presentation

Another important feature of conversion disorders appears to be the distinction between acute and chronic forms of clinical presentation (12,15,16,21,22). The data suggest that these may be two distinct populations with quite different characteristics (Table 8.2).

Patients presenting with an acute conversion or psychogenic pain symptom would predictably give a recent history of a precipitating affectively charged stressful event. Likewise, the predominance of primary gain through the psychological defensive use of the symptom would be expected. If the primary gain is defensively effective, la belle indifférence would be likely. Where the defense is less effective, symptomatic anxiety would be likely. Typically, a past history of conversion symptoms will be unlikely, and the

Table 8.2 Acute and Chronic Forms of Conversion or Psychogenic Pain Disorders

Acute	*Chronic*
Onset recent	Onset distant
Precipitating stressful event apparent and affectively charged	Precipitating event not apparent or vague and lacks affect
Primary gain predominant where conversion symptom serves a clear defensive function	Secondary gain predominant where conversion symptom serves as necessary requirement of sick role
La belle indifférence more likely if conversion defense effective; anxiety if defense not effective	La belle indifférence not apparent as secondary gain requires a focus on the conversion symptom as disabling
Anxiety is predominant affect; symptom may be warding off a psychotic decompensation	Depression is predominant affect; secondary depression features are common
Single conversion symptom common	Multiple conversion symptoms likely, simultaneously or in sequence
Acute form not specific to any personality type or mental disorder	High incidence of occurrence with somatization disorder (Briquet's syndrome) or other dependent personality disorder
Prognosis usually good for spontaneous lasting recovery and for complete recovery with treatment if other major mental disorder is not present	Prognosis usually poor for spontaneous lasting recovery and for complete recovery with treatment

premorbid personality makeup could include a full spectrum of personality types or possible mental disorders. Prognostically, this population fares well with a high incidence of spontaneous recovery, as well as a favorable treatment response, providing that other major mental disorders are not present. A minority of these patients may persist in their symptoms or develop recurrent symptoms with chronicity.

The second form of conversion disorder and by far the most problematic for the physician is the chronic form. In this situation, symptoms have often been present for months or years often with indistinct data as to the circumstances of symptom onset. Precipitating stressful events are vaguely recalled if at all and lacking in affective intensity. Here, secondary gain is central with the symptoms but a necessary requirement for the perpetuation of the sick-role life adjustment. La belle indifférence would be unlikely since the maintenance of secondary gain requires a view of the symptom as disabling. Self-esteem is maintained through suffering and the repeating unsuccessful pursuit of cure. Since conflicts usually arise around issues of chronic dependence and loss, clinical depression is a common observation. In addition, the history is likely to be positive for multiple conversion or psychogenic symptoms. Finally, a relatively high incidence of major dependent personality disorders would be expected, including the somatization disorder, or Briquet's syndrome. For the chronic conversional patient, prognosis for recovery is poor since the secondary gain reinforces the perpetuation of already established maladaptive character defenses.

Other Somatoform Disorders

In addition to conversion disorder and psychogenic pain disorder, two other specific disorders are classified in the *DSM-III* under the category of "somatoform disorders" (7), both of which may present with pain complaints: hypochondriasis and the somatization disorder.

Hypochondriasis is a disorder characterized by a persistent preoccupation on the part of the patient with the most trivial of somatic sensations that the sufferer misinterprets as evidence of a major disease process. Consequently, minor aches or twinges, constipation, minor changes in color or odor of urine, alterations in menstrual flow, blemishes in the skin, common viral infections, and the like may be presumed by the patient to be evidence of a serious or potentially fatal illness. Despite negative medical workups with thoughtful reassurance from physicians that no evidence exists for serious illness, the patient's belief and conviction that serious illness is present persist. Often the intensity of preoccupation is sufficient to impair social or occupational function significantly.

The term *somatization disorder* was introduced in the *DSM-III* (7) in place of what in the past had been referred to in the literature as hysteria, or Briquet's syndrome. Guze (23,24) and his colleagues in St. Louis have been central in establishing this diagnostic category. They have attempted to refine diagnostic validity and specificity for what had been called hysteria in an effort to enhance the quality and reliability of epidemiologic and psychobiologic studies of the syndrome. Some of their findings have suggested that somatization disorder (Briquet's syndrome) and sociopathy may have a common familial origin and seem to share a possible association to childhood hyperactive syndromes and various forms of delinquency. They have suggested that the primary adult syndrome presentation in women is one of somatization disorder, while sociopathic behavior predominates in the male adult.

DSM-III (7) defines the predominant disturbance in somatization disorder as a clear history of multiple physical symptoms or somatic preoccupations that has been present for several years with initial onset prior to the age of thirty. No clear medical explanation can be found to account for the complaints that, in the opinion of the physician, are not under voluntary control. To be significant, each symptom must have been of sufficient severity to result in the utilization of medication, consultation of a physician, or alteration in life pattern. A lengthy checklist of thirty-seven possible somatic complaints has been developed in which at least fourteen must be positive for a female patient and twelve for a male patient to satisfy requirements for the diagnosis. By category, these complaints are divided into the following: a history of being chronically sickly, twelve possible pseudoneurologic complaints, six gastrointestinal complaints, five female reproductive complaints, three psychosexual complaints, four cardiopulmonary complaints, and six pain complaints. Pain complaints specifically noted are pain in the back, joints, extremities, genitals, on urination, and any other pain not explainable medically.

DIAGNOSTIC APPROACH

In a previous publication, the author and his colleagues (3) suggested a diagnostic approach to the patient with chronic pain that incorporated three specific levels of clinical focus, each having diagnostic and therapeutic utility. The first level was that of the peripheral noxious stimulus serving to generate unpleasant afferent sensory input. The next level of pain integration was that of affective pain experience. Here, with persistent unrelenting painful perception unrelieved by efforts to extinguish the pain, a gradually escalating state of distress and dread may result. Moreover, continual pain may interfere with sleep, serving further to impede adaptive abilities and to contribute to progressive feelings of helplessness. In addition, past morbid memories of loss, previous pain experience in self or others, and preoccupation with serious illness or death may contribute to the development of vegetative biological depression. The final level of pain integration is that of coping behavior or pain adaptation. Here, a qualitative determination of the life adaptation made to the reality of pain is the focus. The maintenance of self-esteem, appropriate independent function, and effective interpersonal relationships reflect this adaptation, despite the presence of pain. Excellent indicators of pain adaptation include work, quality of family and sexual relationships, and social pursuits. Of considerable importance is a premorbid evaluation of coping skills in an effort to establish baseline function. Where prepain adaptation was marginal, postpain adaptation would be expected to be poor. Likewise, with secondary gain and conflicted dependence factors reinforcing pain behavior, chronic maladaptive life adjustments are common. Essential to this model is the recognition that the patient experiencing chronic pain may or may not demonstrate pathologic findings at one or more of the levels of pain integration and may or may not benefit from treatment interventions at any one of these levels. The following case report is illustrative:

A forty-two-year-old married white man presented for evaluation of chronic pain with a history of suffering massive crush injuries two years previously in an on-the-job accident in which several tons of lumber fell on him, pinning him to the ground and crushing his pelvis, right arm, and leg. Emergency management included the amputation below the knee of his right leg, massive transfusion, and apparent cardiopulmonary resuscitation. Surgical reconstruction of his right arm and physical rehabilitation after healing of his pelvic fractures followed. He was fitted with a prosthesis. When he sought care at the pain clinic, the only medication provided was acetaminophen, which he used occasionally. He regularly attended outpatient physical therapy, wore a lower back brace, and complained bitterly of chronic pain, particularly involving his lower back with radiation down the right leg to the stump. Psychiatric evaluation revealed a somewhat agitated, depressed appearing, occasionally tearful man. Marked sleep impairment associated with a history of a fifty-pound weight loss over the previous eight months and a loss of sexual interest and potency were attributed by the patient to pain. He also reported continual preoccupation with the injury including intense fantasies of his trauma during the day, as well as recurrent nightmares of the event at night. Since the injury he had not worked and had entirely withdrawn from social activities, spending the majority of his day in bed. He admitted to suicidal ideation "if the pain does not stop." While uneducated, he had been a conscientious, productive father and husband. For pleasure, he had enjoyed hunting and fishing with friends and family. He had not attempted to fish or hunt since his injury, despite many offers from friends, due to fear of falling and further hurting himself.

This case history illustrates the variety and complexity of pathology often encountered. Orthopedic consultation determined that this man's prosthesis was a quarter-inch too long and that, by shortening the prosthesis to the appropriate length, some of the strain on his lower back would be lessened. His pelvis and lumbosacral spine were determined to be stable, and a vigorous physical therapy program was advised. He was placed on doxepin with escalating nightly doses to antidepressant levels. He reported an almost immediate sleep response and great delight that his nightmares were no longer a problem. Over the course of hospitalization, his energy level dramatically improved as did his appetite and interests in activities with friends. Physical strength and walking ability dramatically improved. He was actively involved in a daily biofeedback program and ongoing behavior-oriented group treatment designed to enhance pain management skills. He was also seen daily by his attending psychiatrist and a psychiatric resident for supportive psychotherapy, as well as being actively involved in an integrated nursing program designed to enhance coping skills and pain management. He spent eighteen days in the hospital with outpatient pain clinic follow-up initially at monthly intervals. An interesting point is that, at time of admission, a dexamethasone suppression test was nonsuppressant.

This case illustrates the complexity of chronic pain and the usefulness of considering such a problem from the multiple levels noted previously. Clearly, the different disciplines mentioned approached this patient from one or more of the levels, applying their various diagnostic and therapeutic skills in an integrated effort designed to lessen afferent inputs, to alter the clinically depressed affective state, and/or to enhance specific coping skills through various techniques.

DEPRESSION AND PAIN

While the interrelationship between chronic pain and depression has long been recognized clinically, only in recent years have investigators initiated controlled studies of the relationship. Clinical observations and anecdotal reports in the literature of the late 1960s and early 1970s reported on the usefulness of psychotropic drugs in the treatment of chronic pain, particularly the tricyclic antidepressants (25,26,27,28). With this new application of psychotropic drugs, more and more psychiatrists have become involved in the evaluation of chronic pain patients. Studies have evaluated the frequency of depressive disorders in patients presenting with chronic pain syndromes, as well as the frequency of occurrence of chronic pain syndromes in patients presenting with complaints of depression. The following studies are illustrative.

Ward and associates (29) reported in 1979 the results of a study designed to determine the frequency of occurrence and response to antidepressant treatment of chronic pain in individuals identified as having depressive disorder. They utilized a creative design through the use of a local newspaper advertisement where the Zung scale for depression and anxiety was published and patients meeting criteria for moderate to severe depression and moderate anxiety were invited to respond. Those who answered the ad were then accepted as study subjects only if Hamilton depression ratings and research diagnostic criteria supported a diagnosis of unipolar depression. In this initial study, the authors identified a total of sixteen patients with previously undiagnosed unipolar depression. These sixteen patients were then interviewed to determine the presence or absence of chronic pain, which was defined for the study as pain occurring a minimum of four hours per day, five days per week for at least the previous six months. It is interesting that, while depression was the only patient selection criterion, all sixteen patients met the criteria for chronic pain as well. The most common complaints were headache and back pain. A consistent observation was that the course of the pain symptoms paralleled the course of the depressive illness. The treatment phase of the study included a single-blind one-week course of placebo followed by increasing doses of doxepin for an additional month. In contrast to placebo that was ineffective, doxepin was found to have significant analgesic effects that were intimately associated with antidepressant effects. The authors speculated that the high incidence of pain in these sixteen depressed patients might reflect their selection of anxious depressives as a study population. They felt the study confirmed their hypothesis that pain symptoms associated with depression were improved to the extent that the depression improved with treatment. They suggested that pain symptoms might be considered another vegetative sign of depression.

Schaffer and associates (30) published a report in 1980 designed to evaluate the relationship between chronic pain and depression. They studied twenty consecutive chronic pain patients having at least a six-month history of chronic pain. Patients were evaluated for the presence or absence of medical pathology, presence of significant depression, and presence of relatives with depressive spectrum illness. They were compared to a control group of family practice outpatients presenting for routine medical evaluation without active medical illness. The patients' average age was forty-seven, with eleven women and nine men, mean pain duration of six years, and most predominant complaint of lower back pain. Most patients considered themselves totally disabled, and all felt they had underlying problems. Of the twenty patients, thirteen had no significant medical pathology, two had equivocal pathology, and five had definite organic disease. Of the thirteen with medical pathology, seven had definable depression. Only one of the seven in whom organicity was present or suspected met the criterion for depression. The family history evaluation showed that thirteen of the twenty pain patients had positive family histories of depressive spectrum disorder in one or more of their relatives. Six of the seven depressed pain patients without medical pathology had a positive family history of overt depression, while only three of the patients with organic or suspected organic disorder had a positive family history of depressive spectrum disorder. In contrast, two of the twenty control subjects were clinically depressed, and only three of the controls had a positive family history of depressive spectrum disease. The authors felt that their data suggest that chronic pain patients do have a higher frequency of clinical depression, as well as depressive spectrum disorder in their first-degree relatives as compared to controls. They called for more extensive research and noted that while their numbers were small their data seemed to suggest that a substantial proportion of those patients without contributing medical pathology (30 percent) might be suffering from primary affective disorder.

Pilowski and Bassett (30a), in a 1982 report from the British literature, presented a study of 114 patients with chronic pain who were compared with 53 depressed inpatients. They noted that pain patients tended to be older (forty-five versus thirty-eight), and were more likely to be married and to have large families. Pain patients more commonly attributed their problems with activity and sleep to pain and more often reported impaired motor functions. Pain patients were less dysphoric and had a typical illness behavioral profile that suggested a conversion reaction. They added that the salient feature of the chronic pain patient as with the conversion patient was a denial of emotional disturbance and life problems unrelated to their pain. They observed that the depressed patients more commonly recalled stressful life events in the year preceding onset of the illness while pain patients seemed focused on stressful events often of nine to ten years in the past. The authors argued that this discrepancy distinguishes the depressed patients as more acute in their response to stresses, while with chronic pain a pattern of long-standing unresolved distress over many years is more likely. They felt that the two groups could not be considered as identical and that abnormal illness behavior distinguishes chronic pain patients as a group from depressed psychiatric patients. Last, the authors state that use of illness behavior as a means of coping characterizes the chronic pain population.

Blumer and Heilbronn (31), in another 1982 report, present a compelling argument in support of their contention that chronic pain in the absence of major organic pathology represents a variant of depressive disease. For this they suggest the name "pain prone disorder." In support of their argument they note the consistent absence of a definable peripheral noxious stimulus in the majority of chronic pain patients, suggesting that the pain appears to be perpetuated by central mechanisms. They add that no plausible neurologic theory has been proposed to explain this mechanism and argue that chronic pain is essentially a masked depressive state. They cite their data on 900 patients with chronic pain whom they have seen for evaluation over several years. Of their patients, they report 1.7 women per man, a mean age of pain onset at 39 years, typical duration of pain of 6.5 years at evaluation, twelfth grade average education, and greatest prevalence in the lower middle socioeconomic class (blue-collar workers). They listed the clinical features of the pain prone disorder as the following:

• A somatic focus of complaints exists where pain is usually perceived as continuous in nature. Despite repeated negative examinations, a persistence of hypochondriacal preoccupations and a frequent desire for surgical treatment are common.

• A distortion in self-image is typical, with massive denial of conflicts coupled with idealization of self (the solid citizen) and family relationships. A history of excessive work (workaholic), often beginning in childhood or adolescence, is frequent.

- The presence of depression is a consistent finding characterized by little energy and inactivity in striking contrast to the overactivity preceding pain onset. Anhedonia with an inability to enjoy social activities, leisure, and sexual relationships is frequent. Insomnia, depressive mood, and despair are also common, but appetite is usually well maintained. Characteristically, all of these symptoms are attributed to pain with massive denial of depression.

- Common historical findings include frequent family and personal history of depression and alcoholism. Past abuse, often at the hands of a former spouse, is common as is the history of having a crippled relative and a relative with chronic pain.

The authors contrast 129 chronic pain patients meeting the pain prone disorder criteria with 36 rheumatoid arthritics. The two groups differed significantly in several distinct areas. First, the nature of pain varied, with the chronic pain presenting as sudden onset of continuous pain, often following mild trauma, in contrast to the gradual onset of intermittent arthritic pain without trauma. Second, depressive traits were consistently and significantly more prevalent in the chronic pain patients—particularly, diminished sleep and anhedonia. Third, chronic pain patients showed a significant prevalence of past physical abuse often from a former spouse, a higher incidence of crippled relatives, and a frequent family history of manifest episodic depression or a personal history of depression. None of these findings is common to the arthritic group. The authors argue that the pain prone disorder represents a specific syndrome: a variant of depressive disease that is a distinct entity when compared with a group of patients with well-defined somatic disease (rheumatoid arthritis). They note that the chronicity of the disorder may be related in part to the practice of continued costly and futile physical procedures aimed at correcting a "phantom peripheral source of pain." They argue that clinical recognition of this disorder should greatly enhance early identification and more effective treatment.

To summarize, it seems apparent that the relationship between pain and depression is becoming progressively more focused as an area of psychiatric interest. The frequency of painful disorders presenting in patients with clinical depression is one area of inquiry, the study of which can better define the interplay between affective disorder and painful experience. Depressed patients with chronic pain, however, should in no way be considered as synonymous with chronic pain patients, and caution must be used in making comparisons between these two populations. The question of whether chronic pain is a clinical presentation of masked depression is compelling. Likewise, the suggestion of a characterologically vulnerable population deserves further study. Perhaps a common vulnerable population susceptible both to chronic maladaptive sick-role behavior and depressive illness is the case. Clearly, much is to be learned from further studies.

TREATMENT

As is already apparent, chronic pain is a complex problem and, as such, involves complex treatment considerations. The expertise of a wide variety of medical specialists including neurosurgeons, anesthesiologists, orthopedic surgeons, internists, rheumatologists, neurologists, and others may be actively involved in the effort to manage the chronic pain patient. Modern interdisciplinary treatment of chronic pain is in large part a result of the influence of John Bonica (1), an anesthesiologist at Seattle best thought of as the father of modern chronic pain treatment.

We would hope the psychiatrist will become more directly involved in early evaluation and treatment of chronic pain disorders. While treatment considerations for chronic pain are diffuse, those applicable to the psychiatrist are most typically treatments already being utilized by the psychiatrist in other settings that now are being discovered to be effective in the chronic pain population.

Tricyclic Antidepressants

In 1967, Dalessio (25) suggested that tricyclics might be effective in the treatment of pain syndromes. Mersky and Hessler (26), in 1972, reported a clinical trial involving thirty chronic pain patients where the combination of a phenothiazine, a tricyclic antidepressant, and an antihistamine afforded moderately good pain relief. The following year Taub and Collins (27) suggested the still popular combination of fluphenazine and amitriptyline for the pain of denervation dyssthesia. They reported that thirty-four of thirty-nine patients showed significant benefit, particularly those with postherpetic neuralgia. Double-blind studies showed the efficacy of tricyclics in the management of chronic tension headache (32,33) and migraine headache (34). Additional reports noted the usefulness of tricyclics in specialized settings such as with rheumatoid arthritic pain (35,36,37) and chronic cancer pain (38,39). Singh and Verma (40) reported in the Indian literature that imipramine and amitriptyline were equally effective and clearly superior when compared to chlordiazepoxide in the treatment of patients with chronic intractable pain.

The use of tricyclic antidepressants is now common in pain clinics around the country. While the literature is mixed regarding the choice of antidepressant, antidepressants that are more active in blocking reuptake of serotonin are believed to be more efficacious (29,41,42,43,44). These authors present considerable data supporting the notion that a depletion or perhaps decreased activity of brain serotonin may serve as a common mechanism accounting for both increased pain experience and depressive symptomatology in chronic pain patients. In addition, evidence of a possible interaction between opiates and tricyclics has been suggested (42,43).

The enkephalins and endorphins are naturally occurring opiatelike substances that function as neurotransmitters active at the morphine receptors (43,44). Studies have demonstrated the range of endorphin-mediated analgesic effects. Varied phenomena such as placebo-induced pain relief, acupuncture, and transcutaneous and direct electrical neural stimulation have been linked to endorphin activity (43,44). Such analgesia can be dramatically blocked by the administration of naloxone, a powerful and pharmacologically specific narcotic antagonist. Researchers have shown that serotonin acts to potentiate narcotic analgesia while norepinephrine blocks it (44). Consequently, norepinephrine and serotonin seem to have opposing effects on endorphin-mediated pain regulation in the central nervous system. It has further been observed that increased levels of available dopamine enhance endorphin-mediated analgesia (44). At present, the relationship between serotonin and endorphin analgesia seems most pertinent to the understanding of tricyclic analgesia effects. In addition, serotonin antagonists have been shown to interfere both with opiate- and electrical-stimulation-produced analgesia (44).

Those tricyclics known to block serotonin reuptake and consequently increase systemic serotonin levels would be expected to have analgesic effects. In this country, most of the clinical reports regarding the use of tricyclic antidepressants in chronic pain have referred to either amitriptyline or doxepin, both of which are active serotonergic reuptake blockers (44). Dosage schedules recommended in the earlier literature suggested reasonably small doses of tricyclics but more recent reports (29,31) recommend the use of tricyclics in full antidepressant dose ranges.

Electroconvulsive Therapy (ECT)

ECT has also on occasion been utilized in the treatment of severe chronic pain disorder (45,46,47). In 1957, VonHagen (45) reported eight patients with intractable chronic pain who improved considerably with ECT. Of the eight, six were noted to be depressed. Weinstein et al. (46) reported ten patients selected from a neurologic ward and treated with ECT with no essential change in their perception of pain after they had recovered from the post-ECT confusional syndrome. They felt that ECT was not useful as a treatment method for chronic pain.

Mandel (47) presented a series of six chronic pain patients including one man and five women with a mean age of fifty-four years and without organic substrate for their pain complaints. Five of the six patients had experienced intensified pain complaints with a six- to twenty-four-month history of depressive symptomatology. One was considered psychotically depressed, and all had failed to respond to tricyclic antidepressants. They all met the research criteria for a secondary affective disorder. Unlike those patients reported in the earlier literature where bilateral ECT was utilized, unilateral nondominant ECT was administered. Of the six patients, four responded to ECT with alleviation of depressive symptoms, as well as cessation of chronic pain complaints. Follow-up data acquired at six months for three of the patients and at one year for one substantiated the persistence of pain-free and depression-free functioning. It is interesting that the two nonresponders were the oldest patients in the group (seventy-three and sixty-eight), each with pain duration in excess of twenty years.

Antipsychotics

Antipsychotic agents have been reported to be useful in the management of various pain states. The earlier literature regarding chronic pain often included mixes of antipsychotics with tricyclic antidepressants (26,27,28). Antipsychotics have long been known to potentiate the effects of narcotics. This potentiation is often used clinically in the management of acute pain as, for example, when promethazine is utilized as a potentiator of meperidine. Similar potentiating effects have been effectively used in the management of chronic cancer pain (38). Antipsychotic agents have been shown to possess varying degrees of activity at the opiate receptor (48).

Of clinically available agents, haloperidol seems to possess the most potent analgesic properties as well as narcotic potentiating properties (48,49). To date, however, antipsychotic agents seem useful primarily in the special circumstance of cancer pain or where narcotic treatment is primary. Here, the use of an antipsychotic may enable a reduced narcotic dosage as well as provide a smoother between dose analgesia with improved sleep.

Earlier combined regimens of tricyclics with antipsychotics no longer appear justified for routine chronic pain management. Potential possibility of tardive dyskinesia as a long-term complication of antipsychotics must be weighed in the selection of an antipsychotic for chronic pain management. For the management of cancer pain, tricyclic antidepressants also play a major role (38) and would be utilized clinically prior to the addition of an antipsychotic.

General Principles

Well-established general principles of chronic pain treatment include efforts to avoid narcotic analgesics, efforts to deemphasize pain as a focal topic of preoccupation, and efforts to increase levels of physical activity. Behavior modification techniques and operant conditioning have been well established (31,50,51) as useful in altering maladaptive pain behavior patterns. In addition, efforts toward work rehabilitation, when successful, are often dramatically helpful in enhancing self-esteem with chronic pain patients. Unfortunately, issues of compensation and disability are frequently unavoidable and pose powerful obstacles in the way of recovery to functional work status. Clearly, the direction of psychotherapeutic intervention is one of enhancing self-esteem through independent functioning and deemphasizing secondary gain.

PSYCHOBIOLOGIC MARKERS

It seems clear that growing biologic knowledge in psychiatry will have major impact on the understanding and clarification of mechanisms of pain. For example, Blumer and associates (52) presented a study of twenty consecutive chronic pain patients that examined dexamethasone suppression, as well as REM latency, both thought to be biologic markers for depression. They studied ten male and ten female patients with an average age of forty-five and pain history of 4.3 years. Abnormal REM latency (less than sixty minutes) was demonstrated in eight patients. Also, eight patients demonstrated nonsuppression on the dexamethasone suppression test. Of those patients with reduced REM latency, six were nonsuppressors, while two with normal REM latency were nonsuppressors. Thus, of the twenty patients, ten showed abnormal REM latency and/or dexamethasone nonsuppression. Tricyclic response varied in the two groups where six of the eight nonsuppressors responded to antidepressant treatment while seven of the twelve suppressors did not respond to the antidepressants. Likewise, five of the eight patients with abnormal REM latency responded to treatment, while six of the ten with normal REM latency did not respond. The authors suggest that these data support their argument that pain prone disorder represents a variant of depressive disease.

Finally, Ward and associates (53) presented a report of psychobiologic markers and coexisting pain and depression. In this study, two groups of depressed patients with chronic pain were identified. A nontreatment group of twenty-five was compared to a treatment group of sixteen. Doxepin was the treatment drug. In the treatment group, 87 percent experienced pain relief, and 56 percent of the group experienced complete pain relief. For the nontreatment population, severity of anxiety, severity of depression, and urinary MHPG were found to have significant positive correlation with severity of pain as determined on the McGill pain questionnaire. In the treatment group, doxepin induced pain relief correlated positively with high levels of pretreatment urinary MHPG, high levels of pretreatment anxiety, and with the degree of improvement in depression.

The choice of MHPG as a marker was derived from the work of Goodwin et al. (54), suggesting that most depressions demonstrate low brain turnover of either serotonin or norepinephrine. High levels of urinary MHPG correlate with high levels of available brain norepinephrine, whereas high levels of 5-HIAA in the cerebrospinal fluid correlate with high levels of active brain serotonin. It has been shown that few patients demonstrate low levels of both markers and that when one marker is low, the other marker often tends to be normal or even above normal. Consequently, normal or high levels of urinary MHPG were expected to support the existence of serotonin-depleted depression that was found. The authors present a theory that serotonin inhibits spinal neuronal pain transmission in the paleospinothalamic tract. A serotonin-depleted depression would predictably be associated with spinal serotonin depletion and increased dull burning forms of pain perception. Medications that increase available synaptic serotonin levels would be expected to reverse this situation with both antidepressant and analgesic effects.

These studies are but the beginning of a major revolution in the understanding of mental function. As psychiatry develops progressively sophisticated methods of defining the neurochemistry and neurophysiology of brain function, we will better understand the process of pain as an experience, with increased benefit to patients.

REFERENCES

1. Bonica, J.J. Neurophysiologic and pathologic aspects of acute and chronic pain. *Arch. Surgery* 112:750–761, 1977.
2. Wilson, W.P., and Nashold, B.S., Jr. Pain and emotion. *Postgrad. Med.* 46:183–187, 1970.
3. Maltbie, A.A.; Cavenar, J.O., Jr.; Hammett, E.B.; and Sullivan, J.L. A diagnostic approach to pain. *Psychosomatics* 19:359–366, 1978.
4. Freud, S. Inhibitions, symptoms, and anxiety. In *Complete Psychological Works of Sigmond Freud.* Strachy, J., trans. London: Hogarth Press, 1955, 20:169–172.
5. Rangell, L. Psychiatric aspects of pain. *Psychosomatic Med.* 15:22–37, 1953.
6. Engel, G.L. Psychogenic pain and the pain prone patient. *Am. J. Med.* 26:899–918, 1959.
7. American Psychiatric Association. *Diagnostic and Statistical Manual of Mental Disorders,* 3rd ed. Washington, D.C., 1980.
8. Bishop, E.R., Jr., and Torch, E.M. Dividing "hysteria": A preliminary investigation of conversion disorder and psychalgia. *J. Nerv. Ment. Dis.* 167:348–356, 1979.
9. Chodoff, P., and Lyons, H. Hysteria, hysterical personality, and "hysterical" conversion. *Am. J. Psychiatry* 114:734–740, 1958.
10. Ziegler, F.J.; Imboden, J.B.; and Meyer, E. Contemporary conversion reactions: A clinical study. *Am. J. Psychiatry* 116:901–909, 1960.
11. McKegney, F.P. The incidence and characteristics of patients with conversion reactions: A general hospital consultation service sample. *Am. J. Psychiatry* 124:542–545, 1967.
12. Steffansson, J.G.; Messina, J.A.; and Meyerowitz, S. Hysterical neurosis, conversion type: Clinical and epidemiologic considerations. *Acta Psychiat. Scand.* 53:119–138, 1976.
13. Merskey, H., and Burich, N.A. Hysteria and organic brain disease. *Br. J. Med. Psychology* 48:359–366, 1975.
14. Merskey, H., and Trimble, M. Personality, sexual adjustment, and brain lesions in patients with conversion symptoms. *Am. J. Psychiatry* 136:179–182, 1979.

15. Gatfield, P.D., and Guze, S.B. Prognosis and differential diagnosis of conversion reactions. *Dis. Nerv. System* 23:623–631, 1962.

16. Slater, E.T.O., and Glighero, E. A followup of patients diagnosed as suffering from "hysteria." *J. Psychosom Res.* 9:9–13, 1965.

17. Raskin, M.; Talbott, J.A.; and Meyerson, A.T. Diagnosis of conversion reactions. *JAMA* 197:530–534, 1966.

18. Watson, C.G., and Buranen, C. The frequency and identification of false positive conversion reactions. *J. Nerv. Men. Dis.* 167:243–247, 1979.

19. Engel, G.L. Conversion symptoms. In *Signs and Symptoms of Medical Illness*, McBride, L.M., ed. Philadelphia: J.B. Lippincott Co., 1970, pp. 650–668.

20. Cavenar, J.O., Jr., and Nash, J.L. Narcoanalysis, the forgotten diagnostic aid. *Military Med.* 142:553–555, 1977.

21. Hafeiz, H.B. Hysterical conversion: A prognostic study. *Br. J. Psychiatry* 136:548–551, 1980.

22. Maltbie, A.A. Conversion disorder. In *Signs and Symptoms of Psychiatry*, Cavenar, J.O., Jr., and Brodie, H.K.H., eds. Philadelphia: J.B. Lippincott Co., 1983.

23. Guze, S.B. The validity and significance of the clinical diagnosis of hysteria (Briquet's syndrome). *Am. J. Psychiatry* 132:138–141, 1975.

24. Guze, S.B. The diagnosis of hysteria: What are we trying to do? *Am. J. Psychiatry* 124:491–498, 1967.

25. Dalessio, D.J. Chronic pain syndromes and disordered cortical inhibition: Effects of tricyclic compounds. *Dis. Nerv. System* 28:325–332, 1967.

26. Merskey, H., and Hester, R.A. The treatment of chronic pain with psychotropic drugs. *Postgrad. Med.* 48:584–590, 1972.

27. Taub, A., and Collins, W.F., Jr. Observations on the treatment of denervation dyssthesia with psychotropic drugs: Postherpetic neuralgia, anesthesia dolorosa, peripheral neuropathy. *Adv. Neurol.* 4:309–315, 1974.

28. Kocher, R. Use of psychotropic drugs for the treatment of chronic severe pain. In *Advances in Pain Research and Therapy*, Bonica, J.J., and Albe-Fessard, D., eds. New York: Raven Press, 1976, 1:579–582.

29. Ward, N.G.; Bloom, V.L.; and Friedel, R.O. The effectiveness of tricyclic antidepressants in the treatment of coexisting pain and depression. *Pain* 7:331–341, 1979.

30. Schaffer, C.B.; Donlon, P.T.; and Brittle, R.M. Chronic pain and depression: A clinical and family history survey. *Am. J. Psychiatry* 137:118–120, 1980.

30a. Pilowski, I., and Bassett, D.L. Pain and depression. *Br. J. Psychiatry* 141:30–36, 1982.

31. Blumer, D., and Heilbronn, M. Chronic pain as a variant of depressive disease: The pain prone disorder. *J. Nerv. Ment. Dis.* 170:381–394, 1982.

32. Diamond, S., and Baltes, B.J. Chronic tension headache treated with amitriptyline—A double blind study. *Headache* 11:110–116, 1971.

33. Lance, J.W., and Curran, D.A. Treatment of chronic tension headache. *Lancet* 1:1236–1239, 1964.

34. Gamersall, J.D., and Stuart, A. Amitriptyline in migraine prophylaxis. *J. Neurol. Neurosurg. Psychiatry* 36:684–690, 1973.

35. Gingras, M. A clinical trial of Tofranil in rheumatic pain in general practice. *J. Int. Med. Res.* 4(suppl. 2):41–49, 1976.

36. McDonald, S.W.A. The relief of pain with an antidepressant in arthritis. *Practitioner* 202:802, 1969.

37. Dudley, H.F. The use of psychotropic drugs in rheumatology. *J. International Med. Res.* 4(suppl. 2):15, 1976.
38. Shimm, D.S.; Logue, G.L.; Maltbie, A.A.; and Dugan, S. Medical management of chronic cancer pain. *JAMA* 241:2408–2412, 1979.
39. Gebhardt, K.H.; Beller, J.; and Nisdik, R. *Behandlung des Karzinomschmerzes mit Chlorimipramin (Anafril). Medizinische Klinik* 64:751, 1969.
40. Singh, G., and Verma, H.C. Drug treatment of chronic intractable pain in patients referred to a psychiatry clinic. *J. Indian Med. Assoc.* 56:341–345, 1971.
41. Sternbach, R.A.; Janowsky, D.S.; and Huey, L.Y. Effects of altering brain serotonin activity in chronic pain. In *Proceedings of First International Congress on Pain*, Florence. New York: Raven Press, 1975.
42. Lee, R., and Spencer, P.S.J. Antidepressants and pain: A review of the pharmacological data supporting the use of certain tricyclics in chronic pain. *J. Int. Med. Res.* 5(suppl. 1):146–156, 1977.
43. Fields, H.L. Pain II: New approaches to management. *Ann. Neurol.* 9:101–106, 1981.
44. Hendler, N. The anatomy and psychopharmacology of chronic pain. *J. Clin. Psychiatry* 43:8 (sect. 2), 15–21, 1982.
45. VonHagen, K.O. Chronic intolerable pain—Discussion of its mechanisms and report of eight cases treated with electroshock. *JAMA* 165:773–777, 1957.
46. Weinstein, E.A.; Kahn, R.L.; and Bergman, P.S. Effect of electroconvulsive therapy on intractable pain. *Arch. Neurol. Psychiatry* 81:37–42, 1959.
47. Mandel, M.R. Electroconvulsive therapy for chronic pain associated with depression. *Am. J. Psychiatry* 132:632–636, 1975.
48. Creese, I.; Feinberg, A.P.; and Snyder, S.H. Buterophenone influences on the opiate receptor. *Eur. J. Pharmacol.* 36:231, 1976.
49. Maltbie, A.A.; Cavenar, J.O., Jr.; Sullivan, J.L.; Hammett, E.B.; and Zung, W.W.K. Analgesia and haloperidol: A hypothesis. *J. Clin. Psychiatry* 40:323–326, 1979.
50. Fordyce, W.E. *Behavioral Methods for Chronic Pain and Illness.* St. Louis: C.V. Mosby, 1976.
51. Fordyce, W.E. Learning processes in pain. In *The Psychology of Pain*, Sternbach, R.A., ed. New York: Raven Press, 1978, pp. 49–72.
52. Blumer, D.; Zorick, F.; Heilbronn, M.; and Roth, T. Biological markers for depression and chronic pain. *J. Nerv. Ment. Dis.* 170:425–428, 1982.
53. Ward, N.J.; Bloom, V.L.; Dworkin, S.; Fawcett, J.; Narasimhachari, N.; and Friedel, R.O. Psychobiological markers in coexisting pain and depression: Toward a unified theory. *J. Clin. Psychiatry* 43:8 (sect. 2), 32–39, 1982.
54. Goodwin, F.K.; Cowdry, R.W.; and Webster, M.H. Predictors of drug response in the affective disorders: Toward an integrated approach. In *Psychopharmacology: A Generation of Progress*, Lipton, M.A., DiMascio, A., and Killman, K.E., eds. New York: Raven Press, 1978.

CHAPTER 9

Psychotropic Drug Interactions

William E. Fann,
Wesley M. Pitts,
Manuel Rodriguez-Garcia,
and
Jeanine C. Wheless

Polypharmacy usually refers to the use of more than one drug, taken simultaneously. Serial polypharmacy, however, is also practiced by some clinicians who prescribe one drug after another, often stringing together a parade of psychoactive agents. Problems can arise with serial polypharmacy if drug-free intervals are not allowed because drug interactions can occur even when the drugs are not administered concurrently. For example, metabolites of phenothiazines have been found in patients' urine as long as six months after the drug was discontinued (1), and serious interactions involving MAO inhibitors have been described up to two weeks after the drug was stopped (2). This chapter deals with simultaneous polypharmacy. It is important, however, for clinicians to realize that drug interactions can also occur with serial polypharmacy.

Psychotropic polypharmacy is common. For example, Hemminki (3) reports that 69 percent of new admissions to mental hospitals and outpatient clinics received more than one psychotropic drug, and Fann (4) cites studies that show that 28 to 75 percent of psychiatric patients are treated with more than one psychoactive agent. Swett (5) studied almost 2,600 psychiatric inpatients in six hospitals and discovered that the mean number of drug exposures was 5.1. The numbers of drugs increased with age: patients younger than twenty received 4.2 drugs, whereas those seventy or older were prescribed 7 drugs.

Psychotropic drug usage is not limited to psychiatric patients. At least 10 percent of the American population use medically prescribed psychoactive agents, and psychotropics account for approximately 20 percent of all prescriptions (6). Derogatis et al. (7) report that 51 percent of oncology patients in five major oncology centers were prescribed at least one psychoactive agent, and the overall rate of prescription was two psychotropics per patient per admission. In a survey of all general inpatients of a Boston teaching and referral hospital, 42.8 percent were administered a minimum of one psychotropic medication, with the average patient receiving seven different drugs (8). Thus, psychotropics are widely used and frequently are prescribed in conjunction with other psychoactive compounds and/or medical drugs.

The practice of psychotropic polypharmacy evolved largely from clinical experience rather than from scientifically developed data. Drug combinations reflected physicians' attempts to ameliorate symptoms that did not respond adequately to available drugs used singly (9,10,11,12). Pharmacotherapy typically is initiated with a single medication, and other drugs are subsequently added either to alleviate symptoms for which the first drug is ineffective or to counteract side effects of the first drug. For unremitting symptoms, rather than to increase the initial drug of choice to maximum dosage, physicians frequently add a second drug. The assumption behind this tactic is that smaller doses of two drugs may be more potent therapeutically and less toxic than a high dose of one drug. However, there are no controlled data to support this hypothesis, and combined use of drugs at lower doses may, in fact, result in more side effects (11,12,13). A second fallacy associated with psychiatric polypharmacy is that significantly lower doses of psychotropic drugs are prescribed when used in combination; the tendency, however, is toward prescribing significantly higher doses for combinations of drugs (14).

Sheppard et al. (10) conducted a case history survey of prescription practices among psychiatrists in four states. Despite the fact that the presenting symptoms and course of illness of the hypothetical patient were held constant, diverse treatment preferences were expressed. More than one-third of the sample initiated treatment with a broad array of drug combinations. Of the polypharmacy respondents, 79 percent prescribed two neuroleptics. As the hypothetical patient's condition worsened, the psychiatrists showed less preference for single drug treatment and used more diverse groups of drugs in combination, and the use of so-called maxipharmacy (three or more drugs) emerged. After one year of ineffective pharmacotherapy, combinations of three to six potent neuroleptics were frequently prescribed. Between admission and final stages of treatment, the number of physicians prescribing three or more psychotropics increased elevenfold.

The literature is replete with information on drug interactions, and concern is being expressed about the escalating use of multiple psychotropic drugs. Available data indicate that most combinations are no more effective than single drugs, and scientific evidence supporting the use of drug combinations is lacking (3,11). Merlis et al. (11) report that male (but not female) psychiatric inpatients improved when switched from two psychotropics to two placebos or to one psychotropic and one placebo. Hemminki (3) reviewed fourteen clinical trials on psychotropic polypharmacy and found only three studies indicating that combinations were superior to single drugs or placebo. The author concludes that little evidence from clinical trials defends the frequent use of polypharmacy.

Ayd (13) also has criticized the practice of polypharmacy and demands a more rational approach to drug treatment. Because deleterious drug effects and errors in administration increase in direct proportion to the number of drugs prescribed (13,15), physicians should make every effort to limit the number of drugs used. Unfortunately, many patients require multiple-drug therapy for various medical and psychiatric conditions, and the pejorative connotation of polypharmacy is not always justified (16). With the multiplicity of psychopharmacologic agents now available and the increasing use of poly-pharmacy, the frequency and variety of psychotropic drug interactions are escalating faster than our ability to discover and adequately analyze the causative components. Drug combinations should therefore be viewed as new treatment forms that require research into efficacy, compatibility, dose response factors, side effects, and toxicity (9,10,12). Furthermore, clinicians need to be familiar with pharmacologic principles in order to anticipate and avoid some of the common and serious side effects known to occur during combination drug therapy.

DRUG INTERACTIONS

Although the principles involved in the various drug interactions are simple, drug response is not always predictable. Age, sex, race, and genetic back-ground of the patient can affect drug response (17,18) and disease-diet-drug interplay can modify the results of a drug regimen. Specific adverse drug interactions, however, are well documented. Interactions can occur during absorption, protein binding, metabolism, or excretion; these are called "phar-macokinetic" interactions. In addition, "pharmacodynamic" interactions can occur and include blockade of transport to the site of action of one drug by another and change of drug mediator activity (19,20,21).

Absorption

Gel antacids containing magnesium and aluminum and oral resins interfere with absorption from the gastrointestinal tract of a variety of drugs including antipsychotics and antidepressants. The resulting increase in enzymatic activ-ity lowers blood and tissue levels of the metabolized drug and may result in decreased therapeutic effectiveness. Concomitant administration of an ant-acid and a neuroleptic may reduce efficacy of the antipsychotic by impairing its absorption (15,21,22,23,24). Although the total amount of drug absorbed may not be significantly lessened, the delay in rate of absorption diminishes the amount of drug therapeutically active at any given time (25). Administra-tion of the antacid at least one hour before or two hours after the neuroleptic may avoid the interaction (23).

Cholestyramine, an ion-exchange resin used for treating hypercholesterolemia, also interferes with absorption of psychotropic agents because it binds any drug with an appropriate charge at the pH at which the two coexist in the intestine. Thus, when antacids or oral resins are prescribed, adjustment in dosage of co-administered maintenance therapy is needed (4).

Interaction at the Plasma-Binding Level

Most psychotropic drugs circulating in blood are highly protein bound. When drugs are highly bound, only a small fraction of the circulating compound is free to diffuse to the target receptor site where it exerts its therapeutic effects. Any activity that decreases the plasma binding of the psychotropic may significantly increase the pharmacological actions of the psychotropic. Even small changes in the ratio of bound to free drug may markedly affect its efficacy as well as its potential to cause side effects. For example, only 2 percent of chlorpromazine is reported to be free and pharmacologically active. Displacement of 2 percent of bound chlorpromazine approximately doubles the available drug, doubling the effective dose. Such an interaction has been reported for phenytoin (formerly known as diphenylhydantoin), a drug highly bound to plasma albumin, which can displace other drugs—notably, tricyclic antidepressants and neuroleptics (26,27). Conversely, the psychoactive agent may affect the binding of other compounds like warfarin, thereby altering the pharmacological effects of the second drug.

Altered Metabolism

Hepatic microsomal enzymes responsible for metabolizing drugs can be increased in amount and activity by numerous drugs. The resulting increase in enzymatic activity lowers blood and tissue levels of the metabolized drug (15,28). The barbiturates, and to a lesser extent other sedative-hypnotics and antianxiety agents, are known to stimulate the production and activity of hepatic microsomal enzymes involved in the metabolic degradation of a great many medications (20,29). For example, the barbiturate phenobarbital has been shown to stimulate the metabolism of more than sixty chemicals, including phenothiazines, digitoxin (digitalis), warfarin, and phenytoin (4,19,30). Most anticonvulsants are potent inducers of hepatic microsomal enzymes and enhance metabolism of numerous drugs, including diazepam and nortriptyline (27). Cigarette smoking, chronic ingestion of alcohol, and exposure to chlorinated insecticides such as dicophane (DDT) and lindane can also increase metabolism of other drugs (31).

Through enzyme induction, barbiturates lower plasma warfarin levels. A patient prescribed both drugs simultaneously would require higher doses of anticoagulant to compensate for the increased hepatic activity. Subsequent discontinuation of the barbiturate may result in severe bleeding episodes

(23,28,32,33,34). Patients treated with both a barbiturate and warfarin should have close monitoring of prothrombin times (35).

Although chloral hydrate does not appear to be metabolized by hepatic microsomal enzymes, it can induce the accelerated metabolism of numerous drugs including dicumarol and warfarin and may dangerously lower their therapeutic efficacy (29). Cuinell et al. (36) describe a fatal hemorrhage precipitated by chloral hydrate and bishydroxycoumarin. Sellers at el. (33) report that 1 gram chloral hydrate administered daily for one week increased the hypoprothrombinemic effect of warfarin 40 to 80 percent. For patients on anticoagulant therapy who require a hypnotic, the use of flurazepam is recommended (37).

Hepatic microsomal drug-metabolizing systems are inhibited by tricyclic antidepressants, and the effects of many drugs (propranolol, amphetamine, guanethidine, barbiturates, dicumarol) are prolonged (38,39). For example, tricyclics may impair the metabolism of anticoagulants, raising their serum levels and prolonging their pharmacological half-lives by as much as 300 percent (40). When introducing tricyclics in patients receiving oral anticoagulants, prothrombin levels must be carefully monitored to avoid excessive anticoagulation (41).

Methylphenidate retards liver microsomal metabolism of certain compounds, including anticonvulsants, anticoagulants, antidepressants, and phenothiazines, thereby enhancing blood and tissue levels of the metabolized drug (30,42). Thus, methylphenidate, administered to counteract drug-induced sedation, in reality increases sedation by blocking liver metabolism of the offending drug (4,34). Garretson et al. (30) report that therapeutic doses of methylphenidate inhibit metabolism of antiepileptic agents, raising serum levels such that serum phenytoin reached toxic proportions. Inhibition of the anticoagulant ethyl biscoumatetate by methylphenidate has also been documented (30,43). The dose of anticoagulant and/or anticonvulsant normally should be decreased when methylphenidate is added to the treatment regimen.

Phenothiazines decrease hepatic metabolism and thereby increase plasma levels of propranolol (44) and phenytoin (20). To prevent toxicity, reduced doses are recommended with these combinations.

Cimetidine has been shown to interfere with the metabolism of drugs that are metabolized by hepatic, mixed-function, oxidase systems. Drugs so far demonstrated to undergo this type of hepatic metabolism are antipyrine, warfarin, diazepam, chlordiazepoxide, alprazolam propranolol, theophylline, carbamazepine, phenytoin, and imipramine (93). If normal therapeutic doses of cimetidine are co-administered or administered immediately before intake of any of these drugs, increased serum concentrations result; such an effect is particularly significant for drugs such as phenytoin, warfarin, and theophylline that become toxic if a narrow therapeutic range is exceeded (see also Chapter 1).

A number of drugs interfere with the metabolism of tricyclic antidepressants, altering the steady-state plasma concentration achieved. The effects of barbiturates through enzyme induction on steady-state plasma concentrations are well known (45,46,47). Both chlorpromazine (42,43,48) and antidepressants may be more rapidly metabolized with concomitant use of barbiturates. Conversely, the combined administration of tricyclics and methylphenidate or neuroleptics inhibits metabolism of the antidepressant, increasing plasma concentrations (47,49,50). Alcohol is also an enzyme inducer and appears to interfere with tricyclic metabolism, although this interaction has not been unequivocally established. The deleterious effects, however, of alcohol and tricyclics on psychomotor skills related to driving are well documented, and patients should be warned of this potentially dangerous interaction (47).

Altered Excretion

Lithium carbonate has been demonstrated to be an effective prophylactic agent for the control of bipolar affective disorders. However, lithium has a low therapeutic index, and serious side effects can occur when serum levels exceed the generally accepted safe level of 1.5 to 2 mEq/L. The maintenance of a physiologically normal serum sodium level is of utmost importance in patients treated with lithium. On the one hand, ingestion of large amounts of sodium ion can lead to increased renal clearance of lithium (47). On the other hand, a decrease of serum sodium concentration below normal levels results in selective renal reabsorption of the lithium ion with rapid accumulation of lithium to toxic levels. In patients well controlled on lithium maintenance, the addition of a thiazide diuretic, which produces prompt sodium depletion, can cause the serum lithium to rise by as much as twofold (51), precipitating lithium toxicity (23,52,53,54). In contrast to thiazide diuretics, osmotic diuretics like mannitol increase lithium excretion (41). Accelerated excretion of lithium has also been reported when the compound is used in conjunction with chlorpromazine (55).

A patient maintained on lithium may take a diuretic if the lithium dose is decreased, usually by about half, and if serum lithium levels are carefully monitored. The co-administration of lithium and diuretics is less dangerous when the diuretic is prescribed first. Subsequently, a lower dose of lithium produces a therapeutic serum level (51).

An interaction between lithium and prostaglandin inhibitors has been reported whereby serum lithium levels are elevated by concomitant administration of phenylbutazone or ibuprofen. The mechanism of this effect is thought to be reduced renal clearance of lithium. This is, of course, a potentially serious interaction due to the narrow margin of safety between therapeutic and toxic doses for lithium (56).

An unusual interaction between methyldopa and lithium was described by Byrd (57). The addition of methyldopa was associated with lower serum lithium levels at a higher lithium dose, and signs of lithium toxicity were present. The mechanism of action of the puzzling phenomenon is currently unknown.

Blocked Transport

In 1963, three hypertensive patients treated with guanethidine suffered a loss of blood pressure control when imipramine was added to their treatment regimens (58). Four years later, Mitchell and associates (59) demonstrated in a controlled study tricyclic-induced blockade of the guanethidine effect. The antihypertensive effects of guanethidine and bethanidine appear to depend on their uptake into peripheral nerve terminals via the norepinephrine pump (adrenergic membrane transport system). A number of psychoactive drugs including neuroleptics, tricyclic antidepressants, and sympathomimetic agents also act peripherally to clock synaptic reuptake of norepinephrine and may thereby block synaptic uptake of other drugs transported by the norepinephrine pump. By preventing accumulation of guanethidine and other antihypertensive drugs at their site of action, the hypotensive efficacy of these compounds is reduced or abolished (4,19,23,60,61,62,63,64). In patients whose blood pressure is stabilized on a combination of tricyclic antidepressants or neuroleptics and guanethidine, discontinuation of the tricyclic or neuroleptic can cause significant hypotension—and even hypotensive shock—due to excessive guanethidine action (19,41,65). Conversely, introduction of a tricyclic or neuroleptic in patients on long-term antihypertensive therapy may lead to loss of blood pressure control. The rate of onset of antagonism depends upon the duration of action of the antihypertensive agent. Antagonism may thus occur within several hours with bethanidine but may require several days with guanethidine (41).

Severity of antagonism varies among the psychotropics. Chlorpromazine markedly antagonizes guanethidine. Fann et al. (66) report that the blood pressure of two patients rose to pretreatment levels with the addition of chlorpromazine. Haloperidol and thiothixene have demonstrated lesser effects in blocking the uptake of guanethidine in nerve endings (67). No antagonism of guanethidine has been reported with molindone (68,69), and this may be the neuroleptic of choice for patients who receive concurrent guanethidine for hypertension. The tetracyclic agent mianserin does not appear to interact with the antihypertensive drugs (47,70). If preliminary trials with mianserin are substantiated, mianserin may become the drug of choice in patients on antihypertensive therapy who also require antidepressant medication (41).

The amino acid methyldopa is not transported by the norepinephrine pump, and consequently, its antihypertensive activity is not altered to a clinically significant degree by co-administration of a tricyclic (71,72). Both hypertension and lithium toxicity have been reported with the combined use of methyldopa and lithium, and these medications should not be administered concurrently (57). MAO inhibitors antagonize the antihypertensive effects of guanethidine and methyldopa but potentiate the effects of ganglion-blocking drugs (27). Chouinard et al. (73) report that phenothiazines may potentiate the hypotensive effects of methyldopa; conversely, methyldopa has been reported to augment the effects of haloperidol, leading to toxicity (74,75).

Although the exact pharmacological mechanism is unknown, tricyclic antidepressants have been shown to antagonize the antihypertensive effects of the centrally active agent clonidine (61,62). Briant et al. (62) conducted a double-blind, crossover trial of five hypertensive patients on clonidine. The introduction of desipramine caused an increase of arterial pressure in four patients; in one patient the rise occurred within twenty-four hours, and blood pressure increased to pretreatment levels. Any patient whose blood pressure is controlled with clonidine and who requires therapy for concomitant depression should be carefully monitored if a tricyclic antidepressant is added to the treatment regimen.

Like guanethidine, indirectly acting sympathomimetic amines such as tyramine, phenethylamine, ephedrine, metaraminol, amphetamine, and methylphenidate enter the adrenergic membrane via the norepinephrine pump. Clinical doses of tricyclic antidepressants block the action of these drugs by preventing their synaptic uptake (20,71). If the sympathomimetic has already gained access to the presynaptic neuron, however, the tricyclic alternatively may prolong and potentiate its pharmacologic action by preventing synaptic reuptake of the released sympathomimetic (41). Marked potentiation of the pressor effects of oral and IV tyramine has been demonstrated in patients receiving MAO inhibitors (76).

In contrast to antagonizing the action of indirect acting sympathomimetics, tricyclics have been shown to augment markedly the pressor response of parenteral norepinephrine (four- to eightfold), epinephrine (two- to four-fold), and phenylephrine (two- to threefold) (77). Increased cardiovascular effects occur because the pharmacological effect of tricyclics is to block the reuptake of catecholamines. The result of this interaction may be a hypertensive crisis characterized by sweating, severe headache, hyperthermia, cerebrovascular accident, and even death. In patients taking tricyclics, the dental administration of local anesthetics containing norepinephrine or epinephrine has proved hazardous and even fatal (47,78,79). MAO inhibitors have shown a twofold or greater potentiation of the pressor effect of phenylephrine but no clinically significant potentiation with norepinephrine or epinephrine (77). Therefore, local anesthetics containing norepinephrine or epinephrine should not be hazardous in otherwise healthy patients taking MAO inhibitors. Lithium decreases the pressor effects of infused norepinephrine without significantly altering tyramine sensitivity (80).

Studies suggest that thyroid hormone (L-triiodothyronine, or TSH) potentiates the effects of tricyclic antidepressants, producing a more rapid recovery from depression. A possible explanation for this interaction is that the tricyclic blocks nerve reuptake of norepinephrine while the thyroid hormone enhances catecholamine metabolism or increases receptor sensitivity (43,81,82). Coppen et al. (83), however, in double-blind trials, found no therapeutic effect of TRH administered alone or in combination with amitriptyline. This controversy has not been resolved (also see Chapter 2).

Altered Mediator Activity

A number of dietary substances including certain cheeses, beer, Chianti wine, chicken livers, pickled herring, caviar, yeast extracts, and broad beans have a high content of pressor amines, such as tyramine, that are ordinarily metabolized by MAO enzymes in the liver and intestinal wall. When patients receiving an MAO inhibitor unsuspectingly ingest foods with high tyramine content, however, MAO is inhibited and tyramine accumulates and stimulates the release of norepinephrine from the adrenergic nerve endings. A hypertensive crisis, characterized by precipitous hypertension, throbbing headache, sweating, tachycardia, hyperpyrexia, and sometimes rupture of intracranial vessels and death, may be the result (4,23,34,47,76,81). Although McGilchrist (84) has reported that some dietary precautions have acquired unwarranted and unrealistic importance, it is recommended that patients treated with MAO inhibitors avoid dietary items containing high concentrations of tyramine and other amines. Although tyramine is most notable for causing this interaction, dopamine and tyrosine may also be implicated (27).

MAO inhibitors prevent deamination of catecholamines within the adrenergic neuron. Indirect-acting sympathomimetic amines such as amphetamine and ephedrine can cause the release of large stores of catecholamines. When MAO inhibitors and sympathomimetic agents are administered concurrently, the pharmacologic action of pressor amines is markedly potentiated. Severe headache, hypertension or hypertensive crisis, and cardiac arrhythmias can occur. Most nonprescription cold and allergy medications contain sympathomimetics, and patients treated with MAO inhibitors should be warned against the concurrent use of proprietary drugs that might interact with the inhibitors (4,23,34,43). Ban (19) reports that a patient prescribed an MAO inhibitor suffered a rapid and potentially dangerous increase in blood pressure following the ingestion of an over-the-counter cough medicine containing a small amount of phenylpropanolamine (Propadrine); in contrast, he also describes the successful treatment of severe, therapy-resistant orthostatic hypotension with the combined administration of an MAO inhibitor and cheddar cheese. Although both direct and indirect sympathomimetics have been reported to cause hypertensive crises, direct-acting sympathomimetics do not depend on MAO for metabolic inactivation, and these compounds appear to produce only a mild hypertensive effect when used concomitantly with MAO inhibitors (77). The effects of alcohol, sedative hypnotics, general anesthetics, opiates and phenothiazines have also been reported to be potentiated by MAO inhibitors (85).

PSYCHOTROPIC POLYPHARMACY

Opinions differ on the risks involved in treating depressed patients with combinations of MAO inhibitors and tricyclic antidepressants. Not every patient manifests toxicity when administered an MAO inhibitor and an interacting drug. Depending upon individual susceptibility, dosage, duration of treatment, and other factors, one patient may develop a severe reaction, another only a mild reaction, and another no reaction at all (43).

Some authorities (23,27,34,43), including the FDA, consider the concomitant administration of a tricyclic antidepressant and an MAO inhibitor to be absolutely contraindicated and recommend that at least two weeks elapse after discontinuation of one of these drugs before initiating the other drug. Consequently, coprescription of these drugs has been avoided in the United States due to concern over deleterious reactions. Other investigators, however, suggest that under certain conditions and with due precautions, the use of the combination may be safe and effective in the small percentage of patients in whom adequate trials of a tricyclic or an MAO inhibitor alone have failed (19,86,87,88,89,90). Sethna (88) and Schuckit et al. (89) reviewed the case reports on which this concern with morbidity is based and found no convincing evidence that the tricyclic–MAO inhibitor combination, taken in therapeutic dose and prescribed with caution, was responsible for the side effects reported. Winston (90) concurs, stating that most severe cases reported in the literature were due either to massive overdoses of combined drugs, usually suicide attempts, or to the parenteral administration of imipramine in patients taking MAO inhibitors. He suggests that adverse side effects are directly related to dose and speed of intake and that careful control of these factors may determine the difference between recovery and disaster. In an informal review of 350 outpatients, a record examination of 50 inpatients, and a drug trial with 10 patients, Schuckit et al. (89) found no drug-related morbidity. Athough recognizing the need for further study, these authors conclude that present evidence does not indicate the combined drug regimen to be unsafe.

The coprescription of tricyclics and MAO inhibitors nevertheless remains controversial, and the combination should only be used as a last resort. Extreme caution should be exercised: the patient should be hospitalized, drugs should be oral, small doses and gradual increases of dose should be prescribed, and the use of tranylcypromine, imipramine, and clomipramine should be avoided (see Chapter 2). Also, no data have documented that combinations of antidepressants of the same group are superior to the component drugs used alone (13,19).

Methylphenidate appears to inhibit metabolism of tricyclics and may appreciably increase tricyclic blood levels (43). Seven patients suffering from recurrent refractory psychotic depressive episodes were prescribed combined tricyclics and methylphenidate during a two-week trial. In five patients, striking clinical remission occurred within the trial, and the remaining two patients recovered over a longer period. Thus, methylphenidate may enhance therapeutic effectiveness of tricyclics by markedly increasing blood levels. When the two drugs are administered concurrently, the dose of the tricyclic may need to be decreased (43,91).

Surveys indicate that combinations of a major or minor tranquilizer with an antidepressant comprise between 40 and 50 percent of all polypharmacy regimens (9,92). The most commonly prescribed combination is perphenazine and amitriptyline (10). Phenothiazines and tricyclics are frequently administered in fixed-dose combinations, and although additive anticholinergic effects occur, the risk of serious cholinergic blockade is minor at the fixed doses used (43). While the concurrent use of benzodiazepines and antidepressants has not been found to offer significantly superior therapeutic effects, the combination in some patients may produce mutual enhancement of sedation and anticholinergic side effects. On the one hand, Hansten (43) suggests that adverse interactions between benzodiazepines and antidepressants probably occur in only a small proportion of patients and that any reactions are usually mild. Ban (19), on the other hand, reports that addition of chlordiazepoxide to amitriptyline treatment may intensify rather than ameliorate depressive symptomatology in some patients and that the combination has led to a clinical picture that simulated organic brain damage.

Through enzyme induction, barbiturates increase metabolism of chlorpromazine. During combined use, urinary excretion of chlorpromazine has been reported to be increased (48) while plasma levels have decreased (42). Antipsychotic effects may be diminished, and increased dosage of chlorpromazine may be necessary when the phenothiazine is prescribed concurrently with a barbiturate (43).

No substantial evidence from well-controlled studies indicates that coadministration of antipsychotic medications enhances clinical effectiveness (4,11,13). Combinations of neuroleptics are nevertheless frequently prescribed. In one survey, for example, two neuroleptics comprised one-third of all drug combinations; chlorpromazine and trifluoperazine were the most commonly coprescribed neuroleptics (9). There has been some evidence that addition of nylidrine (Arlidin), a central vasodilator; methyl-p-tyrosine, a tyrosine hydroxylase inhibitor; and methyldopa (Aldomet), a dopa-decarboxylase inhibitor, may potentiate the therapeutic effect of neuroleptics (19).

SUMMARY

Psychotropic polypharmacy developed and continues largely out of clinical experience. Physicians have prescribed combinations of drugs in the hope of alleviating clinical symptoms resistant to single medications. Although some drug combinations are desirable and efficacious, most are of limited usefulness and are potentially hazardous. Drug interactions can occur by changes in absorption, excretion, metabolism, or plasma protein-binding effects as well as by blocked transport and changes in drug mediator activity. Some drug interactions produce clinical responses directly contrary to those intended; consequently, it is vital that physicians understand pharmacologic principles when prescribing more than one drug. Because interactions among most drugs are unknown or only partially known, polypharmacy should be regarded primarily as investigational.

Despite the fact that current evidence indicates that most drug combinations are no more effective than drugs used singly, many physicians continue to prescribe polydrug regimens. The rationale behind this practice is that lower doses of two drugs may be more potent therapeutically and may cause fewer side effects than higher doses of one drug. Surveys of prescribing trends, however, indicate that doses of drugs used in combination tend to be higher than doses of the same drugs used individually. Furthermore, two drugs, even at lower doses, appear to cause more side effects than a higher dose of a single drug. Until further research clarifies possible drug interactions, physicians should limit the number of psychotropic drugs administered simultaneously.

REFERENCES

1. Goodman, L.S., and Gilman, A. *The Pharmacological Basis of Therapeutics*, 5th ed. New York: Macmillan, 1975.
2. *Physicians Desk Reference*, 31st ed. Oradell: Medical Economics Co., 1977.
3. Hemminki, E. Polypharmacy among psychiatric patients. *Acta Psychiatr. Scand.* 56:347–356, 1977.
4. Fann, W.E. Some clinically important interactions of psychotropic drugs. *Southern Med. J.* 66:661–665, 1973.
5. Swett, C. Patterns of drug use in psychiatric inpatient wards. *J. Clin. Psychiat.* 40:464–468, 1979.
6. Parry, H.J.; Balter, M.B.; Mellinger, G.D.; Cisin, I.H.; and Manheimer, D.I. National patterns of psychotherapeutic drug use. *Arch. Gen. Psychiatry* 28:769–783, 1973.
7. Derogatis, L.R.; Feldstein, M.; Morrow, G.; Schmale, A.; Schmitt, M.; Gates, C.; Murawski, B.; Holland, J.; Penman, D.; Melisarato, S.N.; Enelow, A.J.; and Adler, L.M. A survey of psychotropic drug prescription in an oncology population. *Cancer* 44:1919–1929, 1979.
8. Salzman, C. Psychotropic drug use and polypharmacy in a general hospital. *Gen. Hosp. Psychiatry* 3:1–9, 1981.
9. Sheppard, C.; Collins, L.; Fiorentino, D.; Fracchia, J.; and Merlis, S. Polypharmacy in psychiatric treatment: I. Incidence at a state hospital. *Curr. Ther. Res.* 11:765–774, 1969.
10. Sheppard, C.; Beyel, V.; Fracchia, J.; and Merlis, S. Polypharmacy in psychiatry: A multi-state comparison of psychotropic drug combinations. *Dis. Nerv. Sys.* 35:183–188, 1974.
11. Merlis, S.; Sheppard, C.; Collins, L.; and Fiorentino, D. Polypharmacy in psychiatry: Patterns of differential treatment. *Am. J. Psychiatry* 126:1647–1651, 1970.

12. Prien, P.F.; Klett, C.J.; and Caffey, E.M. Polypharmacy in the psychiatric treatment of elderly hospitalized patients: A survey of 12 Veterans Administration hospitals. *Dis. Nerv. Sys.* 37:333–336, 1976.
13. Ayd, F.J. Rational pharmacotherapy: Once-a-day drug dosage. *Dis. Nerv. Sys.* 34:371–378, 1973.
14. Fracchia, J.; Sheppard, C.; Canale, D.; Ruest, E.; Cambria, E.; and Merlis, S. Combination of dosage levels of the same psychotropic drugs, used singly and in combination. *J. Am. Ger. Soc.* 23:508–511, 1975.
15. Robinson, D.S. Pharmacokinetic mechanisms of drug interactions. *Postgrad. Med.* 57:55–62, 1975.
16. Shader, R.I. Problems of polypharmacy in depression. *Dis. Nerv. Sys.* 38:30–34, 1976.
17. Osol, A. *Remington's Pharmaceutical Sciences*, 16th ed. Easton, Pa.: Mack Publishing Co., 1980.
18. Vesell, E.S. Pharmacogenetics. In *Drug Therapy from The New England Journal of Medicine*, Koch-Weser, J., ed. Boston: Mass. Medical Society, 1976.
19. Ban, T.A. Drug interactions with psychoactive drugs. *Dis. Nerv. Sys.* 36:164–166, 1975.
20. Gualtieri, C.T., and Powell, S.F. Psychoactive drug interactions. *J. Clin. Psychiatry* 39:720–729, 1978.
21. Fann, W.E.; Davis, J.M.; Janowsky, D.S.; and Schmidt, D. The effect of antacids on blood levels of chlorpromazine. *Clin. Pharmacol. Ther.* 14:135, 1973.
22. Fann, W.E.; Davis, J.M.; Janowsky, D.S.; and Schmidt, D. Chlorpromazine: Effects of antacids on its gastro-intestinal absorption. *J. Clin. Pharmacology* 13:388–390, 1973.
23. Hussar, D.A. Review of some significant drug interactions. *Pa. Med.* 79:37–41, 1976.
24. Fann, W.E. Interactions of psychotropic drugs in the elderly. *Postgrad. Med.* 53:182–186, 1973.
25. Greenblatt, D.J.; Shader, R.I.; Harmatz, J.S.; Franke, K.; and Koch-Weser, J. Influence of magnesium and aluminum hydroxide mixture on chlordiazepoxide absorption. *Clin. Pharmacol. Ther.* 19:234–239, 1976.
26. Koch-Weser, J., and Sellers, E.M. Drug interactions with coumarin anticoagulants. *N. Engl. J. Med.* 285:487–498, 1971.
27. Van Praag, H.M.; Lader, M.H.; Rafaelson, O.J.; and Sachar, E.J. *Handbook of Biological Psychiatry*. Part V. Drug Treatment in Psychiatry—Psychotropic Drugs. New York: Marcel Dekker, 1981.
28. MacDonald, M.G., and Robinson, D.S. Clinical observations of possible barbiturate interference with anticoagulation. *JAMA* 204:97–100, 1968.
29. Harvey, S.C. Hypnotics and sedatives. In *The Pharmacological Basis of Therapeutics*, Goodman, L.S., and Gilman, A., eds. New York: Macmillan, 1975.
30. Garretson, L.K.; Perel, J.M.; and Dayton, P.G. Methylphenidate interaction with both anticonvulsants and ethyl biscoumacetate. *JAMA* 207:2053–2056, 1969.
31. Drug interactions. *Lancet* 1:904–905, 1975.
32. Levy, G.; O'Reilly, R.A; Aggeler, P.M.; and Keech, G.M. Pharmacokinetic analysis of the effect of barbiturate on the anticoagulant action of warfarin in man. *Clin. Pharmacol. Ther.* 11:372–377, 1970.
33. Sellers, E.M., and Koch-Weser, J. Potentiation of warfarin-induced hypoprothrombinemia by chloral hydrate. *N. Engl. J. Med.* 282:827–831, 1970.

34. Kaufmann, J.S. Drug interactions involving psychotherapeutic agents. In *Drug Treatment of Mental Disorders*, Simpson, L.L., ed. New York: Raven Press, 1976.

35. Hicks, R.; Dysken, M.W.; Davis, J.M.; Lesser, J.; Ripeckyj, A.; and Lazarus, L. The pharmacokinetics of psychotropic medication in the elderly: A review. *J. Clin. Psychiatry* 42:374–385, 1981.

36. Cuinell, S.A.; Odessky, L.; Weiss, M.; and Dayton, P.G. The effect of chloral hydrate on bishydroxycoumarin metabolism: A fatal outcome. *JAMA* 197:366–368, 1966.

37. Udall, J.A. Clinical implications of warfarin interactions with five sedatives. *Am. J. Cardiol.* 35:67–71, 1975.

38. Kato, R.; Chiesara, E.; and Vassanelli, P. Mechanism of potentiation of barbiturates and meprobamate actions by imipramine. *Biochem. Pharmacol.* 12:357–364, 1963.

39. Pond, S.M.; Graham, G.G.; Birkett, D.J.; and Wade, D.N. Effects of tricyclic antidepressants on drug metabolism. *Clin. Pharmacol. Ther.* 18:191–199, 1975.

40. Vesell, E.S.; Passananti, T.; and Greene, F.E. Impairment of drug metabolism in man by allopurinol and nortriptyline. *N. Engl. J. Med.* 283:1484–1488, 1970.

41. Risch, S.C.; Groom, G.P.; and Janowsky, D.S. Interfaces of psychopharmacology and cardiology. Part one. *J. Clin. Psychiatry* 42:23–34, 1981.

42. Curry, S.H.; Davis, J.M.; Janowsky, D.S.; and Marshall, J.H.L. Factors affecting chlorpromazine plasma levels in psychiatric patients. *Arch. Gen. Psychiatry* 22:209–215, 1970.

43. Hansten, P.D. *Drug Interactions*. Philadelphia: Lea & Febiger, 1972.

44. Vestal, R.E.; Kornhauser, D.M.; Hollifield, J.W.; and Shand, D.G. Inhibition of propranolol metabolism by chlorpromazine. *Clin. Pharmacol. Ther.* 25:19–24, 1979.

45. Alexanderson, B.; Price-Evans, D.A.; and Sjoqvist, F. Steady-state plasma levels of nortriptyline in twins: Influence of genetic factors and drug therapy. *Br. Med. J.* 4:764–768, 1969.

46. Ballinger. B.J.; Presly, A.; Reid, A.H.; and Stevenson, I.H. The effects of hypnotics on imipramine treatment. *Psychopharmocologia* 39:267–274, 1974.

47. Burrows, G.D., and Norman, T.R. Psychotherapeutic drugs: Important adverse reactions and interactions. *Drugs* 20:485–493, 1980.

48. Forrest, F.M.; Forrest, I.S.; and Serra, M.T. Modification of chlorpromazine metabolism by some other drugs frequently administered to psychiatric patients. *Biol. Psychiatry* 2:53–58, 1970.

49. Gram, L.F., and Overo, K.F. Drug interaction: Inhibitory effect of neuroleptics on metabolism of tricyclic antidepressants in man. *Br. Med. J.* 1:463–465, 1972.

50. Gram, L.F.; Reisby, N.; Ibsen, I.; Nagy, A.; Dencker, S.J.; Bech, P.; Petersen, G.O.; and Christiansen, J. Plasma levels and antidepressant effect of imipramine. *Clin. Pharmacol. Ther.* 19:318–324, 1976.

51. Sandifer, M.G. The hypertensive psychiatric patient: Pharmacologic problems. *J. Clin. Psychiatry* 39:700–702, 1978.

52. Macfie, A.L. Lithium poisoning precipitated by diuretics. *Br. Med. J.* 1:516–517, 1975.

53. Himmelhoch, J.M.; Forrest, J.; Neil, S.; and Detre, T.P. Thiazide-lithium synergy in refractory mood swings. *Am. J. Psychiatry* 134:148–152, 1977.

54. Jefferson, J.W., and Kalin, N.H. Serum lithium levels and long-term diuretics use. *JAMA* 241:1134–1136, 1979.

PSYCHOTROPIC DRUG INTERACTIONS   205

55. Sletten, I.; Pichardo, J.; Korol, B.; and Gershon, S. The effect of chlorpromazine on lithium excretion in psychiatric subjects. *Curr. Ther. Res.* 8:410–446, 1966.

56. Ragheb, M.; Ban, T.A.; and Buchanan, D. Interaction of indomethacin and ibuprofen with lithium in manic patients under a steady-state lithium level. *J. Clin. Psychiatry* 41:397–398, 1980.

57. Byrd, G.J. Methyldopa and lithium carbonate: Suspected interaction. *JAMA* 233:320, 1975.

58. Leishman, A.W.D.; Matthews, H.L.; and Smith, A.J. Antagonism of guanethidine by imipramine. *Lancet* 1:112, 1963.

59. Mitchell, J.R.; Arias, L.; and Oates, J.A. Antagonism of the antihypertensive action of guanethidine sulfate. *JAMA* 202:973–976, 1967.

60. Jefferson, J.W. A review of the cardiovascular effects of toxicity of tricyclic antidepressants. *Psychosom. Med.* 37:160–179, 1975.

61. Von Zwieten, P.A. Interaction between centrally acting hypotensive drugs and tricyclic antidepressants. *Arch. Int. Pharmacodyn. Ther.* 215:12–30, 1975.

62. Briant, J.W.; Reid, J.L.; and Dollery, C.T. Interaction between clonidine and desipramine in man. *Br. Med. J.* 1:522–523, 1973.

63. Stafford, J.R., and Fann, W.E. Drug interactions with guanidinium antihypertensives. *Drugs* 13:57–64, 1977.

64. Cocco, G., and Ague, C. Interactions between cardioactive drugs and antidepressants. *Eur. J. Clin. Pharmacol.* 11:389–393, 1977.

65. Myer, J.F.; McAllister, C.K.; and Goldberg, L.I. Insidious and prolonged antagonism of guanethidine by amitriptyline. *JAMA* 213:1487–1488, 1970.

66. Fann, W.E.; Janowsky, D.S.; Davis, J.M.; and Oads, J.A. Chlorpromazine reversal of the antihypertensive action of guanethidine. *Lancet* 2:236–237, 1971.

67. Janowsky, D.S.; El-Yousef, M.K.; Davis, J.M.; and Fann, W.E. Antagonism of guanethidine by chlorpromazine. *Am. J. Psychiatry* 130:808–810, 1973.

68. Gilder, D.A.; Fain, W.; and Simpson, L.L. A comparison of the abilities of chlorpromazine and molindone to interact adversely with guanethidine. *J. Pharmacol. Exp. Ther.* 198:255–263, 1976.

69. Simpson, L.L. Combined use of molindone and guanethidine in patients with schizophrenia and hypertension. *Am. J. Psychiatry* 136:1410–1414, 1979.

70. Burgess, C.D.; Turner, P.; and Wadsworth, J. Cardiovascular responses to mianserin hydrochloride: A comparison with tricyclic antidepressant drugs. *Br. J. Clin. Pharmacol.* 5:215–285, 1978.

71. Mitchell, J.R.; Cavanaugh, J.H.; Arias, L.; and Oates, J.A. Guanethidine and related agents. III. Antagonism by drugs which inhibit the norepinephrine pump in man. *J. Clin. Invest.* 49:1596–1604, 1970.

72. Simpson, F.O. Antihypertensive drug therapy. *Drugs* 6:333–363, 1973.

73. Chouinard, G.; Pinard, G.; Prenoveau, Y.; and Tetreau, H.L. Alpha methyldopa-chlorpromazine interaction in schizophrenic patients. *Curr. Ther. Res.* 15:60–72, 1973.

74. Thornton, W.E., and Pray, B.J. Combination drug therapy in psychopharmacology. *J. Clin. Pharmacol.* 15:511–517, 1975.

75. Thornton, W.E. Dementia induced by methyldopa with haloperidol. *N. Engl. J. Med.* 294:1222, 1976.

76. Horwitz, D.; Lovenberg, W.; Engelman, K., and Sjoerdsma, A. Monoamine oxidase inhibitors, tyramine, and cheese. *JAMA* 188:1088–1110, 1964.

77. Boakes, A.F.; Laurence, D.R.; Teoh, D.C.; Barar, F.S.K.; Benidikter, L.T.; and Prichard, B.N.C. Interaction between sympathomimetic amines and antidepressant agents in man. *Br. Med. J.* 1:311–315, 1973.

78. Verrill, P.J. Adverse reactions to local anaesthetics and vasoconstrictor drugs. *Practitioner* 218:380–387, 1975.

79. Goldman, U. Local anaesthetics containing vasoconstrictors. *Br. Med. J.* 1:175, 1971.

80. Davis, J.M., and Fann, W.E. Lithium. *Ann. Rev. Pharmacol.* 11:285–303, 1970.

81. Prange, A.J.; Wilson, I.C.; Knox, A.; McClane, T.K.; and Lipton, M.A. Enhancement of imipramine by thyroid stimulating hormone: Clinical and theoretical implications. *Am. J. Psychiatry* 127:191–199, 1970.

82. Earle, B.U. Thyroid hormone and tricyclic antidepressants in resistant depression. *Am. J. Psychiatry* 126:1667–1669, 1970.

83. Coppen, A.; Montgomery, S.; Peet, M.; Bailey, J.; Marks, V.; and Woods, P. Thyrotropin-releasing hormone in the treatment of depression. *Lancet* 2:433–434, 1974.

84. McGilchrist, J.M. Interactions with monoamine-oxidase inhibitors. *Br. Med. J.* 3:591–592, 1975.

85. Greenblatt, D.J., and Shader, R.I. Drug interactions in psychopharmacology. In *Manual of Psychiatric Therapeutics*, Shader, R.I., ed. Boston: Little, Brown, 1975, pp. 269–279.

86. Spiker, K.G., and Pugh, D.D. Combining tricyclic and monoamine oxidase inhibitor antidepressant. *Arch. Gen. Psychiatry* 33:828–830, 1976.

87. Ponto, L.B.; Perry, P.J.; Liskow, B.I.; and Seaba, H.H. Drug therapy reviews: Tricyclic antidepressants and monoamine oxidase inhibitor combination therapy. *Am. J. Pharm.* 34:954–961, 1977.

88. Sethna, E.R. A study of refractory cases of depressive illness and their response to combined antidepressant treatment. *Br. J. Psychiatry* 124:265–272, 1974.

89. Schuckit, M.; Robins, E.; and Feighner, J. Tricyclic antidepressants and monoamine-oxidase inhibitors. *Arch. Gen. Psychiatry* 24:509–514, 1971.

90. Winston, F. Combined antidepressant therapy. *Br. J. Psychiatry* 118:301–303, 1971.

91. Wharton, R.N.; Perel, J.M.; Dayton, P.G.; and Malitz, S. A potential clinical use for methylphenidate with tricyclic antidepressants. *Am. J. Psychiatry* 127:1619–1625, 1971.

92. Fracchia, J.; Sheppard, C.; and Merlis, S. Combination medications in psychiatric treatment: Patterns in a group of elderly hospital patients. *J. Am. Ger. Soc.* 19:301–307, 1971.

93. Miller, D.D., and Macklin, M. Cimetidine-imipramine interaction: A case report. *Am. J. Psychiatry* 140:351–352, 1983.

CHAPTER 10

Psychiatric Complications of Nonpsychiatric Drugs

Donald R. Ross,
J. Ingram Walker,
Tim Covington,
and
Joseph Cools

Approximately 3 percent of patients who receive medications develop psychiatric symptoms secondary to those medications (1). These symptoms vary from mild reactions (irritability, insomnia, drowsiness, nightmares) to full-blown delirium (confusion, visual hallucinations, paranoid delusions) or an affective syndrome (major depressive episode or mania). Drugs may cause these symptoms due either to dose-related toxicity, an idiosyncratic response in the patient, or through other mechanisms (folic acid depletion, changes in receptor sensitivity).

An important factor that must be considered when evaluating psychiatric symptomatology caused by drugs is the premorbid mental state of the patient. Preexistent chronic organic brain syndrome (dementia), even when subtle, predisposes to toxic delirium from many drugs. A past history of depression or schizophrenia may indicate a biologic susceptibility to these diseases and make it more likely that the patient will develop the same clinical syndrome under the biochemical influence of certain medications. Finally, the patient's personality structure and his or her characteristic way of handling stress will help to shape the psychiatric manifestations that are finally observed.

This chapter looks only at nonpsychiatric drugs. Specifically, the anti-anxiety agents, antidepressants, antipsychotics, hallucinogens, lithium, narcotics, psychostimulants, and sedative-hypnotics are not discussed.

ANESTHETIC AGENTS

Gaseous anesthetics are rarely the cause of an organic brain syndrome because of their rapid excretion. Anoxia during anesthesia is a more likely cause of postoperative organic brain syndrome. Halothane has been implicated in several cases of postoperative depression (2). Ketamine is a general anesthetic given IV or IM that has a 12 percent incidence of visual hallucinations that occur as the patient awakens (emergence reaction). The hallucinations may be accompanied by agitated behavior and confusion and commonly last for several hours (3).

Local anesthetics such as lidocaine, cocaine, and procaine can cause severe reactions if absorbed in sufficient amounts through mucous membranes or inadvertent IV administration (4). They act as central nervous system stimulants and cause restlessness, anxiety, confusion, headache, vomiting, palpitations, hyperpyrexia, and hypertension. Convulsions and death may occur.

ANTI-INFECTIVES

Antibacterial agents are associated with a variety of psychiatric side effects. Sulfonamides commonly cause drowsiness, irritability, headache, insomnia, and a mild depression. Ataxia and peripheral neuritis are also common. Rarely, sulfonamides have been associated with major depressive reactions, psychosis, and confusional states (5). Penicillin, when given IV or intrathecally, may cause an acute delirium. Procaine penicillin has most commonly been implicated, and one-third of the patients affected have additional symptoms of severe anxiety, palpitations, hypertension, and hallucinations (Hoigné syndrome) (6). Carbenicillin and ticarcillin may cause neurotoxicity manifest as lethargy, neuromuscular irritability, hallucinations, asterixis, and seizures (large IV doses). Patients with renal failure are particularly at risk. Certain agents used to treat gram-negative infections have been reported to cause both delirium and depressive reactions (chloramphenicol, nalidixic acid, and nitrofurantoin).

Antituberculous drugs are often used in combination, and therefore, it is difficult to identify individual drug effects. Isoniazid is frequently used in isolation to suppress tuberculosis and has been associated with symptoms of irritability, belligerence, and paranoia, which may progress to a schizophreniform psychosis or an acute confusional state (7). Symptoms of paresthesia, anxiety, and muscle twitching may precede the psychosis by days or weeks and should alert the physician to lower the dose (8). Pyridoxine does not prevent this syndrome. Cycloserine is also associated with anxiety, delirium, and schizophreniform psychosis (9). Both drugs can activate psychotic episodes in schizophrenic patients. Ethionamide has been reported to cause lethargy, depression, and suicidal ideation (1). Iproniazid is used infrequently but should be remembered as the original MAO inhibitor used as an antidepressant in psychiatry. Its use may occasionally result in euphoria and a manic state (1).

The antifungal agent amphotericin B is given IV for systemic infections and can cause a delirium (10). Griseofulvin is an oral medication used to treat fungal infections of nails, hair, and skin. It may produce fatigue, irritability, and insomnia or occasionally may be responsible for a major depressive episode (1).

Antiparasitic agents (chloroquine, quinacrine, niridazole, thiabendazole) have been associated with delirium characterized by agitated and bizarre behavior, hallucinations, paranoid delusions, and manic or depressive symptoms. One patient developed an acute psychosis within two hours of a single 1 gram dose of chloroquine (11). Alternatively, a gradual personality change and amnestic-confabulatory syndrome may develop (12).

ANTICHOLINERGICS

Anticholinergic drugs are widely used in medicine. They are routinely used as an antisialagogue premedication in anesthesia (atropine); are effective treatment for cardiac arrhythmias such as sinus bradycardia and atrial fibrillation (atropine); counteract the extrapyramidal symptoms caused by antipsychotic medications and Parkinson's disease (benztropine, biperiden, trihexyphenidyl); work as an antispasmodic for gastrointestinal cramping (propantheline); and are used in ophthalmology for pupillary dilation and cycloplegia (atropine, homatropine, cyclopentolate). The antihistaminic drugs also have significant anticholinergic properties and produce similar toxic symptomatology. Many over-the-counter hypnotics contain 0.125 to 0.25 mg of scopolamine per tablet (Compoze, Quiet World, Sleep-Eze, Sominex). Finally, the common plants belladonna and Jimson weed have anticholinergic properties when ingested. Besides their medical use, anticholinergics are frequently abused on the street and in prisons.

Delirium complicates the use of anticholinergic drugs when patients become toxic. Patients may be excited, restless and agitated, or somnolent. Visual hallucinations and mental confusion are common, especially in the elderly. In higher concentrations, convulsions and coma may occur. Death is rare and usually secondary to other properties of the ingested substance (e.g., the arrhythmogenic properties of tricyclic antidepressants) (13).

Anticholinergic delirium can be identified by the characteristic peripheral effects of these drugs. Fever, tachycardia, elevated blood pressure, dry skin (including axillae) and dry mouth, sluggish and dilated pupils, and decreased or absent bowel sounds are classic. Each of these can be predicted on the basis of cholinergic blockade.

Treatment of anticholinergic poisoning involves emptying the stomach and supporting vital functions. If sedation is necessary, a nonanticholinergic antipsychotic (haloperidol) may be used. Parenteral physostigmine (1 to 2 mg IM or IV, which may be repeated in 20 minutes) can reverse the delirium, but it has its own complications (nausea, increased bronchial secretions), and it is a matter of clinical judgment whether or not it is indicated. The delirium and peripheral symptoms clear over twenty-four hours.

ANTICONVULSANTS

The anticonvulsant drugs cause a generalized slowing of mental processes. In toxic doses, sedation, confusion, ataxia, slurred speech, and nystagmus regularly occur. Since therapeutic serum levels of these drugs are close to toxic levels, these symptoms are commonly seen in clinical practice. These drugs may also cause hallucinations (visual, auditory, or tactile), delusions (grandiose or paranoid, often fragmented or poorly systematized), or affective symptoms (mania, depression, or rage reactions) in toxic doses or as idiosyncratic responses (14).

Phenytoin and phenobarbital are frequently used to treat grand mal epilepsy. Besides the symptoms listed previously, phenytoin may interfere with folic acid metabolism and produce a folic acid deficiency. Some patients who are lethargic and confused on phenytoin respond to folic acid replacement (1). Phenobarbital may produce a paradoxical excited state with agitation and hyperactivity, most commonly seen in pediatric and geriatric populations. In addition, the abrupt discontinuation of phenobarbital may produce a severe withdrawal syndrome resembling delirium tremens (15).

Ethosuximide is primarily used to treat petit mal epilepsy. Occasionally this drug may cause manic symptomatology with euphoria, irritability, and hyperactivity. At other times a severe depressive reaction with suicidal ideation may result (16).

Phenacemide, marketed for use in psychomotor epilepsy, is rarely used because of its frequent neurotoxic reactions. Psychosis, manic states, depression, or aggressive outbursts have been reported (1).

Clonazepam is a benzodiazepine derivative that has been useful in treating petit mal, akinetic, and myoclonic seizures. It has been associated with rage reactions, perhaps due to disinhibition of higher cerebral functions. This drug also may produce a withdrawal syndrome typical of other benzodiazepines (16).

ANTIHYPERTENSIVES

It is estimated that 15 to 20 percent of the adult population in the United States has hypertension. Many of the drugs prescribed to treat hypertension have a small but real incidence of depression associated with their use (17). Patients with previous depressive episodes are more vulnerable to this effect (18).

Reserpine and related rauwolfia alkaloids act by depleting catecholamine stores. In doses above 0.5 mg per day, severe endogenous depression is common (more than 20 percent). Insomnia, nightmares, and agitation may precede the depression, and suicide has been reported in several cases (19).

Methyldopa produces depression in 6 percent of cases (20). Fatigue, weariness, and nightmares are more common complaints.

Guanethidine, hydralazine, and clonidine have each been associated with symptoms of fatigue and drowsiness and with isolated cases of depression (13).

Propranolol is a peripheral β-blocker with unknown central actions. Although it is seemingly rare, depression has been clearly documented with as small a dose as 80 mg per day (21). Paranoid reactions have also been reported (5).

Diuretics probably have no psychiatric side effects other than those resulting from electrolyte imbalances (hyponatremia, hypokalemia) or dehydration (1). Weakness, confusion, and delirium are common sequelae of these states.

NONSTEROIDAL ANTI-INFLAMMATORY AGENTS

Indomethacin frequently produces psychiatric symptoms. Headache has been reported in 50 percent of patients taking this drug (1). Delirium with nightmares, hallucinations, paranoia, depersonalization, and agitation is seen at times with therapeutic doses. Depression may result from prolonged use (22).

Phenylbutazone may produce an agitated delirium in high doses. Convulsions and coma may supervene. Headache and depression are common with more moderate doses (1).

Sulindac has been reported to cause paranoia, rage reactions, and personality change in five patients (23,24).

ANTINEOPLASTIC AGENTS

Most antineoplastic agents do not cross the blood-brain barrier and do not cause psychiatric symptoms. Methotrexate used to treat leukemic meningitis has been reported to produce a delirium-dementia syndrome characterized by progressive impairment of consciousness and permanent intellectual deficits in some cases (25). The inflamed meninges allow entry of the drug into the cerebrospinal fluid. The mental changes may be secondary to an acute folic acid deficiency since methotrexate is a folate antagonist.

Vincristine and vinblastine have also been associated with neurotoxic effects. Depressed affect and somnolence a few days after treatment are commonly reported (1). Hallucinations and impairment of consciousness are sometimes seen with high doses (26).

Asparaginase has been reported to cause a delirium with confusion, bizarre behavior, and paranoid ideation in several cases (27).

ANTIPARKINSON AGENTS

Parkinson's disease involves a degeneration of nigrostriatal pathways and results in symptoms of tremor, rigidity, and bradykinesia. In many patients, the movement disorder is accompanied by a slowly progressive dementia. Because of the degree of disability and the poor prognosis, depressive reactions are common psychiatric sequelae of parkinsonism.

Levodopa, usually in combination with a peripheral decarboxylase inhibitor (carbidopa), is currently the mainstay of treatment of parkinsonism. Levodopa crosses the blood-brain barrier and augments the supply of precursor for the neurotransmitters dopamine and norepinephrine. The most common side effects are nausea and vomiting (50 percent) and choreoathetotic dyskinesias (50 percent) (28). Psychiatric symptoms complicate the use of this drug in approximately 20 percent of patients (29). The most frequent psychiatric manifestation is a dose-related delirium. Variable degrees of confusion, nightmares, visual hallucinations, paranoid delusions, and agitation are reported (30). Delirium is most common in those patients with an underlying dementia (31). A decrease in dosage usually brings the delirium under control. The addition of levotryptophan may also be of some benefit.

Affective syndromes caused by levodopa are also reported. An improvement in mood commonly accompanies the amelioration of physical disability brought about by the drug. This is not a true drug effect. Hypomanic episodes and severe depressive reactions due to levodopa occur in 2 percent of cases (32). Patients with preexisting bipolar affective disorder are particularly vulnerable to the precipitation of hypomania.

Bromocriptine is a dopamine agonist that has psychiatric side effects similar to those of levodopa. The delirium produced by bromocriptine, however, may last up to six weeks after the drug is discontinued (33).

Amantadine is an antiviral agent that has empirically been found to be useful in parkinsonism. When used in combination with anticholinergic drugs, amantadine has produced nightmares, visual hallucinations, and delirium (34). Again, those patients with preexisting dementia are most vulnerable.

CARDIAC DRUGS

Digitalis glycosides are estimated to be the fourth most prescribed drugs in the United States (14). Toxic serum levels are close to therapeutic levels, and clinical toxicity is common. Mild toxicity includes symptoms of nausea and vomiting, visual disturbances (yellow vision, white halos around dark objects), cardiac conduction abnormalities, painful neuralgias, nightmares, irritability, anxiety, and fatigue (14). More severe toxicity predisposes to malignant arrhythmias and may produce a delirium with visual hallucinations, paranoia, euphoria, belligerence, and confusion (35). Psychiatric symptoms are more frequent in the elderly and those with poor cerebral circulation. Electrolyte imbalances and cerebral anoxia must also be considered in evaluating a delirious patient who is taking digitalis (13).

Disopyramide is used in treating various arrhythmias. It has been reported to produce a delirium with agitation, hallucinations, paranoia, and panic in three patients shortly after they had begun treatment (36,37,38).

Procainamide is another antiarrhythmic with psychiatric morbidity. Moderate doses have been accompanied by mild depression and fatigue, while higher doses have been associated with psychotic depression (39).

HORMONES

Corticosteroids are endogenously produced by the adrenal cortex but are also exogenously administered for their anti-inflammatory and other properties. In 5 percent of patients, serious psychiatric sequelae result from the use of these drugs. Delirium and manic psychosis (with euphoria, decreased sleep, hyperactivity, and grandiose or paranoid delusions) are the most common syndromes. Only rarely does a severe depression result from exogenous corticosteroids. (This is in contrast to a 20 percent incidence of depression in idiopathic Cushing's syndrome) (40). The psychiatric side effects are usually dose related and are uncommon with oral doses of prednisone below 40 mg per day or equivalent doses of other steroids (4).

For some conditions like systemic lupus erythematosus, it is difficult to determine whether the delirium is due to the underlying disease process (cerebritis) or the steroid treatment. In such cases it is reasonable to increase the steroid dose rapidly and observe. If the psychiatric symptoms worsen, a reduction of steroids is called for; if they improve, the higher dose should be maintained (41). Adrenocorticotrophic hormone (ACTH) can be responsible for the same symptoms (delirium and mania), presumably because it stimulates the production and release of endogenous corticosteroids (42).

Thyroid hormone is used as replacement therapy in patients with hypothyroidism. If it is given in excess, symptoms of hyperthyroidism occur, including tachycardia, agitation, excessive perspiration, tremor, exaggerated startle response, hyperactive deep tendon reflexes, and heat intolerance. The patient may feel panicky or chronically anxious and may be misdiagnosed as having generalized anxiety disorder. If a patient acutely overdoses on thyroid hormone, the syndrome of thyroid storm may develop (fever, extreme tachycardia, dehydration, delirium) (1). Antithyroid medications (propylthiouracil, methimazole, carbimazole, radioactive iodine) may produce an acute hypothyroid state with delirium (myxedema madness) (1).

The psychiatric complications of oral contraceptives have been controversial. Six percent of women on oral contraceptives develop depression (43). Arguments have been put forth that estrogen (via pyridoxine deficiency) (44), progesterone (via increased MAO activity) (45), or psychodynamic factors are primarily responsible (46). Oral contraceptives seem to ameliorate the symptoms of premenstrual tension (irritability, depression, impulsivity) in a high percentage of patients (47).

Hypoglycemic agents (insulin, sulfonylureas) have the potential to lower serum glucose below the normal range. Acute or subacute hypoglycemia results in confusion, headache, cold and clammy skin, and impairment of consciousness. Repeated episodes over time may result in dementia and personality change (1).

NONNARCOTIC ANALGESICS

Aspirin is frequently involved in intentional overdoses and accidental poisonings. Signs of mild salicylate toxicity include headache, dizziness, tinnitus, nausea, sweating, thirst, lassitude, and drowsiness. Higher serum levels may produce skin eruptions, acid base disturbances (respiratory alkalosis and metabolic acidosis), and a central nervous system syndrome referred to as "salicylate jag." This consists of a restless delirium with garrulity, incoherent speech, and hallucinations. Convulsions, coma, and death are possible sequelae (14).

Phenacetin has also been reported to cause lethargy, mild depression, or delirium, but it is usually taken in combination with other drugs (aspirin, phenobarbital) that could account for these psychiatric symptoms (48).

Propoxyphene in high doses has been associated with confusion and auditory hallucinations (5). Pentazocine produces a transient euphoria (high) when injected IV. Chronic use or overdose may produce nightmares, hallucinations, racing thoughts, and paranoid delusions. A feeling of detachment and depersonalization is also frequently reported (49).

Carbamazepine is used in the treatment of trigeminal neuralgia. It has properties similar to the tricyclic antidepressants and may produce a toxic delirium (1).

MISCELLANEOUS

Aminocaproic acid, used to inhibit fibrinolysis, has been reported to cause an acute delirium with vivid hallucinations following bolus injection (50).

Antihistamines have significant central anticholinergic effects. Drowsiness is extremely common, and agitated delirium with overdose has been reported (51).

Baclofen, a centrally active skeletal muscle relaxant, may cause drowsiness and confusion during treatment. Abrupt withdrawal has been associated with nightmares, hallucinations, and delirium (52).

Cimetidine, a histamine H_2 receptor blocker, is used in the treatment of peptic ulcer disease and other hyperacidity states. Hallucinations, delusions, and delirium have been reported with high doses (53,54). Elderly patients with impaired renal function are at greater risk.

Disulfiram blocks acetaldehyde dehydrogenase, interfering with ethanol metabolism and producing a toxic build-up of acetaldehyde if ethanol is consumed. This accumulation of acetaldehyde results in aversive symptoms such as flushing, severe headache, vomiting, chest pain, vertigo, weakness, anxiety, and hypotension (14). Disulfiram is used to discourage chronic alcoholics from drinking. Besides the unpleasant disulfiram-alcohol reaction, disulfiram may produce mild side effects of fatigue and a decline in sexual potency. Dosages larger than 0.25 gm per day may produce a confused, somnolent, and disoriented patient. Disulfiram may also exacerbate psychotic symptoms (hallucinations, delusions, bizarre behavior) in schizophrenic patients (55,56). There is some thought that this may be secondary to the inhibition of dopamine-β-hydroxylase and a build-up of dopamine in the limbic system (13).

A second set of psychiatric complications with disulfiram involves the build-up of the metabolite carbon disulfide. This may result in symptoms of depression or delirium along with direct neurotoxicity (parkinsonism, choreoathetosis, thalamic syndrome, or peripheral neuropathy). Carbon disulfide toxicity requires chronic ingestion of high doses of the drug. Treatment is immediate discontinuation of disulfiram to prevent permanent neurological damage (57).

Methysergide, used in the prophylaxis of migraine headache, may occasionally produce delirium with hallucinations or symptoms of depersonalization (58).

Metrizamide, a contrast material injected intrathecally, has also been associated with delirium (confusion, disorientation, hallucinations) (59).

REFERENCES

1. Peterson, G.C. Organic mental disorders induced by drugs or poisons. In *Comprehensive Textbook of Psychiatry*, 3rd ed., Freedman, A.M., and Kaplan, H.I., eds. Baltimore: Williams and Wilkins, 1980, pp. 1437–1451.
2. Davison, L.A.; Steinhelber, J.C.; Eger, E.I.; and Stevens, W.C. Psychological effects of halothane and isoflurane anesthesia. *Anesthesiology* 43:313–324, 1975.
3. Dundee, J.W.; Knox, J.W.; Black, G.W.; Moore, J.; Pandit, S.K.; Bovill, J.; Clarke, R.S.; Love, S.H.; Elliott, J.; and Coppel, D.L. Ketamine as an induction agent in anesthetics. *Lancet* 1:1370–1371, 1970.
4. Miller, R.R., and Greenblatt, D.J. *Drug Effects in Hospitalized Patients*. New York: John Wiley and Sons, 1976.
5. Drugs that cause psychiatric symptoms. *Med. Letter* 23:9–12, 1981.
6. Thompsett, R. Pseudoanaphylactic reactions to procaine penicillin G. *Arch. Int. Med.* 120:565–567, 1967.
7. Kiersch, T.A. Toxic organic psychoses due to isoniazid therapy. *U.S. Armed Forces Med. J.* 5:1353–1359, 1954.
8. Organick, A.B. Toxic psychosis due to isoniazid. *Am. Rev. Tuberc. Pulm. Dis.* 79:799–804, 1959.

9. Lewis, W.C. Psychiatric and neurological reactions to cycloserine in the treatment of tuberculosis. *Dis. Chest* 32:172–182, 1957.
10. Winn, R.E.; Bower, J.H.; and Richards, J.F. Acute toxic delirium: Neurotoxicity of intrathecal administration of amphotericin B. *Arch. Int. Med.* 139:706–707, 1979.
11. Bomb, B.S.; Bedi, H.K.; and Bhatnagar, L.K. Chloroquine psychosis. *Trans. Royal Soc. Trop. Med. Hyg.* 69:523, 1975.
12. Torrey, E.F. Chloroquine seizures. *JAMA* 204:867–870, 1968.
13. Davies, D.M., ed. *Textbook of Adverse Drug Reactions.* New York: Oxford University Press, 1981.
14. Goodman, L.S., and Gilman, A., eds. *The Pharmacological Basis of Therapeutics,* 6th ed. London: Macmillan, 1980.
15. Smith, D.E., and Wesson, D.R. Phenobarbital technique for treatment of barbiturate dependence. *Arch. Gen. Psychiatry* 24:56–60, 1971.
16. Woodbury, D.M.; Penry, J.K.; and Pippenger, C.E., eds. *Antiepileptic Drugs.* New York: Raven Press, 1972.
17. Quetsch, R.M.; Achor, R.W.P.; Litin, E.M.; and Faucett, R.L. Depressive reactions in hypertensive patients. *Circulation* 19:366–375, 1959.
18. Muller, J.C.; Pryor, W.W.; Gibbons, J.E.; and Orgain, E.S. Depression and anxiety occurring during rauwolfia therapy. *JAMA* 159:836–839, 1955.
19. Goodwin, F.K., and Bunney, W.E. Depression following reserpine: A reevaluation. *Semin. Psychiatry* 3:435–448, 1971.
20. Granville-Grossman, K.G., ed. *Recent Advances in Clinical Psychiatry,* 4:199. London: Churchill Livingstone, 1982.
21. Petrie, W.M.; Maffucci, R.J.; and Woosley, R.L. Propranolol and depression. *Am. J. Psychiatry* 139:92–94, 1982.
22. Gotz, V. Paranoid psychosis with indomethacin. *Br. Med. J.* 1:49, 1978.
23. Thornton, T.L. Delirium associated with sulindac. *JAMA* 243:1630–1631, 1980.
24. Kruis, R., and Barger, R. Paranoid psychosis with sulindac. *JAMA* 243:1420, 1980.
25. Kay, H.E.; Knapton, P.J.; O'Sullivan, J.P.; Wells, D.G.; Harris, R.F.; Innes, E.M.; Stuart, J.; Schwartz, F.C.; and Thompson, E.N. Encephalopathy in acute leukemia associated with methotrexate therapy. *Arch. Dis. Child* 47:344–354, 1972.
26. Holland, J.F.; Scharlau, C.; Gailani, S.; Krant, M.J.; Olson, K.B.; Horton, J.; Shnider, B.I.; Lynch, J.J.; Owens, A.; Carbone, P.P.; Colsky, J.; Grob, D.; Miller, S.P.; and Hall, T.C. Vincristine treatment of advanced cancer: A cooperative study of 392 cases. *Cancer Res.* 33:1258–1264, 1973.
27. Moure, J.M.B.; Whitecar, J.P., Jr., and Bodey, G.P. Electroencephalogram changes secondary to asparaginase. *Arch. Neurol.* 23:365–368, 1970.
28. Sweet, R.D., and McDowell, F.H. Five years treatment of Parkinson's disease with levodopa. *Ann. Int. Med.* 8:456–463, 1975.
29. Celesia, G.G., and Barr, A.N. Psychosis and other psychiatric manifestations of levodopa therapy. *Arch. Neurol.* 23:193–200, 1970.
30. Shader, R.I., ed. *Psychiatric Complications of Medical Drugs.* New York: Raven Press, 1972, p. 149.
31. Sweet, R.D.; McDowell, F.H.; Feigenson, J.S.; Loranger, A.W.; and Goodell, H. Mental symptoms in Parkinson's disease during chronic treatment with levodopa. *Neurology* 26:305–310, 1976.
32. Goodwin, F.K.; Murphy, D.L.; Brodie, H.; Keith, H.; and Bunney, W.E. Levodopa: Alterations in behavior. *Clin. Pharm. Ther.* 12:383–396, 1971.

33. Calne, D.B.; Williams, A.C.; Neophytides, A.; Plotkin, C.; Nutt, J.G.; and Teychenne, P.F. Long-term treatment of parkinsonism with bromocriptine. *Lancet* 1:735–738, 1978.
34. Schwab, R.S.; England, A.C., Jr.; Poskanzer, D.C.; and Young, R.R. Amantadine in the treatment of Parkinson's disease. *JAMA* 208:1168–1170, 1969.
35. Beller, G.A.; Smith, T.W.; Abelmann, W.H.; Haber, E.; and Hood, W.B., Jr. Digitalis intoxication. *N. Engl. J. Med.* 284:989–997, 1971.
36. Falk, R.H.; Nisbet, P.A.; and Gray, T.J. Mental distress in patient on disopyramide. *Lancet* 1:858–859, 1977.
37. Padfield, P.L.; Smith, D.A.; Fitzsimons, E.J.; and McCruden, D.C. Disopyramide and acute psychosis. *Lancet* 1:1152, 1977.
38. Ahmad, S.; Sheikh, A.I.; and Meeran, M.K. Disopyramide-induced acute psychosis. *Chest* 76:712, 1979.
39. McCrum, I.D., and Guidry, J.R. Procainamide-induced psychosis. *JAMA* 240:1265–1266, 1978.
40. Michael, R.P., and Gibbons, J.L. Interrelationships between the endocrines and neuropsychiatry. *Int. Rev. Neurobiol.* 5:243–302, 1963.
41. Medical Research Council. Treatment of systemic lupus erythematosus with steroids. *Br. Med. J.* 2:915–920, 1961.
42. Clarke, L.D. Preliminary observations on mental disturbances occurring in patients under therapy with cortisone and ACTH. *N. Engl. J. Med.* 246:205–216, 1952.
43. Editorial. Depression and oral contraception. *Br. Med. J.* 4:127–128, 1970.
44. Adams, P.W.; Rose, D.P.; Folkard, J.; Wynn, V.; Seed, M.; and Strong, R. Effect of pyridoxine hydrochloride (vitamin B$_6$) upon depression associated with oral contraceptives. *Lancet* 1:897–904, 1973.
45. Grant, R.H.E., and Pryse-Davies, J. Effect of oral contraceptives on depressive mood changes and on endometrial monoamine oxidase and phosphatases. *Br. Med. J.* 3:777–780, 1968.
46. Wallach, E.E., and Garcia, C.R. Psychodynamic aspects of oral contraception. *JAMA* 203:927–931, 1968.
47. Moos, R.H. Psychological aspects of oral contraceptives. *Arch. Gen. Psychiatry* 19:87–94, 1968.
48. Prescott, C.F. Anti-inflammatory agents and drugs used in rheumatism and gout. In *Side Effects of Drugs*, Dukes, M.N.G., ed. Amsterdam: Associated Science Publishers, 1978, pp. 91–104.
49. Kane, F.J., and Pokorny, A. Mental and emotional disturbance with pentazocine (Talwin) use. *South. Med. J.* 68:808–811, 1975.
50. Wysenbeek, A.J.; Sella, A.; Blum, I.; and Yeshurun, D. Acute delirious state after amino caproic acid administration. *Clin. Toxicol.* 14:93–95, 1979.
51. Nigro, S.A. Toxic psychosis due to diphenhydramine hydrochloride (benadryl). *JAMA* 203:301–302, 1968.
52. Skausig, O.B., and Korsgaard, S. Hallucinations and baclofen. *Lancet* 1:1258, 1977.
53. Menzies-Gou, N. Cimetidine and mental confusion. *Lancet* 2:928, 1977.
54. Adler, L.E.; Sadja, L.; and Wilets, G. Cimetidine toxicity manifested as paranoia and hallucinations. *Am. J. Psychiatry* 137:1112–1113, 1980.

55. Knee, S.T., and Razani, J. Acute organic brain syndrome: A complication of disulfiram therapy. *Am. J. Psychiatry* 131:1281–1282, 1974.
56. Rainey, J.M. Disulfiram toxicity and carbon disulfide poisoning. *Am. J. Psychiatry* 134:371–378, 1977.
57. Davidson, M., and Feinleib, M. Carbon disulfide poisoning: A review. *Am. Heart J.* 83:100–114, 1972.
58. Persyko, I. Psychiatric adverse reactions to methysergide. *J. Nerv. Ment. Dis.* 154:299–301, 1972.
59. Schmidt, R.C. Mental disorders after myelography with metrizamide and other water-soluble contrast media. *Neuroradiology* 19:153–157, 1980.

CHAPTER 11

Psychodynamic Factors Affecting Biomedical Psychiatric Therapeutics

Jesse O. Cavenar, Jr.,
Mary G. Cavenar, and
J. Ingram Walker

All human interactions involve both conscious and unconscious psychodynamics, and the rendering of biomedical psychiatric treatments is no exception. There are, in all situations, dynamic issues in the person who is rendering the treatment, in the patient who is receiving the treatment, and in their mutual interaction. Whether one chooses the psychoanalytic terms of *transference reactions* and *countertransference reactions* or other descriptive terms matters little.

THE PLACEBO EFFECT

In attempting to discuss the psychodynamic issues involved, it is beneficial to understand first the placebo effect that biomedical psychiatric treatments may have. A rather narrow and restricted definition of placebo is an inactive substance or procedure which is administered in order to satisfy the patient's symbolic need for active treatment or used in controlled studies to help determine the efficacy of an active substance or procedure. (1). A broader view of the placebo is taken by Shapiro (2), who defines it as follows:

> [A]ny therapeutic procedure which is given deliberately to have an effect, or unknowingly has an effect on a patient, symptom, syndrome, or disease, but which is objectively without specific activity for the condition being treated. The therapeutic procedure may be given with or without conscious knowledge that

219

the procedure is a placebo, may be an active (non-inert) or non-active (inert) procedure, and includes, therefore, all medical procedures no matter how specific—oral and parenteral medication, topical preparations, inhalants, and mechanical, surgical, and psychotherapeutic procedures. The placebo must be differentiated from the placebo effect which may or may not occur, and which may be favorable or unfavorable. The placebo effect is defined as the changes produced by placebos. The placebo is also used to describe an adequate control in research. (p. 73)

The placebo effect has been clearly documented in the treatment of many disease processes. At times, it is impossible to differentiate the placebo effect from a spontaneous remission or change in the disease process, but in other cases, the placebo effect can be differentiated. There are reports of placebos affording relief of angina pectoris (3), rheumatoid arthritis (4), hypertension (5), peptic ulcer (6), headache (7), hay fever (8), and other illnesses involving diverse systems throughout the body. One investigator has reported that 35.2 ± 2.2 percent of a large group of patients will benefit from placebo treatment (7).

The placebo effect of psychoactive drugs has been studied extensively. Loranger and associates (9) noted that in drug research three types of phenomena can be viewed as placebo effect: (1) the changes produced in a person by the set, suggestibility, or expectations of taking a medication; (2) the perceived changes in a person or patient believed by an observer or evaluator to represent change when, in fact, the patient is no different than he or she was initially; and (3) a type of reasoning that considers most or any changes that follow the administration of a placebo as being placebo effect. They suggest that those who use the latter reasoning fail to appreciate that changes may occur in persons due to either endogenous or environmental events that by chance temporally coincide with the administering of a placebo. To illustrate their thesis, a drug investigation using 120 hospitalized psychiatric patients was done. Participating physicians, nurses, and patients were told that a new tranquilizer and a new energizer were to be tested when, in fact, both substances were placebos. With subjective methods of evaluation, 53 to 80 percent of patients were found to benefit from the so-called drugs. The tendency to attribute improvement to what were believed to be active drugs demonstrated clearly the placebo effect and illustrated the difficulty of comprehending studies that are not double-blind, controlled studies. Given that this is true with clinical drug trials, it still leaves open the question of the placebo effect on the individual patient given any psychobiological treatment.

The milieu in which treatment takes place or a drug is administered may markedly influence the patient's response to that treatment or drug. Rashkis and Smarr (10) have shown improvement in up to 80 percent of patients with schizophrenia in response to the increased attention provided by a special research unit, and a common clinical observation is to see a depressed patient improve markedly when removed from a stressful situation and hospitalized in a facility where people in the immediate environment evidence an interest and are supportive. Clinicians frequently hear anecdotal reports from marijuana users concerning the different effects that the same marijuana may produce, depending upon the environment in which the drug is used, the expectation of the smoker, the mental set of the smoker, and various other psychological parameters. Thus, there seems to be little question that the milieu can have a pronounced influence on the response to a procedure, treatment, or drug.

One of the most important determinants of the placebo effect appears to be the physician-patient relationship. Shapiro (2) noted that an emotionally meaningful physician-patient relationship allows the transfer of the patient's concerns and worries to a recognized healer and scientist. In psychoanalytic terminology, it could be said that early, embryonic transference reactions and the beginnings of both the therapeutic and working alliance are of primary importance in determining the nature and extent of the placebo reaction. It has long been recognized that transference reactions may begin with the initial telephone call to the physician's office, before any personal contact has taken place. Lesse (11) has noted that the largest number of possible placebo reactions are obtained in those individuals who have a strong desire for and expectancy that relief from particular signs and symptoms will occur as the consequence of a specific drug or procedure.

In addition to these hopes and expectations from the patient, the attitudes, hopes, expectations, and feelings about a particular treatment or drug by the physician are of extreme importance. These attitudes and biases of the physician are communicated to the patient on both a conscious and unconscious level, and the physician's enthusiasm or, conversely, disdain for a particular treatment is readily perceived by the patient.

The most positive placebo effect is created in the patient when the physician has faith in the treatment or drug he or she is prescribing. For example, one of the authors had a positive experience with a particular psychotropic drug early in residency training and, as a result, has a positive attitude and faith in that particular drug. When that drug is prescribed, the patients appear uniformly to obtain a positive response, yet in discussions with colleagues, it is clear that they have little faith in that drug and obtain very poor therapeutic results. There is little question that the physician's belief and faith in the drug, which is communicated to the patient, therefore accounts for the positive experience with the drug.

Benson and Epstein (12) note that in recent years the placebo effect has been viewed with disdain due to the placebo's being used as a control in drug trials to test the efficacy of new drugs. They raise a very challenging question when they wonder whether a new drug that produces an effect equal to placebo should be disregarded; instead, they suggest that the placebo effect and its physiology be further investigated.

PSYCHODYNAMIC AND PSYCHOANALYTIC PRINCIPLES

Rarely is a patient given a psychobiological treatment without being given psychotherapy of some type also. Even though at times a formal psychotherapy is not planned, a therapeutic and a working alliance are formed and resistances are encountered. Most drug therapies or other biologic therapy programs, including ECT, thus entail an amount of psychotherapy.

It is helpful to comprehend certain basic psychotherapeutic principles and concepts of psychoanalytic theory and thought to understand the psychodynamic considerations in psychobiological treatments. The mental apparatus is divided, according to psychoanalytic structural theory, into three major groups: the id, ego, and superego. All mental processes occurring in the mind can be conceptualized as occurring in one of the three groups of functions. While the id, ego, and superego are referred to as psychic structures, it is important to realize that they do not correspond to any specific type of anatomical structure. The functional groups are referred to as structures because it has been repeatedly observed that, once established early in an individual's life, the functions included in the group tend to be organized in a repetitive, automatic, persistent manner and to change very slowly, if at all, throughout that individual's life.

The id is that portion of the mental apparatus that gives psychic representation to the instinctual forces originating in the biological function of the individual. The drives are motivational forces that initiate behavior; by mechanisms that are not understood, biological forces achieve a psychic representation in the mind and are then named, in psychoanalytic and psychodynamic theory, as drives. While multiple forces exist in the id, Freud broadly conceived of the drives as being either aggressive or sexual. The id is totally unconscious and out of the individual's awareness; id functions operate according to the primary process and pleasure principle.

The primary process is best illustrated by the manifest dream structure. In the manifest dream, distortions in time sequence, logical progression, and cause and effect may occur; negatives and contradictions may exist, without conflict, and displacement, condensation, and symbolism are common. Primary process thought is characteristic of the thinking process of young children or infants.

The pleasure principle holds that the drives seek immediate and direct gratification regardless of the reality of external forces. Various drives will vary in intensity from time to time, but the stronger the drive, the greater will be the pressure for discharge in order to reduce the drive tension. As noted, the id drives are totally unconscious and cannot be directly observed. However, derivatives of the drives are closer to consciousness and can be observed in an individual's preconscious and conscious thoughts, behaviors, and feelings.

The superego is that portion of the mental apparatus that judges the other mental functions critically in terms of right and wrong, punishment or reward, or good and bad. The superego is made up of conscious, pre-conscious, and unconscious elements. The conscious and preconscious elements are at times called one's conscience. The more unconscious aspects of the superego are responsible for the more primitive and archaic considerations of punishment and reward. The superego is formed by the incorporation and internalization of parental standards and attitudes of right and wrong; while such internalizations occur from infancy onward, the child's attempts to resolve oedipal conflicts by identification with the parents is of crucial importance in the formation of the superego. Another component of the superego is the ego ideal, which is composed of the ideals the individual strives to attain.

The ego is that group of mental processes that functions to perceive and recognize various forces from both internal and external sources that may impinge on the individual. The ego must integrate, assimilate, and synthesize these various functions and then execute activities necessary to maintain a state of both internal and external adaptation. Ego functions include memory, thought, motor functions, perceptions, and judgment. The ego operates according to the reality principle, as opposed to the pleasure principle of the id, as discussed earlier. Thus, the ego must assess the total forces impinging on the individual and then arrive at an action or judgment that has the greatest benefit for the individual in the long term. Ego functions are in accord with the secondary process mode of functioning in which logic, cause and effect, contradictions, negations, and time are recognized. The secondary process mode of functioning is clearly more reality oriented than the primary process described earlier.

From this discussion of id, ego, and superego, it becomes apparent that contradictory psychological forces may be present in the mind at any time and that intrapsychic conflict may arise. There may also be conflict between the individual and the external environment. Most often, there is a combination of such conflicts so that conflict may exist between the individual and his or her environment that is also related to an intrapsychic conflict. For example, an id drive seeking immediate and direct gratification may be in conflict with a superego prohibition against the expression of the drive. The same id drive may also be in conflict with the ego because of the ego's recognition of a real or fantasied danger arising from the gratification of the id drive; gratification or discharge of the drive may be in conflict with the reality principle and the external environment. There can also be conflict between the ego and the external environment in terms of the demands the environment places on the individual and in terms of the individual's ego attempting to alter the external reality so that it is in keeping with the wishes of the individual. Still other conflictual situations may involve the superego making such excessive demands that the individual's ego is unable to withstand the pressure. Clearly, any number of conflictual situations may arise from conflict among internal structures or between internal structures and external reality.

The major function of the ego is to maintain both a state of internal adaptation and adaptation between the individual and his or her environment. The nature and intensity of the internal forces are constantly shifting and changing, as are external environmental factors. Thus, the equilibrium and adaptation maintained by the ego is not a static, fixed, rigid state but a constantly changing, dynamic, fluid one. If the dynamic equilibrium is not maintained, signal anxiety is the result until the dynamic equilibrium can be restored. The ego mechanisms of defense are important functions that play a crucial role in the initial establishment of equilibrium, the maintenance of equilibrium, and the restoration of the equilibrium if the balance has been upset or shifted by either internal or external forces. The defense mechanisms are unconscious ego functions and, if fully successful, prevent the individual from becoming aware of the drive that is being defended against or of experiencing overt anxiety. Examples of such defense mechanisms include denial, introjection, projection, intellectualization, isolation of affect, regression, displacement, and other similar mechanisms.

According to psychoanalytic and psychodynamic theory, psychopathology and the development of psychological symptoms result from disturbances in the mental processes involved in this dynamic, changing psychological equilibrium. An individual may be functioning at a reasonable level of adaptation and be in a dynamic equilibrium or homeostasis and then experience intensification of an id drive, an increase in superego force, a change in the ego's integrative or adaptive capacity, or a marked change in external reality. The dynamic homeostasis may be disrupted so that there is a threat of the return of the unconscious drive into conscious awareness; this drive is seeking discharge and thus brings the threat of superego condemnation or a threat of danger as perceived by the ego.

The danger situations perceived by the ego are primitive primary process fantasies that were experienced in childhood and then repressed; since these fantasies have been repressed, they continue to be viable unconsciously. The fantasies include things such as bodily destruction, castration anxiety, sadistic and masochistic fantasies, violent physical punishment, feelings of inferiority or inadequacy, and many others, depending upon the individual's past experiences and childhood fantasies. As these repressed conflicts and fantasies approach conscious awareness, the individual's anxiety will increase; various ego functions intensify to attempt to establish a dynamic steady state in order to avoid the discomfort of anxiety and to prevent the danger situation from reaching conscious awareness. On the one hand, if the ego functions are successful, the anxiety disappears and the homeostasis is restored. On the other hand, if prompt resolution does not occur, other ego mechanisms must be utilized, and previous defenses must be strengthened. A new level of adaptation is attempted, with a compromise taking place in which there is partial gratification of the drive in a disguised form and at the same time a partial satisfaction of both ego and superego demands toward that drive. This new level of adjustment and compromise may have as a manifestation the neurotic symptom. In the neurotic symptom one may find various mixtures of the drive, or the drive derivative, and the defenses and condemnations or prohibitions against the drive.

PSYCHOTHERAPIES

Since psychotherapy systems are logical extensions of the preceding description of psychopathology and symptom formation, it is important that this information be understood. This section presents a description of the two major types of psychotherapies and then it discusses studies describing the psychodynamic issues of psychobiological treatments with these psychotherapies. For convenience, it is best to conceptualize a spectrum of psychotherapy ranging from supportive psychotherapy at one polar extreme to intensive, insight-oriented psychotherapy at the other polar extreme. While it is theoretically easy to distinguish the two polar extremes, it should be recognized that in clinical practice there is frequently a large zone in the center between the extremes in which the therapist may choose to use both support and insight, depending upon many different variables including factors within the patient, the reality circumstance, the training of the physician or therapist, and the availability and efficacy of medical psychiatric treatments.

Supportive Psychotherapy

Those patients for whom supportive psychotherapy is the psychotherapeutic treatment of choice are those individuals who are felt to be suffering primarily from a biologically determined illness or who can maximally benefit from limited involvement and participation in the psychotherapeutic process. The psychotherapeutic treatment is aimed at symptom relief or amelioration without expectation or anticipation of changing the basic character structure. With such a patient, the therapist must realize that efforts to change or alter the symptoms rapidly may in fact make the patient much worse and produce a worse level of adaptation. For example, one woman had a conversion symptom in which her arms were tightly locked across her chest; with the inspiration of well-meaning friends, she rapidly became capable of moving her arms and killed her mother. Clearly, her symptom was serving a defensive purpose and was needed to defend against the id drive. In other individuals, the goal of supportive therapy is to help the individual over an acute crisis in his or her life, again without attempting to change the character patterns.

In supportive psychotherapy, the technique involves allowing the patient to maintain repression and to deal with issues that are preconscious or conscious. No attempt is made to explore unconscious conflicts or to bring those conflicts to conscious awareness. Thus, the patient is encouraged to talk about current concerns and worries, and the therapist has the opportunity to offer support, guidance, and suggestion. One therapeutic task for the therapist in supportive psychotherapy is to recognize the defenses that are currently being utilized by the patient, to determine how these defenses might be strengthened or made more effective, and to attempt to determine what other defenses might be re-introduced or introduced to the patient. The goals of the strategy are to aid the patient's ego in defense.

The therapist attempts to reduce the conscious and preconscious conflict by many different techniques; at times, it may be useful and necessary for the therapist to assume certain ego functions for the patient until he or she is capable of assuming the functions. Such a technique may repeat a parent-child relationship from the patient's past and should be given up as soon as the patient is capable of assuming those functions. A therapist who takes over certain ego functions for the patient must do so with a thorough knowledge of the patient's dynamics and psychological conflicts because otherwise, it may tend to regress the individual further.

In supportive therapy, the patient is encouraged to identify with the therapist. This is accomplished by the therapist's taking an active role in helping the patient seek solutions to his or her difficulties and by maintaining a positive rapport and relationship with the patient. As the therapist is more open with his or her own thoughts and feelings and demonstrates to the patient how he or she thinks about and approaches problems and conflicts, an identification with the therapist is encouraged.

In supportive therapy, the positive relationship and rapport are based on conscious thoughts and feelings. Any distortions of the relationship based on the patient's past experience with parents or other significant persons are corrected as rapidly as possible so that the focus of the therapeutic relationship can be on conscious, reality-based interactions between therapist and patient. However, derivatives of drives may be gratified without exploring the deeper unconscious meaning of the drive; the focus remains on the realistic, conscious situation and the problems at hand.

Most of the therapeutic work that is done with the superego in supportive psychotherapy consists of attempting to enable the patient to identify with the therapist and, thereby, either to soften the superego if it is too harsh or to reinforce aspects of the superego if impulsive behavior is taking place.

Insight Psychotherapy

Insight psychotherapy is a more complicated psychotherapeutic undertaking than supportive psychotherapy. The main goals of insight therapy are to help the patient achieve greater self-awareness and self-understanding and to effect some degree of personality change. The main avenue to achieving these goals is through making conscious those conflicts that have been unconscious, with the patient then achieving a better integration of these conflicts. In general, once the patient has an awareness of the conflicts, he or she can then exercise a greater freedom of choice about what he or she may choose to do in a particular situation. Other goals include psychological development toward psychosexual maturity, increased anxiety tolerance, and ego expansion so that more reality-principle functioning may be present and more appropriate drive satisfaction may be obtained. A resolution of major unconscious conflict with more freedom, unhampered by neurotic processes, is an overall goal.

Psychoanalysis is the most intensive form of insight psychotherapy, and a discussion of psychoanalysis is beyond the scope of this chapter. However, psychoanalytic principles are used in less intensive types of insight psychotherapy, and we use that type of psychotherapy for comparison with supportive psychotherapy.

Patients for whom insight psychotherapy is the treatment of choice are those individuals who are felt to be capable of change, to be able to achieve some self-understanding, and to have the ego capacity to participate actively in the treatment process. The goal of therapy is not symptom relief or amelioration, and the symptoms may not be an area of direct discussion. Instead, psychotherapists feel that if the unconscious conflicts can be understood and worked through, many of the symptoms will disappear without direct confrontation. The degree and depth of bringing unconscious and preconscious material to conscious awareness will vary, depending upon the intensity of the therapeutic endeavor.

Resistances and defenses are interpreted and worked with at appropriate times in the treatment in order to reduce the defenses so that previously unconscious material may come to conscious awareness. Thus, the patient may gradually become aware of id drives, ego defenses and patterns, and superego manifestations; he or she learns not only what was being defended against but also about the defense. During the course of interpreting and working with the patient's resistances and defenses, exacerbations of anxiety may be present as unconscious material threatens to become conscious. As an aspect of the psychotherapeutic technique, the therapist attempts to keep the anxiety or other psychological symptoms at levels that do not exceed the patient's tolerance.

As noted, one goal of insight therapy is to bring unconscious conflict to conscious awareness. The therapist attempts to reestablish and recreate earlier conflicts that have created neurotic conflict and attempts to do this in a manner that will have emotional meaning for the patient. One major method of doing this is via the transference. Transference is a type of displacement in which the individual unconsciously and unknowingly displaces to a person in his or her current life various feelings, attitudes, responses, and drives that had their origin in relationships in the individual's earlier life. This displacement is out of conscious awareness and thus allows the individual to experience reactions toward the therapist that are not founded in the reality of the current relationship but are a product of the patient's unconscious internal psychic life. After becoming consciously aware of the conflict via the transference, the patient is afforded another opportunity to resolve the conflict that he or she could not handle at an earlier point in his or her life.

To facilitate the formation of the transference feelings, the therapist does not actively intervene, advise the patient, or offer solutions as might be done in supportive therapy; instead, he or she maintains a neutral stance and encourages the patient to seek his or her own solutions as he or she develops more self-understanding and insight. By the same token, the therapist wants to remain as anonymous as possible to permit the full development of transference fantasies. The more realistic information the patient knows about the therapist, the more difficulty the patient may have in allowing his or her fantasies and drives to reach consciousness. As the therapist becomes a transference object for the patient, it is important that the therapist maintain a neutral role and that the therapy continue in a relative abstinence of gratification of the drives or drive derivatives by the therapist. The technique of insight-directed therapy might be seen as a relative frustration of drive and drive derivatives in the treatment situation in order to enhance the development of a transference situation in which conflicts may become conscious.

Psychobiological Treatments

Various investigators have made efforts to comprehend the effects of psychoactive drugs on psychiatric illness from the perspective of psychoanalytic psychology and structural theory. Specifically, efforts have been made to understand the pharmacologic effect on id drives or derivatives of the id drives, on ego defensive patterns, on the superego, and on the narcissistic balance of the individual. In addition, other efforts have attempted to understand the symbolic meaning of a psychobiological treatment in the context of both a supportive and insight-oriented psychotherapy and to understand the alterations that a psychobiological treatment may cause in the transference relationship. This section reviews these studies and then discusses their potential impact on a treatment situation.

Sarwer-Foner (13, 14) noted that the effects of a given drug are not always consistent. He attempted to explain these differences as arising from the influence of the drug upon the ego defenses so that variations among an individual's array of ego defenses would determine differences in response to a drug. He noted four specific situations in which tranquilizing drugs had a deleterious effect: (1) In male patients attempting to repress feminine impulses, repression may be challenged by the restriction of mobility, fatigue, and enervation that the drug might cause; (2) patients with hypochondriacal concerns may find the side effects or effects of the tranquilizers an additional threat to their efforts to maintain somatic integrity; (3) depressed patients become worse when tranquilizers increase psychomotor retardation; and (4) some patients interpret the administration of medication as a sexual assault and respond with increased defensiveness.

Winkelman (15) studied the effect of drugs on both id and ego functions in patients in psychotherapy. He suggested that the tranquilizers decreased id impulses and, while initially improving ego function, gradually impaired it. He believed that drugs could improve reality testing, strengthen defenses, and aid the ego in achieving some distance from psychic pain.

Azima and associates (16, 17) also studied drug actions from a psychoanalytic standpoint, and they believed that the drugs affected instinctual drives and energies. They considered the aggressive drive energy alteration to be more significant than the libidinal energy alterations.

Perhaps the most comprehensive works on relating drug action to psychic structure have been the contributions by Ostow (18, 19). While others have maintained for many years that psychoactive drugs should not be used in patients in insight-oriented psychotherapy or psychoanalysis, Ostow feels that psychoactive agents lend themselves to use in psychoanalysis or intensive psychotherapy for several reasons. First, the therapy is gentle and does not disrupt ego function and, thus, does not interfere with interpretation or damage transference. Second, when properly used, drugs may facilitate the psychotherapeutic work. Third, Ostow suggests that drugs can be used to achieve quickly, though temporarily, the same therapeutic influence that is achieved more slowly, but more permanently, through psychological treatment. By this Ostow means a redistribution of psychic energy within the psychic apparatus. He suggests that this is the common ground whereby psychoanalytic therapy and pharmacotherapy can be compared and coordinated with each other.

Whereas other psychoanalysts and psychotherapists have been concerned that the prescribing of a drug would distort or influence the transference, Ostow does not agree. He suggests that the alternatives to the prescribing of a drug, like hospitalization, are more disruptive. Further, he feels that it is essential only that all transactions between the therapist and patient be controlled and deliberate so that fantasy can be distinguished from reality; as long as this criterion is met, the transference should not be unduly disrupted. Ostow suggests that drug therapy can in fact reconstitute a fragmented ego so as to make psychoanalysis or insight-directed therapy possible for patients who would otherwise be too ill to participate in the therapy. While drug therapy is often not necessary in psychoanalysis or insight-directed therapy, it can be helpful to the patient and the therapist in the occasional acute exacerbations of illness that may occur during therapy.

Ostow is of the opinion that psychoactive drugs have an effect upon the ego's supply of libido, or sexual drive energy, and that the clinical changes from the drugs can be accounted for as a result of variations in the ego's supply of libido; that is, ego function varies sensitively with the amount of psychic energy available to it. He has developed a scale for ego libido that can be used clinically to assess the patient (see Table 11.1).

Ostow suggests that fluctuations between positions four and seven are normal, while positions three and eight raise the suspicion of disease and two

Table 11.1 Scale of Ego Libido

Position	Criterion
0	Profound, inert melancholia or catatonia
1	Delusional melancholia
2	Vigorous self-condemnation and pessimism
3	Guilt, pessimism, and primary self-observation
4	Self-orientation, feeling of enervation
5	Showing no other indicators distinctly
6	Object orientation
7	Moderate object striving with optimism
8	Pronounced object striving, perhaps with anxiety or with tertiary self-observation
9	Ideas of reference but with adequate reality testing
10	Delusional mania or schizophrenia

and nine are definitely pathological. He discusses in detail clinical syndromes such as melancholia, mania, schizophrenia, delirium, obsessive-compulsive neurosis, hysteria, and addictions to demonstrate how he prescribes drugs either to raise or lower the ego libido level. Further, he makes the point that no physician can select or adjust the dosage of medication other than the treating psychiatrist because no other physician is in a position to know the level of ego libido. The interested reader is referred to his books for a detailed analysis of his theory on specific clinical syndromes.

Clinically, interactions between the prescribing and taking of drugs are part of the therapist-patient relationship and, thus, may be invested by the patient with a variety of conscious and unconscious meanings. In the therapeutic situation, it is not vital that the clinician clearly delineate the psychological effect from the pharmacological effect as long as the desired result is being obtained. For some patients, consulting a physician for a psychological problem is much like consulting a physician for a strictly medical disorder; they expect the prescribing of a medication and may be consciously and/or unconsciously disappointed if medication is not prescribed. The prescribing of a medication that does provide immediate relief of the symptoms may make the physician appear omnipotent and will demonstrate concern for and understanding of the patient. Clearly, this can be of great advantage in building a positive relationship and working alliance. Conversely, if the medication prescribed does not produce symptomatic relief or causes serious side effects, it may be destructive to the formation of a positive relationship and working alliance.

Some patients who would benefit greatly from drug therapy are hesitant to take drugs of any type; some such patients, particularly obsessive-compulsive patients, will proudly announce that they have not taken a pill of any type in years. The unconscious fear in such patients appears to be that their dependence needs will become conscious if gratified by oral medication; they must be encouraged to take medication that is of potential benefit to them. Still other patients have fears of becoming addicted to the medication, and most often a straightforward discussion of this fear will aid in alleviating their anxiety.

The unconscious transference implications of the prescribing of a psychobiological treatment are important and, in fact, may determine the patient's conscious response to the therapeutic situation. If the treatment is successful, reduces unpleasant feeling states, and provides the patient a sense of well-being, the physician who prescribed the treatment is associated unconsciously with persons from the patient's early life who cared for him or her in that manner. Via this transference implication, the drug effect may be increased. In contrast, if the drug produces unpleasant side effects, the physician may be seen unconsciously as a sadistic tormentor from the patient's past. Clinically, one may see a patient respond differently to the same drug at different points in time, either responding positively to a drug that previously produced no effect or, conversely, obtaining no response to a drug that previously provided amelioration of symptoms. While some of this variation may be due to drug effect, it may also be related to transference and unconscious fantasies.

For example, a schizophrenic patient was receiving IM antipsychotic medication every two weeks. The female nurse administered the injection for several months, and the patient's symptoms were well controlled by the medication. Abruptly, the patient had an exacerbation of psychotic symptoms, demanded that the injections be stopped, and attempted to discuss his sexual feelings for the nurse with his male therapist. He agreed to receive the injection only if it were given by the male therapist. His psychotic symptoms were again well controlled for several months; however, he then refused to have the injection administered by the male therapist but agreed to permit the female nurse to administer the injection. He then discussed at length with the nurse his concerns about the male therapist's homosexual tendencies. It appeared that in this individual, the administering of the medication was sexualized and alternated between heterosexual and homosexual fantasies, depending upon who was giving the injection. More significantly, he had symptomatic exacerbations primarily depending upon his transference fantasies rather than the pharmacologic effect of the drug.

The drug prescribed by the physician may come to represent the physician; in very regressed, psychotic patients, this may be a conscious fantasy. One psychotic patient remarked that when he felt empty, alone, frightened, or dejected, he could simply take his bottle of medication from his pocket, see the physician's name on the label, and feel a renewed strength as if the physician were there with him. To this patient, the medication served much the same purpose as a child's favorite blanket; it was a transitional object that provided comfort in the absence of the real object. In nonpsychotic patients, the same unconscious fantasy may be present, and the taking of the medication may fulfill an unconscious drive to incorporate the physician. Such positive transference and fantasy gratification may serve to aid the patient in identifying with the physician and his or her strength.

For those patients who are hesitant to accept psychological explanation or in whom feelings of closeness with the therapist create intense anxiety, the prescribing of medication may provide an avenue through which the patient can displace any benefits that are being obtained from the interaction with the physician. Some patients need such a convenient source of displacement until they can develop enough psychological mindedness to appreciate psychodynamic issues; still other patients will never be able to understand or acknowledge any benefit except from the medication.

With these general comments, it is important to understand the specific implications of the treatment in both insight-oriented and supportive psychotherapy.

Implications in Supportive Psychotherapy

Medical psychiatric therapies are commonly prescribed with supportive psychotherapy, with the physician and the patient having tacitly agreed, in a number of instances, that the patient's symptoms are largely biological in origin, or can, in large measure, best be treated by currently available medical therapies. The general strategy and overall principles are in keeping with the goals of supportive psychotherapy—namely, to deal with the realistic situation, to maintain a positive rapport and relationship with the patient, to reduce psychic conflict and strengthen defenses, and to reestablish a dynamic equilibrium. The unconscious transference responses are permitted to remain unconscious and do not become a matter for scrutiny and understanding.

Psychobiological treatments are given more frequently with supportive psychotherapy, and such action supports the concept of the physician as a powerful healing figure and also aids in the formation of a positive rapport. The personality and drives, or drive derivatives, of the particular patient are again important in determining the manner in which the medication is prescribed and instructions are given. If, for example, on the one hand the patient is a passive-dependent individual, it may be advisable to give the drug on a several-times-per-day basis in order to gratify the dependence. On the other hand, if the individual has reaction formations against underlying dependence needs, it may be advisable to give the medication once per day in order not to challenge the defense against the dependence. If the patient is the type of individual who needs to feel in control of all situations, it may be advisable to permit the patient more or less to control the medication time schedule or to take it as necessary. In contrast, if the patient is an individual who wants and needs a large amount of external direction, it may be advisable to suggest strongly specific times to take the medication. The predominant emphasis must continually take into account a strengthening of defenses, partial drive gratification, and the establishment of a positive rapport and working relationship.

Implications in Insight Psychotherapy

By the act of undertaking intensive, insight-oriented psychotherapy, the therapist and patient have tacitly agreed that the patient's symptoms are largely psychogenic in origin and that they are approaching and treating the patient's difficulties by freeing the patient from unconscious conflicts. However, at times, some patients will experience too much anxiety to function effectively in the treatment situation or will experience severe sleep disturbance or other symptoms that can most rapidly and effectively be treated by a psychoactive drug. Prior to prescribing a drug, the therapist must consider that he or she is beginning an active manipulation of the treatment and is departing from the role of a neutral observer. The administering of the drug usually will involve the gratification of an unconscious drive, or drive derivative, and this may be deleterious or advantageous, depending upon several circumstances. If, for example, the patient has a drive or wish to defeat the therapist, the prescribing of a drug may unconsciously mean to the patient that he or she has defeated the therapist. In addition, the effect of the drug may make mobilization of unconscious conflict more difficult. Paradoxically, one goal of insight-oriented psychotherapy is to increase the patient's anxiety and frustration tolerance; with the prescribing of a drug, the therapist is increasing the anxiety tolerance by pharmacological means instead of insight. While some therapists would believe that the transference would be contaminated to the degree that further work would be significantly compromised, still others, like Ostow (19), would suggest that as long as the reality of the situation was separated from the fantasies of the situation, no significant harm had been done.

If a patient in insight-oriented psychotherapy requires or would benefit from a psychobiological treatment, some therapists prefer to refer the patient to a colleague for the prescribing of the treatment. This would be done with the reasoning that such a referral would not contaminate the transference and working alliance with the therapist. Other therapists like Ostow (19) feel that the treating therapist is the only person in a position to comprehend the total situation and to know what treatment is indicated and would therefore prescribe the medical psychiatric treatments as well.

SUMMARY

This chapter has attempted to summarize psychodynamic and psychoanalytic issues that may be involved in the administering of medical psychiatric treatments. In order to administer medical psychiatric treatments most effectively, the physician-patient relationship, placebo effect, the type of psychotherapy that is being provided, the nature of the patient's personality structure, and other relevant psychodynamic parameters must always be considered as important therapeutic factors.

REFERENCES

1. *Dorland's Illustrated Medical Dictionary.* Philadelphia: W.B. Saunders, 1974.
2. Shapiro, A.K. Factors contributing to the placebo effect: Their implications for psychotherapy. *Am. J. Psychother.* 18:73–88, 1961.
3. Amsterdam, E.A.; Wolfson, S.; and Gorlin, R. New aspects of the placebo response in angina pectoris. *Am. J. Cardiol.* 24:305–306, 1969.
4. Traut, E.F., and Passarelli, E.W. Placebos in the treatment of rheumatoid arthritis and other rheumatic conditions. *Ann. Rheum. Dis.* 16:18–21, 1957.
5. Grenfell, R.F.; Briggs, A.H.; and Holland, W.C. Antihypertensive drugs evaluated in a controlled double-blind study. *South. Med. J.* 56:1410–1416, 1963.
6. Backman, H.; Kalliola, H.; and Ostling, G. Placebo effect in peptic ulcer and other gastroduodenal disorders. *Gastroenterologia* 94:11–20, 1960.
7. Beecher, H.K. The powerful placebo. *JAMA* 159:1602–1606, 1955.
8. Baldwin, H.S. How to evaluate a new drug. *Am. J. Med.* 17:722–727, 1954.
9. Loranger, A.W.; Prout, C.T.; and White, M.A. The placebo effect in psychiatric drug research. *JAMA* 176:920–925, 1961.
10. Rashkis, H.A., and Smarr, E.R. Psychopharmacotherapeutic research: A triadistic approach. *Arch. Neurol. Psychiatry* 77:202–209, 1957.
11. Lesse, S. Placebo reactions in psychotherapy. *Dis. Nerv. Syst.* 23:313–319, 1962.
12. Benson, H., and Epstein, M.O. The placebo effect: A neglected asset in the care of patients. *JAMA* 232:1225–1227, 1975.
13. Sarwer-Foner, G. Psychoanalytic theories of activity-passivity conflicts and of the continuum of ego defenses. *Arch. Neurol. Psychiat.* 78:413, 1957.
14. Sarwer-Foner, G. Some therapeutic aspects of the use of neuroleptic drugs in schizophrenia, borderline states, and in the short term psychotherapy of the neuroses. In *The Dynamics of Psychiatric Drug Therapy*, Sarwer-Foner, G., ed. Springfield, Ill.: Charles C Thomas, 1960.
15. Winkelman, N.W. Chlorpromazine and prochlorperazine during psychoanalytic psychotherapy: Theoretical formulations concerning the ego, energy relationships, anxiety, and the psychic therapeutic process. In *The Dynamics of Psychiatric Drug Therapy*, Sarwer-Foner, G., ed. Springfield, Ill.: Charles C Thomas, 1960.
16. Azima, H. Psychodynamic and psychotherapeutic problems in connection with imipramine intake. *J. Mental Science* 101:74, 1961.
17. Azima, H.; Azima, F.; and Durost, H. Psychoanalytic formulations of effects of reserpine on schizophrenic organization. *Arch. Gen. Psychiatry* 1:662, 1959.
18. Ostow, M. *Drugs in Psychoanalysis and Psychotherapy.* New York: Basic Books, 1962.
19. Ostow, M. *The Psychodynamic Approach to Drug Therapy.* New York: Van Nostrand Reinhold, 1979.

PART III

Future Directions

CHAPTER 12

Future Directions for Biological Exploration of Psychiatric Disorders

Richard Jed Wyatt
and
Daniel R. Weinberger

The period from the mid- to late 1950s was a time of great change in psychiatry. The unifying theory of psychoanalysis was at its peak of popularity, behavior modification techniques were formally being introduced, and deinstitutionalization programs were beginning. Most important, however, for both the treatment of and research into the causes of the major psychiatric disorders, efficacious psychotropic drugs were introduced. Since that time, the treatment benefits of the psychotropic drugs have been widely publicized and discussed. Less well known is how important these agents have been for increasing our basic understanding of the disorders they treat. Although there was a relative profusion of drugs—neuroleptics, tricyclic antidepressants, MAO inhibitors, anxiolytics, and lithium—there was no knowledge of their mechanism of action, and the then current notions about the etiologies of psychiatric disorders could not be easily adapted to explain the results these drugs produced.

New ideas developed. Investigations examining the new psychotropic agents were like finding a glove on the street; if the researchers could learn about the contours of the inside of the glove, they might be able to say something about the hand it fits. Immediately, researchers began to ask questions about what systems the new psychotropic drugs altered. For example, because the agents have profound effects on the monoamines, the amine (norepinephrine and serotonin) hypotheses of mood disorders and the dopamine hypothesis of schizophrenia developed. More recently, based on the mechanism of action of the benzodiazepines, the GABA hypothesis of anxiety was proposed.

Given the hypothesis-generating power of these drugs and their profound effects on neurotransmitters, much of the research in biological psychiatry since the 1950s has focused on the synapse. The synapse, the fragile communication center at the juncture of two neurons, has been thought to be the Achilles heel of the brain. Dysfunction at synapses was thought to be responsible for a number of psychiatric disorders. Research in biological psychiatry since the late 1950s has concentrated on this Achilles heel and could be called the era of psychosynaptology.

Prior to the era of psychosynaptology, however, biological psychiatry centered on more traditional neurochemical, neurophysiological, and neuroanatomical approaches. For the most part, work on the synapse replaced these research interests. While investigation of the synapse continues today, a number of recently developed techniques are returning psychiatric attention to earlier areas of inquiry. These technological innovations present the opportunity to examine subtle brain structure and function as never before. These new techniques allow for both static and dynamic in vivo investigation of patients and appropriate reference groups. In the sections that follow, we describe some of these techniques, how they are being used, and how they might be used in the future.

TESTING A SYNAPTIC HYPOTHESIS (THE DOPAMINE HYPOTHESIS OF SCHIZOPHRENIA) USING COMPUTED TOMOGRAPHY TO DICHOTOMIZE PATIENTS

Since Jacobi's and Winkler's 1927 use of pneumoencephalography (1), investigators have described large cerebral ventricles in the brains of schizophrenic patients (for review, see 2). These findings gained relatively little notice until recently, when large ventricles were again reported using computed tomography (CT) (Figure 12.1). Even the first CT scan study (3) in schizophrenic patients, which reported large ventricles with almost no overlap between patients and controls, generated considerable skepticism from the medical community. Over fifteen subsequent controlled studies (reviewed by 4) also demonstrated that there appears to be at least a subgroup of schizophrenic patients with large ventricles. Two reported controlled studies (5,6), however, have not found this difference.

While it is possible that the large ventricles are due to some aspect of being schizophrenic such as hospitalization or medication treatment, the available evidence suggests that these factors are not relevant. Indeed, three studies (7,8,9) found several first-break patients with large ventricles whose exposure to medications and hospitals was minimal at the time of their CT scan.

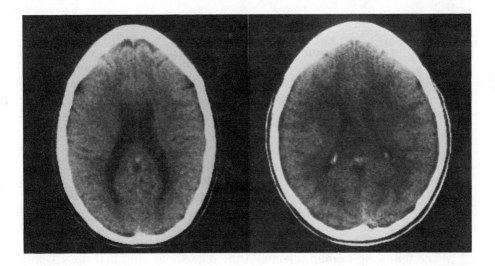

Figure 12.1 CT Scan from Normal (left) and Large (right) Ventricle Schizophrenic Patients.

Type I and Type II Schizophrenia

Crow (10) suggests that two overlapping schizophrenic syndromes may be related to the finding that some patients have normal and some have abnormal CT scans. Type I (with normal scans) is typified by paranoid schizophrenia, good prognosis schizophrenia, schizophreniform psychosis, and reactive psychosis. Type II (large ventricle patients) resembles simple schizophrenia or defect-state schizophrenia. In between these two types and overlapping with them is hebephrenic schizophrenia. Although at times the type II syndrome may coexist with type I, Crow proposes that type II patients are usually at first type I. Crow also postulates that type I schizophrenia is related to a functional excess (our words) of dopamine. A functional excess of dopamine, however, could mean several pathological conditions: too much dopamine, increased dopamine turnover and neuronal firing, increased receptor activity, or increased transduction of the message at the receiving neuron. But, in fact, Crow's group (11), as well as others (reviewed by 12), have found increased neuroleptic binding sites (presumably reflecting dopamine receptor number) in the brains of some schizophrenic patients who have come to autopsy. They have, furthermore, correlated these post mortem findings with clinical evidence of the type I syndrome in the same sample of patients.

The Dopamine Hypothesis

The hypothesis that schizophrenia might be caused by a functional excess of dopamine has been one of the predominant themes in schizophrenia research for a number of years. While there is considerable indirect support of the dopamine hypothesis, testing it directly has been difficult. Thus, a refinement of the hypothesis based on dichotomization of patients into those with functional excesses of dopamine and those without is most welcome.

There are a number of possible variants of this refinement (13). One of these is that only the patients with normal ventricles have an overactive dopamine system; alternatively, perhaps the patients with large ventricles have a relatively underactive dopamine system. Inadequate dopaminergic function could be due to a specific dysfunction of a part of the dopamine system or it could be due to a more generalized process, which is reflected neuroanatomically by the large ventricles.

The following examines some of the data suggesting that the CT scan data can be used to divide patients into meaningful subgroups with regard to dopamine function.

Negative Symptoms and Dopamine

Over the years, a number of clinicians have wrestled with the issue of what the primary alteration is in schizophrenic patients. To some clinicians, it has made sense to divide the symptoms into positive (delusions, hallucinations, formal thought disorder, and bizarre behavior) as well as negative symptoms or defect state (affective flattening, alogia, avolition, impaired attention, and impoverished thinking). This division was first used by Hughlings Jackson (14) (not with regard to schizophrenia) and has been amplified by Andreasen et al. (15). In Johnstone et al.'s (3) original CT study, they noted that there were more negative symptoms in the large ventricle patients than in the normal ventricle group. Andreasen et al. (16) also found more negative and fewer positive symptoms in their large ventricle group compared with their normal ventricle schizophrenic patients. Affective flattening and formal thought disorder, however, were about equally prominent in both groups. Finally, Takahashi et al. (17), in a multihospital study in Japan, found a relationship between atrophy and nonproductive symptoms.

There is some reason to believe that this defect state is not just due to an absence of dopamine's involvement in defect schizophrenia but to a relatively underactive dopamine system. The first piece of evidence for this comes from our knowledge of Parkinson's disease that presents with a number of negativelike symptoms and is due to a loss of neurons in the nigrostriatal dopamine system. A delayed outcome of the flulike epidemic of the last part of the 1920s, which often led to Economo's encephalitis, was Parkinson's syndrome. It is of some interest to read descriptions of Economo's encephalitis.

In Economo's encephalitis (18), or encephalitis lethargica, there was a hypokinetic state. There was often a striking psychological deterioration that Economo called "psychic torpor." Hohman (19) states that the stuporous reactions were mistaken for schizophrenia, but he differentiates it from schizophrenia because of the schizophrenic patients' ability to use their voluntary nervous system and the presence of tremor and rigidity in the encephalitic patients. Grossman (19) cited the preference, in some patients, to be left alone, restlessness, inability to concentrate, and lack of interest in their surroundings as late sequelae. This was also recognized by *DSM-II* (20), which described some patients who lived through the disease as having "apparent indifference to persons and events ordinarily of emotional significance, such as the death of a family member" (p. 27). While many of these patients had a loss of brain dopamine, they had destruction of nondopaminergic brain structures as well.

Another piece of evidence comes from experience with neuroleptic medications. Akinesia, a neuroleptic side effect, usually thought to consist of decreased gestures, shortened stride, and rigid posture, has been described by Klein et al. (21) as also being a behavioral state. There may be a lack of spontaneous speech, apathy, and lack of goal directedness, all of which are corrected by lowering the neuroleptic doses or possibly by using antiparkinsonian medications. These negative symptoms appear to be the result of dopamine blockade.

Another area producing supporting evidence for negative symptoms being associated with a loss of dopamine comes from animal studies. Rats given the neurotoxin 6-hydroxydopamine lose their dopamine neurons. If the lesion is made unilaterally into the dopamine neuronal ascending bundles, the animal develops a syndrome that has been called unilateral sensory neglect; there is a profound deficit in orienting toward sensory stimulation on the side opposite the lesion. It is thought that this deficit is due neither to a primary motor nor sensory defect but to a failure in a sensory motor integrating mechanism (22). Wise (23), in fact, believes, based on studies of neuroleptics given to rats, that there is "a selective attenuation of motivational arousal which is (a) critical for goal-directed behavior, (b) normally induced by reinforcers and associated environmental stimuli, and (c) normally accompanied by the subjective experience of pleasure" (p. 39). He likens this neuroleptic-(antidopaminergic) induced behavior to human anhedonia.

Prolactin Response to Dopamine Agonists

The secretion of prolactin appears to be under dopaminergic control in the tuberoinfundibular system so that increased dopaminergic function decreases prolactin release and decreased function increases prolactin release. Thus, dopamine agonists like bromocriptine decrease prolactin release and are used clinically for this purpose. Likewise, neuroleptic agents, which block dopamine receptors, increase prolactin release (24). A number of investigators have attempted to examine brain dopamine function by measuring resting prolactin serum concentrations and have come to the conclusion that no evidence of an abnormality exists in schizophrenia. However, Kleinman et al. (25) divided their unmedicated chronic schizophrenic patient sample into those with large ventricles and those with normal-size ventricles. The resting prolactin concentrations were inversely correlated with the thought disorder syndrome on the brief psychiatric rating scale consistent with the dopamine hypothesis. This was found, however, only in patients with small ventricles. The patients with large ventricles had no significant correlation between their resting serum prolactin concentrations and thought disorder, while the patients with normal ventricles had a significant inverse correlation ($r = -.72$). As a group, the patients with normal ventricles had slightly greater thought disorder as measured on the brief psychiatric rating scale than the large ventricle group. Since the thought disorder syndrome on the rating scale consists primarily of positive symptoms, this difference might be expected from Crow's prediction.

The inverse correlation of prolactin with thought disorder suggests that, in the normal ventricle patients, dopaminergic function is related to the positive symptoms of the disorder. The absence of a correlation in the large ventricle patients makes it seem unlikely that these patients have a hyperdopaminergic system.

Growth Hormone Response to Dopamine Agonists

GH secretion is controlled in part by dopamine activity, and one way of examining a potential dopamine deficit is by looking at dopamine's influence over GH secretion in schizophrenia. During daytime hours, GH secretion can be increased by dopamine agonists. During sleep, however, GH release appears to be independent of dopamine control (26) and peaks shortly after sleep onset. Therefore, if the dopamine system is dysfunctional in some schizophrenic patients, we might expect to find normal sleep-related GH function with abnormal dopamine-related GH release. Unfortunately, the data are confusing.

Vigneri et al. (27), for example, studied three chronic schizophrenic patients and found them to have normal GH responses to insulin (insulin-related GH response is mediated, at least in part, by dopamine) but relatively constant GH concentrations at night with no peak at sleep onset. Murri et al. (28) had similar nighttime GH findings in four chronic schizophrenic patients. In contrast, Syvälahti and Pekkarinen (29) studied ten chronic schizophrenic patients (duration of illness one to twenty years) and five patients with epilepsy who were given substantial doses of antipsychotic medication. As a group, the schizophrenic patients were not different than the epileptic patients in the pattern of their peak GH response to sleep. If anything, four of the schizophrenic patients had high peak responses. Although as a whole, the sleep-related GH data are meager and inconsistent, the Syvälahti and

Pekkarinen study is consistent with existence of a normal or even slightly hyperactive sleep-related GH relationship.

The daytime dopamine agonist studies are only slightly more consistent than the sleep studies. Ettigi et al. (30) administered 0.75 mg apomorphine to seventeen chronically hospitalized schizophrenics whose chronic neuroleptic therapy had been withdrawn for from two to fifteen weeks. Compared with a group of twenty-one control men (nine hospitalized alcoholics and twelve normals), the schizophrenics had lower apomorphine-stimulated GH responses (11.9 versus 20.8).

Tamminga et al. (31) found a blunted peak GH response in nine drug-free chronic schizophrenics (four with tardive dyskinesia, five without) compared with twelve controls given 500 mg of L-dopa orally. Also, there was a trend toward a decrease in GH response to 0.75 mg (subcutaneously) of apomorphine in schizophrenic patients.

Rotrosen et al. (32) found a bimodal distribution (some patients having very high and some very low) to apomorphine (0.5 mg subcutaneously) for peak GH response in a group of twenty-five chronic and subchronic male schizophrenics compared with sixteen controls. The patients had been taken off neuroleptics seven days prior to testing.

Meltzer et al. (24) gave 0.75 mg of apomorphine subcutaneously to fifteen normal controls and to fourteen schizophrenic patients. GH response was significantly higher in patients ill less than four years compared with those ill longer than four years. The controls' GH response tended to be in the middle.

Thus, it appears that some chronic schizophrenic patients have little GH response to dopamine agonists. Some chronic schizophrenics also appear to have an intact sleep-related GH system. If patients with large ventricles are found to have a blunted GH response to dopamine agonists but normal sleep GH, it would suggest these patients have a dysfunctional dopaminergic system. What is needed is a study in which a series of patients is examined for CT scan abnormalities, as well as sleep-related and dopamine agonist GH function.

Apomorphine

Apomorphine is a short-acting dopamine agonist. If given in small enough doses, it should act on the presynaptic dopamine receptor and decrease that neuron's firing rate. At slightly higher doses, apomorphine acts on the postsynaptic receptor and behaves as if it were dopamine. Thus, it is not surprising to find reports that apomorphine may make schizophrenic patients better (33,34,35), worse, or unchanged (36). In one preliminary study (37), a small dose of apomorphine (0.01 mg/kg subcutaneously) was given to ten chronic schizophrenic patients who also had CT scans. Of the six patients with abnormal CT scans, none became worse. Three of the four patients with normal scans became worse. If confirmed in a larger study, this would suggest that at least some schizophrenics with abnormal CT scans respond differently to apomorphine than normal CT scan patients. Which response is abnormal is of course unclear. Unfortunately, also, the data on the psychologic effects of apomorphine in nonschizophrenic individuals are minimal. Information that is available, however, suggests that apomorphine does not induce a schizophrenic-like psychosis (reviewed in 38).

The Jeste et al. study (37) suggests that increasing dopamine activity compounds the psychotic symptoms only of patients with normal ventricles. The production of increased symptomatology in the normal ventricular schizophrenic patients could either be due to some intrinsic characteristics of the patients or to the fact that the neuroleptic therapy the patients had received produced a dopamine receptor supersensitivity that did not occur in patients with large ventricles.

Response to Neuroleptics

Only a small number of studies have examined response to neuroleptic drugs in light of knowledge about ventricular size. In the first such study, Weinberger et al. (39) examined ten chronic schizophrenic patients with large ventricles and ten similar patients with normal-size ventricles. The patients were admitted to the study because they had poor responses to a variety of treatment modalities and were willing to undergo research protocols. Brief psychiatric rating scales were filled out by nurses at the end of a four-week drug-free period and at the end of eight weeks of neuroleptic treatment. The ten patients with normal-size ventricles improved on their scores by a mean of 27.5 units, while the patients with large ventricles essentially had no change (an improvement of 0.3 unit).

A larger unpublished study by this same group (Weinberger et al.) has validated the original finding. Similarly, a study by Schulz et al. (9) found a greater response to neuroleptics in a normal-size-ventricle group of schizophrenic patients than in a group with large ventricles. It will be of considerable importance to determine how generalizable this finding is to other groups of schizophrenic patients.

If confirmed in other schizophrenic patient populations, these findings may have theoretical implications. For example, they can support the notion (10) that patients with normal ventricles have a disorder closely linked to dopaminergic activity and that the neuroleptics, by blocking the brain's dopamine receptors, decrease symptoms. The corollary of this interpretation is that the patients with large ventricles do not have a dopamine-related disorder. Against this notion is the variety of different diseases where there is a favorable response to neuroleptics and in which no primary abnormality in dopamine metabolism seems likely. These include Huntington's chorea, dementias, affective disorders, insomnia, and even anxiety disorders. It would seem that by toning down the dopaminergic system in these disorders and, perhaps, in schizophrenia, the symptoms are less floridly expressed. It does not mean, however, that the primary deficit is dopaminergic (40).

Blinking

Spontaneous eye blinking appears, in part, to be under dopaminergic control. Spontaneous blinking is markedly decreased in patients with Parkinson's disease and, in fact, is a hallmark of the disorder. In both humans and rhesus monkeys, pharmacological agents that promote dopaminergic function increase eye blinking, and agents that decrease dopaminergic function decrease eye blinking (41).

Unobtrusive monitoring of eye blinks may be a good index to central nervous system dopaminergic function. Karson et al. (42), monitoring eye blinks, found a significant increase in blink rate in a group of forty-three unmedicated chronic schizophrenic patients compared with thirty-nine age-matched normals. When the patients were placed on neuroleptics, their spontaneous blink rate decreased from thirty-one to twenty-four blinks per minute. After the schizophrenic patients were divided into those with large ventricles (ten patients) and those with normal-size ventricles (thirty-three patients), the patients with the large ventricles were found not to have a decrease in blink rate when placed on neuroleptics, while the normal-size-ventricle patients decreased from thirty-one to twenty-three blinks per minute. The failure of the large ventricle patients to suppress their blinking as might be expected with dopamine blockade suggests that the dopaminergic function in these patients is abnormal.

Discussion

The ability to use CT scans to subgroup schizophrenic patients has led to some preliminary testing of two refined dopamine hypotheses of schizophrenia. Certainly with these more refined hypotheses in hand, more specific testing can take place in the future. The ability to distinguish clearly patients who have normal-size and large ventricles presents research leverage that was not previously available. The same leverage is available for testing other notions about psychiatric disorders. As described in the following section, the CT scanner is just the first of what promises to be many new developments that will increase our knowledge of what the living brain looks like and how it functions in health and disease.

NEWER WAYS OF SEEING THE BRAIN

The radiologist, using a CT scan, might be compared with the gross anatomist who examines the size, shape, and relationship of brain structures but only guesses at their qualitative and quantitative functions. Since the 1920s, numerous radiographic techniques have been developed to overcome the static nature of the information the gross anatomist, the histologist, and by extension, the CT scan can produce. Innovations for the examination of the dynamic nature of the brain are positron emission tomography (PET) scanners, nuclear magnetic resonance (NMR) spectrometry, and cortical electrical mapping.

Positron Emission Tomography

The feature that most prominently distinguishes PET from conventional X-rays and the CT scan is the internal location of the radiation source. With PET, instead of the radiation coming from outside the head, the radiation comes from within the head, and with proper biochemical and physiological skills, the experimenter can manipulate the source of radiation to examine specific areas of interest. Thus, chemical probes can be targeted at specific sites within the brain or be differentially metabolized by different parts of the brain, providing information about brain function never before available. Using CT scan technology and mathematics, investigators can produce an image of any transverse section—horizontal, sagittal, or coronal. The imaging of the internal radiation emissions depends upon the special properties of annihilation radiation that result when positrons are absorbed in matter. For example, 18-fluorine has an unstable nucleus due to a deficiency of neutrons and emits a positive electron or positron (beta+) (see Figure 12.2). The emitted positron

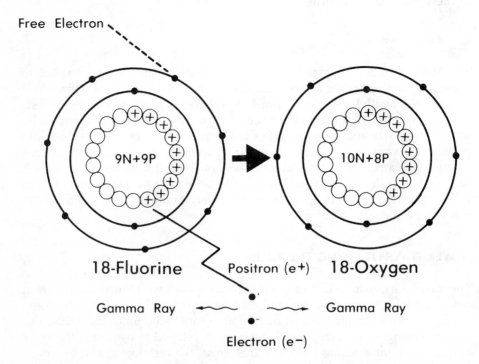

Figure 12.2 Decay of 18-Fluorine to 18-Oxygen by Positron Emission. The Positron Interacts with an Electron with Annihilation of Their Combined Mass. The Energy of Annihilation Is Released as Gamma or X-rays.

travels 2 to 6 mm before losing its energy. As the positron slows down, it collides with an electron (beta−). This collision results in an annihilation of their combined mass. The energy of annihilation is converted into two photons or gamma rays traveling at a 180-degree angle from each other. The high energy of these photons allows them to penetrate easily through tissue. The distance traveled by the positron before annihilation, however (approximately 2 mm for 18-fluorine), defines the ultimate resolution of the image. Thus, for 18-fluorine, regardless of the quality of the machine, the resolution can never be better than the distance it takes the 18-fluorine positron to decay.

The two gamma rays produced by the annihilation of the positron are detected by two of many gamma ray collectors (Figure 12.3) positioned in a ring that encircles the head. Since the motions of the gamma rays are in exactly opposite directions from one another, the detectors are electronically programmed to make counts only of two gamma rays colliding with the detectors at the same time (coincidence counting), 180 degrees apart.

PET is especially appealing to psychiatry, given a variety of developments. Here, we cite some of the most important, many of which are preliminary or problematic and are being refined.

1. Brain physiologists have begun asking appropriate and testable questions related to normal and diseased brains. For example, as discussed in the section on CT scanning, one of the leading hypotheses of schizophrenia is the dopamine hypothesis. Direct testing of this hypothesis has been very difficult. The closest direct test has come from researchers using autopsied brains of deceased schizophrenics and controls. For the most part, these studies have found an increase in the number of neuroleptic binding sites in the brains of schizophrenics compared with controls. This finding has usually been interpreted as reflecting an increased number of dopamine receptors in

COINCIDENCE DETECTION

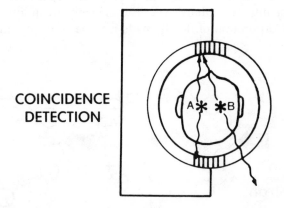

Figure 12.3 Coincidence Detection of Gamma Rays Produced by Annihilation of Positron. Gamma Rays, which Travel in an 180-Degree Direction from One Another, Collide with Gamma Ray Detectors at the Same Time (A) and Are Counted. The Gamma Ray Emitters at (B) Are Not Counted Because One Gamma Ray Misses the Detector.

the brains of schizophrenics. Unfortunately for the interpretation of these studies, most schizophrenic patients who come to autopsy have been given neuroleptics for prolonged periods of time during their life. Since there is considerable animal evidence that chronic neuroleptic use increases the number of binding sites for neuroleptics, it is difficult to determine if the autopsy findings of increased neuroleptic binding sites are primary or secondary to neuroleptic use in this disorder. It would be ideal to examine the number of neuroleptic binding sites prior to a patient ever receiving a neuroleptic. With PET scanners, investigators are trying to use 18-fluorine-labeled neuroleptics for this purpose. If schizophrenic patients who have never been given neuroleptics have more binding of 18-fluorine spiroperidol than other psychotic patients or normals, it would suggest that the autopsy finding of increased binding sites might be related to the cause rather than being secondary to the disorder.

A preliminary example of this kind of study was done by Comar et al. (43) who gave 11-carbon-labeled chlorpromazine (11-carbon, like 18-fluorine, is a positron emitter) to a group of twenty-two schizophrenic patients. There was no comparison group, and the primary result of the study was to demonstrate very rapid uptake of chlorpromazine throughout the brain with no specific brain site taking up more neuroleptic than another. Future studies, with better neuroleptic ligands, will undoubtedly give greater detail and allow discrimination among various patients and controls.

2. The cyclotrons and linear accelerators required for the production of positron-emitting radionuclides (Figure 12.4) are becoming smaller and inexpensive enough to purchase and operate in selected medical environments. At best, however, these machines are still relatively large, clumsy, and expensive to purchase and operate. Undoubtedly, many further refinements will be made that will make them attractive for both research and general clinical use.

3. The developing science of rapidly incorporating the positron-emitting isotope into radiopharmaceuticals is being streamlined. This process requires the incorporation of newly made isotopes into pharmaceuticals in a

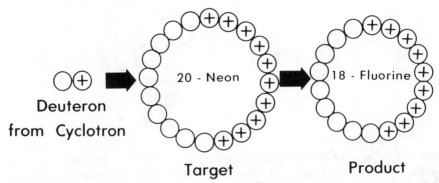

Figure 12.4   Production of 18-Fluorine from a 20-Neon Target in a Cyclotron Using Deuteron Bombardment.

sterile environment within a few minutes. (The physical half-life of 18-fluorine is 110 minutes and that of 11-carbon is only 20 minutes.)

In the Comar et al. (43) study using 11-carbon-labeled chlorpromazine, it took thirty-five minutes for the synthetic process of chemically coupling the 11-carbon into chlorpromazine after the 11-carbon was produced in a cyclotron by proton bombardment of nitrogen gas. Since almost two half-lives had elapsed, this meant that only about one-fourth of the original 11-carbon remained at the time of injection into the patients.

4. Detection systems for monitoring the state of the positron-emitting radiopharmaceuticals are being perfected. Most of the available detection systems, however, give reliable data only when brain volumes of 10 cm^3 are examined.

5. Mathematical models have been developed to determine the source of the radiopharmaceutical decay within the brain and for reconstructing brain images. These models use similar mathematics to that used by CT scanners. Unfortunately, most of the software is of a proprietary nature and not easily available to the scientist.

6. Mathematical modeling has been worked out to give the absolute value of metabolism of some substances. This modeling has been relatively well designed in the 2-deoxyglucose method, primarily by Dr. Louis Sokoloff and colleagues at the National Institute of Mental Health (44), and other systems are still being developed. Even with the 2-deoxyglucose method, there is considerable argument about some of the assumptions made (45,46).

7. Sophisticated computers exist that can use these models to restructure the data in a truly quantitative and regional manner. The amount of data and its manipulation for each PET scan is vast, and on-line computers allowing for such analysis are too costly for most laboratories. Eventually, though, the cost of machines that can analyze such large data bases will decrease. Also, sufficient user experience and intelligent software that will selectively collect and analyze data will have to be developed.

8. Statistical and display techniques to interpret the data are being developed and improved. This is a very primitive science that largely depends on development in the areas discussed in points one through seven. Some excellent attempts have been made by Buchsbaum et al. (47) (Figure 12.5).

In addition to the problems cited, only a small number of radionuclides possess the requisite properties suitable for use by this scanning procedure. A radionuclide must be capable of being incorporated into biologically interesting material without appreciable alteration of the function of that material. The radionuclide also must decay with a short half-life so that the dose of radiation is low and repeat studies can be performed.

To date, the most widely used radionuclide has been 18-fluorine-labeled 2-deoxy-D-glucose to determine regional glucose consumption. Because of the deoxy group, this form of glucose cannot be metabolized past phosphorylation through the action of hexokinase and is thus trapped in the cells of the brain (Figure 12.6). The amount of tracer 18-fluorine-2-deoxyglucose

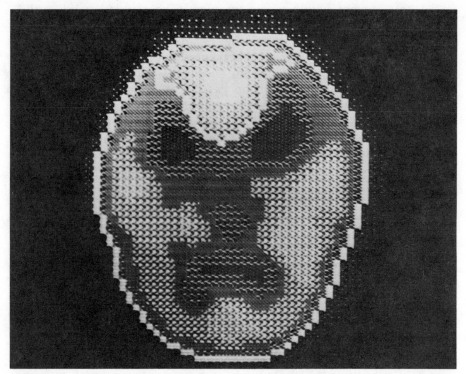

Figure 12.5 PET Scan Using 18-Fluorine-2-Deoxyglucose in Schizophrenic Patient. Scan Is through Thalamus, Splenum, Cingulate Gyrus Anteriorally, and Calcarine Sulcus Posteriorly at Mid-ventricular Level. Lighter Area Indicates Greater Utilization. Computer Has Outlined (White Posterior Line) Area (Calcarine Sulcus) of Greatest Glucose Use. (Courtesy of Monte Buchsbaum, M.D., University of California, Irvine.)

accumulated in the cells is proportional to the metabolic activity of the cell. The metabolic activity, in turn, can be determined from the number of positrons emitted from the brain region of interest.

Several important problems exist with the 2-deoxyglucose method, perhaps the most important being that it takes forty to sixty minutes for the

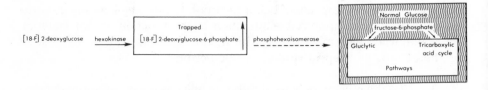

Figure 12.6 Metabolism of 18-Fluorine-2-Deoxyglucose in the Brain. 2-Deoxyglucose Becomes Trapped and Builds up Because It Cannot Be Metabolized by Phosphohexoisomerase. The Amount of 2-Deoxyglucose Built Up in a Given Time Period Reflects the Rate of Glucose Metabolism.

unmetabolized substance to clear the blood and tissue. Current scanning techniques require waiting for this to occur. Therefore, transient phenomena cannot be examined, and even subtle changes in brain activity during this long time span can greatly alter the results.

While solutions to the technical problems continue to be pursued, funding for PET scanners presents its own hurdles. It is estimated that the cost of developing a center containing all the necessary parts ranges from $5 to $10 million, with very large sustaining costs. A single 2-deoxyglucose study in a single patient costs approximately $5,000. While no center, which also includes psychiatric patients available for study, has been a complete success, there appear to be several centers on the verge of contributing new knowledge about psychiatric disorders using the PET scan.

Nuclear Magnetic Resonance

Probably of ultimately greater practical utility, compared with either the CT or the PET scan, is NMR imaging. NMR imaging will be less costly than the PET scan, will not produce the exposure to radiation that is inherent in both CT and PET scanners, will give considerably better resolution than the PET scan, and in some cases, will give better resolution than the CT scan. A form of contrast media can be used to enhance the NMR image, and it is possible that tracers can be developed so that the scan gives dynamic information similar to the PET scan and unlike the CT scan. The only risk is the unknown effect, if any, of passing magnetic and radiofrequency energy through the brain.

NMR is a technique for measuring the magnetic properties of individual atomic nuclei. Although first developed by Block and Purcell, who were awarded the 1952 Nobel Prize in Physics for their work, and used for the last thirty years by analytic chemists, NMR's application to medicine is still in its infancy. It appears, nevertheless, to have greater sensitivity for detecting soft-tissue differences than X-ray techniques like the CT scan. This is particularly valuable for brain imaging where distinguishing between gray and white matter and separating brain nuclei are important (Figures 12.7 and 12.8). Change of tissue structure such as occurs in malignancies, degenerative diseases, atrophy, and in loss of blood supply should also be detectable on NMR scans. Finally, because NMR is not subject to bone artifacts like CT scanners are, it will be much easier to see areas surrounded by bone, such as the posterior fossa and spinal cord.

In addition to the greater resolution of some soft tissue than is available from the CT scan, NMR may eventually offer the opportunity to study the dynamics of specific chemical constituents of the brain, as well as exogenously introduced substances. Furthermore, it should be possible to measure the amount of blood flow through the major vessels of the brain. To a great extent, the ultimate power of NMR to give us new details about the living brain is only limited by its considerable expense and the ingenuity of engineers in designing more sophisticated scanners.

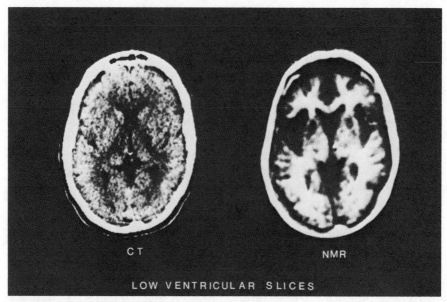

Figure 12.7 The Ventricular System Is Seen Equally Well in Both CT and NMR. In Addition, the Central White Matter, Basal Ganglia, Thalamus, and Cortex Are Better Demarcated on NMR. [Reproduced with permission from R.E. Steiner and *Lancet* (Doyle, F.H., et al., July 11, 1981, pp. 53–57).]

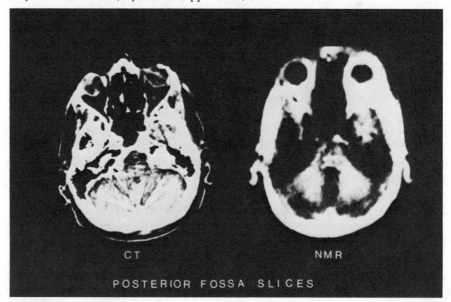

Figure 12.8 The Fourth Ventricle Is Seen Both on CT Scan and NMR. Surrounding the Fourth Ventricle, the Pons, Middle Cerebellar Peduncle, and Vermis of Cerebellum Are Seen More Clearly on NMR. [Reproduced with permission from R.E. Steiner and *Lancet* (Doyle, F.H., et al., July 11, 1981, pp. 53–57).]

NMR scanning makes use of the natural imbalance of the nucleus of certain atoms. A number of atoms of interest to the biologist (1-hydrogen, 13-carbon, 19-fluorine, and 31-phosphorus) have nuclei with properties that make them useful in NMR. Also, ions like manganese (Mn^{++}), with their free electrons, significantly change the properties of the atoms around them so that they can be used as tracers.

Fortunately, nuclear physicists make it possible for others to understand their abstract notions by simplifying them in a concrete fashion. Thus, to understand NMR, we may think of the large subatomic particles—protons and neutrons—as spinning around their own axes. As each large subatomic particle spins around its own axis, like a flywheel, momentum is created. As long as the momentum of the protons is paired, the momentum of the neutrons is paired, and secondarily, if the momentum of the protons is paired with the momentum of the neutrons, the atom does not spin. However, in atoms where these particles are not paired, the whole nucleus can be thought of as spinning. As the nucleus spins, it produces a weak magnetic field, and the nucleus becomes a magnet.

Ordinarily, the dipole (or nuclear magnet) orients itself in a random fashion. In a strong external magnetic field, however, the nuclear magnets behave like a compass and align themselves with the force of the strong magnetic field. The direction in which the nuclei point is by convention called the Z-axis. There is another important quality of nuclei for NMR. Nuclei whose axis is pulled from the vertical (off the Z-axis) will move around the vertical axis in a motion defining a cone; i.e., the nucleus precesses. This cone-shaped movement or precession is analogous to the spinning of a child's top around a point on the floor as it begins to wind down. In NMR, this precession is produced by a second magnetic field of a specific frequency—in the radio band—that matches the frequency of precession of the nuclei. The second magnetic field, or radio frequency, is applied at right angles to the Z-axis. Since each species of nuclei requires its own specific radio frequency to produce precession, a preselected type of nucleus can be observed by choosing the proper radio frequency. Because hydrogen is the most abundant nucleus that has a resonance but also requires the least powerful magnets, it is the species that has been primarily used for biological research.

So far, we have discussed how the nucleus can be perturbed. But how do we know what is happening in the nucleus? What we want to determine is where a species of nucleus is and how many nuclei are present. To do this the radio frequency, or force perpendicular to the Z-axis, is produced as a pulse so that the nucleus precesses for only a brief period of time. The nucleus absorbs the radio frequency energy causing the precession, and as the precession stops or the nucleus returns to the Z-axis, the nucleus gives off this energy.

The time it takes the nucleus to return to its previous state of equilibrium is called the relaxation time. By measuring various aspects of the relaxation time, the structure of the molecules and their environment can be determined. Refinements can be made by perturbating the normal relaxation time by adding additional radiofrequency pulses within the relaxation period.

In the future, because 31-phosphorus has good NMR properties, quantification of the brain's high-energy phosphates should be possible. Important molecules such as adenosine diphosphate (ADT) and adenosine triphosphate (ATP) will be measured. In the more distant future, nonradioactive fluorine may be tagged to tracer molecules in a manner similar to what can now be done with radioactive fluorine in the PET scanner. Unlike the PET scanner, however, NMR does not produce radiation and should be safer for use in children and in experiments where repeat studies are required.

A pioneer in brain imaging, William Oldendorf, in his elegant book titled *The Quest for an Image of Brain* (48), described the potential of NMR as follows: "The capabilities of our 'inner space' interrogation would correspond to those of our existing outer space interrogation and allow living regional chemical analysis. With these developments, NMR imaging could be to clinical *in vivo* biochemistry as radiology is to anatomy and nuclear medicine is to physiology" (p. 145).

Cortical Mapping of Electrophysiological Activity

Electroencephalographers and psychophysiologists have been measuring the brain's electrical activity since Berger's first description of the EEG (49). Researchers have made a number of attempts both to standardize quantitative techniques (50) and to devise methods for managing the enormous amounts of data available from the EEG. Several researchers have derived computer-assisted techniques for making topographical maps of EEG and event-related potentials, also called evoked potentials, usually using color as a third dimension to express intensity. These maps lend themselves to both visual inspection and statistical analysis such as significance probability mapping (51) and multivariate discriminant analysis.

These techniques use the standard international ten to twenty scalp EEG electrodes and an equal number of EEG amplifiers. The data are recorded on an FM analog tape recorder for subsequent digitalization and computer analysis.

Several studies of relevance to psychiatry have used this technique. For example, Mendelson et al. (52) found that sleep stages were not uniform across the cortex during sleep. Stage 1 sleep (very light sleep) and REM, or dreaming, sleep were the most uniformly distributed over the cortex. Delta (slow wave) power increases at the vertex in stage 1 that, with successive non-REM sleep stages, both progresses in power and enlarges radially to the intraparietal sulcus posteriorly and the superior frontal gyrus anteriorly (Figure 12.9). Thus, this measure of deep sleep falls over the head almost like a sleeping cap.

In another study, Morihisa et al. (53), using a technique with the acro-

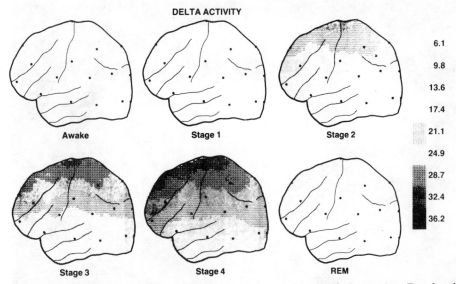

DELTA ACTIVITY

Awake   Stage 1   Stage 2

6.1
9.8
13.6
17.4
21.1
24.9
28.7
32.4
36.2

Stage 3   Stage 4   REM

Figure 12.9 Progressive Increase in Vertex Delta Activity with Increasing Depth of Sleep. (Courtesy of Wallace B. Mendelson, M.D., NIMH, and Monte Buchsbaum, M.D., University of California, Irvine.)

nym BEAM (brain electrical activity mapping), examined the resting EEG of eleven unmedicated treatment-resistant chronic schizophrenic patients and eleven normal controls. Their most striking finding was the presence of increased bifrontal delta activity (Figure 12.10). To put this in perspective, other EEG studies in schizophrenic patients, including one of Itil et al. (54), have found increased amounts of slow delta. Furthermore, preliminary studies indicate there may be decreased frontal lobe cerebral blood flow in some schizophrenic patients compared with controls (55). Also, there are several observations using PET that schizophrenic patients may have relatively lower glucose utilization in the frontal lobes (47,56). Whether or not schizophrenic patients have a frontal lobe abnormality, of course, will require considerably more investigation.

SUMMARY

It has been said that creativity is a function of ignorance of the literature. Some of the current ideas (such as enlarged cerebral ventricles in some schizophrenic patients) in biological psychiatric research have been in the literature for fifty or more years. Certainly, the finding of abnormal brain structure in schizophrenia is not new. Both the thirty-year-old notion that schizophrenia is the graveyard of neuropathologists and the mushrooming science of synaptology have, until recently, distracted most researchers from

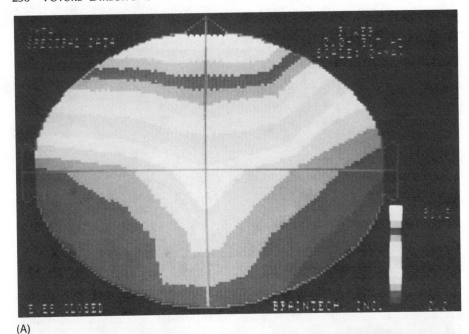

(A)

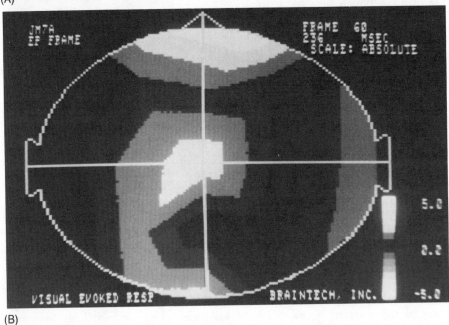

(B)

Figure 12.10 Brain Electrical Activity Maps (BEAM) of a Patient with Schizophrenia. (A) This Image Demonstrates the Topography of the Delta Range of an EEG Spectral Analysis. The Gray Scale Topography Indicates that Delta Activity is Greatest Frontally. (B) This Image Demonstrates the Topography of a Positive Wave at 236 msec from an Evoked Potential Using Light Flashes as Stimuli. (Courtesy of John Morihisa, M.D., NIMH, and Frank Duffy, M.D., Harvard University.)

examining functional anatomy of the brain in the major psychiatric disorders. With the powerful new techniques that have become available in the last few years and with the even more powerful techniques that will soon be available, psychiatric researchers will begin to examine the brain in light of old questions.

In the years ahead, we expect to see a dramatic change in psychiatric research. While synaptology has given us much more solid information on how the brain works, it has not told us the etiology of a psychiatric disorder. Treatment largely remains empirical. Ultimately, more rational treatments or, preferably, prevention will require basic understanding of the etiology of an illness. It is possible that the requisite insights will come from new techniques applied to persistent and fundamental questions.

REFERENCES

1. Jacobi, W., and Winkler, H. *Encephalographische studien an chronisch schizophrenen.* Arch. Psychiat. Nervenkr. 81:299–332, 1927.
2. Weinberger, D.R., and Wyatt, R.J. Cerebral morphology in schizophrenia: *In vivo* studies. In *Schizophrenia as a Brain Disease*, Henn, F., and Nasrallah, H., eds. London: Oxford University Press, forthcoming.
3. Johnstone, E.C.; Crow, T.J.; Frith, C.D.; Husband, J.; and Kreel, L. Cerebral ventricular size and cognitive impairment in chronic schizophrenia. *Lancet* 2:924–926, 1976.
4. Weinberger, D.R.; Wagner, R.I.; and Wyatt, R.J. Neuropathological studies of schizophrenia: A selective review. Submitted for publication.
5. Mundt, C.H.; Radii, W.; and Gluck, E. *Computerotomographische Untersuchungen der Liquorraume an chronisch schizophrenen Patienten.* Nervenarzt 51:743–748, 1980.
6. Jernigan, T.L.; Zatz, L.M.; Moses, J.A.; and Berger, P.A. Computerized measures of cerebral atrophy in schizophrenics and normal volunteers. *Arch. Gen. Psychiat.* 39:765–770, 1982.
7. Weinberger, D.R.; DeLisi, L.E.; Perman, G.P.; Targum, L.; and Wyatt, R.J. Computed tomography in schizophreniform disorder and other acute psychiatric disorders. *Arch. Gen. Psychiat.* 39:778–783, 1982.
8. Nybäck, H.; Wiesel, F.A.; Berggren, B.M.; and Hindmarsh, T. Computed tomography of the brain in patients with acute psychosis and in healthy volunteers. *Acta Psychiat. Scand.* 65:403–414, 1982.
9. Schultz, S.C.; Sinicrope, P.; Koller, M.; Kishore, P.; and Friedel, R.O. Treatment response and ventricular brain ratio in young schizophrenic patients. Presented at the annual meeting of the Society for Biological Psychiatry, Toronto, May 1982, p. 75.
10. Crow, T.J. Positive and negative schizophrenia symptoms and the role of dopamine. *Br. J. Psychiat.* 139:251–254, 1981.
11. Owen, F.; Crow, T.J.; Poulter, M.; Cross, A.; Longden, J.; and Riley, A. Increased dopamine-receptor sensitivity in schizophrenia. *Lancet* 1:223–226, 1978.
12. Wyatt, R.J.; DeLisi, L.E.; Jeste, D.V.; Kleinman, J.E.; Luchins, D.J.; Potkin, S.G.; and Weinberger, D.R. Biochemical and morphological factors in schizophrenia. In *Psychiatry, 1982 Annual Review*, Grinspoon, L., ed. Washington, D.C.: American Psychiatric Association, 1982, pp. 112–153.

13. Chouinard, G., and Jones, B.D. Evidence of brain dopamine deficiency in schizophrenia. *Can. J. Psychiat.* 24:661–667, 1979.
14. Hughlings Jackson, J. *Selected Writings*, Taylor, J., ed. London: Hodder & Stoughton, 1931.
15. Andreasen, N.C.; Smith, M.R.; Jacoby, C.G.; Dennert, J.W.; and Olsen, S.A. Ventricular enlargement in schizophrenia: Definition and prevalence. *Am. J. Psychiat.* 139:292–296, 1982.
16. Andreasen, N.C.; Olsen, S.A.; Dennert, J.W.; and Smith, M.R. Ventricular enlargement in schizophrenia: Relationship to positive and negative symptoms. *Am. J. Psychiat.* 139:297–302, 1982.
17. Takahashi, R.; Inabi, Y.; Inanga, K.; Kato, N.; Kumashiro, H.; Nishimura, T.; Okuma, T.; Otsuki, S.; Sakai, T.; Sato, T.; and Shimazono, Y. CT scanning and the investigation of schizophrenia. In *Third World Congress of Biological Psychiatry*, Jansson, B., Perris, C., and Struwe, G., eds. Amsterdam: Elsevier-North Holland, forthcoming.
18. Economo, C.F. *Encephalitis Lethargica: Its Sequelae and Treatment.* Neuman, K.O., ed. and trans. London: Oxford University Press, 1931.
19. Association for Research in Nervous and Mental Diseases. *Report on the Papers and Discussions of the Investigation on Acute Epidemic Encephalitis (Lethargic Encephalitis).* New York: Paul B. Hoeber, 1921.
20. *Diagnostic and Statistical Manual of Mental Disorders*, 2nd ed. Prepared by the Committee on nomenclature and statistics of the American Psychiatric Association. Washington, D.C.: American Psychiatric Association, 1968.
21. Klein, D.F.; Gittelman, R.; Quitkin, F.; and Rifkin, A. *Diagnosis and Drug Treatment of Psychiatric Disorders: Adults and Children.* Baltimore: Williams and Wilkins, 1980.
22. Siegfried, B., and Bures, J. Conditioning compensates the neglect due to unilateral 6-OHDA lesions of substantia nigra in rats. *Brain Res.* 167:139–155, 1979.
23. Wise, R.A. Neuroleptics and operant behavior: The anhedonia hypothesis. *Behav. Brain Sci.* 5:39–87, 1982.
24. Meltzer, H.Y.; Busch, D.; and Fang, V.S. Hormones, dopamine receptors and schizophrenia. *Psychoneuroendocrinology* 6:17–36, 1981.
25. Kleinman, J.E.; Weinberger, D.R.; Rogol, A.D.; Bigelow, L.B.; Klein, S.T.; and Wyatt, R.J. Relationships between plasma prolactin concentrations and psychopathology in chronic schizophrenia. *Arch. Gen. Psychiat.* 39:655–657, 1982.
26. Mendelson, W.B. The clock and the blue guitar: Studies of human growth hormone secretion in sleep and waking. *Int. Rev. Neurobiol.*, in press.
27. Vigneri, R.; Pezzino, V.; Squatrito, S.; Calandra, A.; and Maricchiolo, M. Sleep-associated growth hormone (GH) release in schizophrenia. *Neuroendocrinology* 14:356–361, 1974.
28. Murri, L.; Cerone, G.; Feriozzi, F.; Mencini, G.M.; and Nurzia, A. *Effectto del triptofano sull'oromone somatogropo durante il son no in schizofrenici.* Boll. Soc. Ital. Biol. Sper. 49:1490–1495, 1973.
29. Syvälahti, E., and Pekkarinen, A. Serum growth hormone levels in schizophrenic patients during sleep. *J. Neurol. Trans.* 40:221–226, 1977.
30. Ettigi, P.; Nair, N.P.V.; Lal, S.; Cervantes, P.; and Guyda, H. Effect of apomorphine on growth hormone and prolactin secretion in schizophrenic

patients, with or without oral dyskinesia, withdrawn from chronic neuroleptic therapy. *J. Neurol. Neurosurg. Psychiat.* 39:870–876, 1976.

31. Tamminga, C.A.; Smith, R.C.; Pandey, G.; Frohman, L.A.; and Davis, J.M. A neuroendocrine study of supersensitivity in tardive dyskinesia. *Arch. Gen. Psychiat.* 34:1199–1203, 1977.

32. Rotrosen, J.; Angrist, B.; Gershon, S.; Paquin, J.; Branchey, L.; Oleshansky, M.; Halpern, F.; and Sachar, E.J. Neuroendocrine effects of apomorphine: Characterization of response patterns and application to schizophrenia research. *Br. J. Psychiat.* 135:444–456, 1979.

33. Bleuler, E. *Dementia Praecox or the Group of Schizophrenias*, Zinkin, J., and Lewis, N.D.C., trans. New York: International University Press, 1950, p. 486.

34. Corsini, C.U.; Del Zompo, M.; Manconi, S.; Cranchetti, C.; Mangoni, A.; and Gessa, G.L. Sedative, hypnotic, and antipsychotic effects of low doses of apomorphine in man. *Adv. Biochem. Pharmacol.* 16:645–648, 1977.

35. Tamminga, C.A.; Schaffer, M.H.; Smith, R.C.; and Davis, J.M. Schizophrenic symptoms improve with apomorphine. *Science* 200:567–568, 1978.

36. Hollister, L.E. Experiences with dopamine agonists in depression and schizophrenia. In *Apomorphine and Other Dopaminomimetics*, Corsini, G.U., and Gessa, G.L., eds. New York: Raven Press, 1981, 2:57–64.

37. Jeste, D.V.; Zalcman, S.; Weinberger, D.R.; Bigelow, L.B.; Klinman, J.E.; Rogol, A.; Gillin, J.C.; and Wyatt, R.J. Apomorphine response and subtyping of schizophrenia. *Progress in Neuropsychopharmacology*, submitted for publication.

38. Lal, S. Clinical studies with apomorphine. In *Apomorphine and Other Dopaminomimetics*, Corsini, G.U., and Gessa, G.L., eds. New York: Raven Press, 1981, 2:1–12.

39. Weinberger, D.R.; Bigelow, L.B.; Kleinman, J.E.; Klein, S.T.; Rosenblatt, J.E.; and Wyatt, R.J. Cerebral ventricular enlargement in chronic schizophrenia: Association with poor response to treatment. *Arch. Gen. Psychiat.* 37:11–14, 1980.

40. Wyatt, R.J., and Torgow, J.S. A comparison of equivalent clinical potencies of neuroleptics as used to treat schizophrenic and affective disorders. *J. Psychiat. Res.* 13:91–98, 1976.

41. Karson, C.N.; Freed, W.J.; and Kleinman, J.E. Spontaneous eye blink rates and dopaminergic systems. *Brain*, in press.

42. Karson, C.N.; Freed, W.J.; Kleinman, J.E.; Bigelow, L.B.; and Wyatt, R.J. Neuroleptics decrease blinking in schizophrenic subjects. *Biol. Psychiat.* 16:679–682, 1981.

43. Comar, D.; Zarifian, E.; Verhas, M.; Soussaline, M.; Maziere, G.; Berger, H.; Loo, H.; Cuche, H.; Kellershohn, C.; and Deniker, P. Brain distribution and kinetics of ^{11}C-chlorpromazine in schizophrenics: Positron emission tomography studies. *Psychiat. Res.* 1:23–29, 1979.

44. Sokoloff, L.; Reivich, M.; Kennedy, C.; DesRosiers, M.H.; Patlak, C.S.; Pettigrew, K.D.; Sakurada, O.; and Shinohara, M. The (^{14}C) deoxyglucose method for the measurement of local cerebral glucose utilization: Theory, procedure, and normal values in the conscious and anesthetized albino rat. *J. Neurochem.* 28:897–916, 1977.

45. Sacks, W.; Schechter, D.C.; and Sacks, S. A difference in the in vivo cerebral production of (1-^{14}C) lactate from D-(3-^{14}C) glucose in chronic mental patients. *J. Neurosci. Res.* 6:225–236, 1981.

46. Sacks, W.; Sacks, S.; Badalamenti, A.; and Fleischer, A. A proposed method for the determination of cerebral regional intermediary glucose metabolism in humans in vivo using specifically labeled ^{11}C-glucose and positron emission transverse tomography (PETT). I. An animal model with ^{14}C-glucose and rat brain autoradiography. *J. Neurosci. Res.* 7:57–69, 1982.

47. Buchsbaum, M.S.; Ingvar, D.H.; Kessler, R.; Waters, R.N.; Cappelletti, J.; van Kammen, D.P.; King, A.C.; Johnson, J.L.; Manning, R.G.; Flynn, R.W.; Mann, L.S.; Bunney, W.E.; and Sokoloff, L. Cerebral glucography with positron emission tomography. *Arch. Gen. Psychiat.* 39:251–259, 1982.

48. Oldendorf, W.H. *The Quest for an Image of Brain.* New York: Raven Press, 1980.

49. Berger, H. *Uber das Elektrenkephalogramm des Menschen I. Arch. Psychiat. Nervenkr.* 87:527–571, 1929.

50. Roy, John E.; Karmel, B.Z.; Corning, W.C.; Easton, P.; Brown, D.; Ahn, H.; John, M.; Harmony, T.; Prichep, L.; Toro, A.; Gershon, I.; Bartlett, F.; Thatcher, R.; Kaye, H.; Valdes, P.; and Schwartz, E. Neurometrics. *Science* 196:1393–1410, 1977.

51. Duffy, F.H.; Bartrels, P.H.; and Burchfiel, J.L. Significance probability mapping: An aid in the topographic analysis of brain electrical activity. *Electroencephalogr. Clin. Neurophysiol.*, in press.

52. Mendelson, W.B.; Buchsbaum, M.S.; Duncan, W.C.; Coppola, R.; Kelso, J.; and Gillin, J.C. Topographical cortical mapping of EEG sleep stages in normal subjects. *Sleep Res.* 10:140, 1981.

53. Morihisa, J.M.; Duffy, F.H.; and Wyatt, R.J. Brain electrical activity mapping (BEAM) in schizophrenic patients. Submitted for publication.

54. Itil, T.M.; Saletu, B.; and Davis, S. EEG findings in chronic schizophrenics based on digital computer period analysis and analog power spectra. *Biol. Psychiat.* 5:1–13, 1972.

55. Ingvar, D.H., and Franzen, G. Abnormalities of cerebral blood flow distribution in patients with chronic schizophrenia. *Acta Psychiat. Scand.* 50:425–462, 1974.

56. Farkas, T.; Wolf, A.P.; and Cancro, R. The application of ^{18}F-deoxy-2-glucose and positron emission tomography in the study of psychiatric conditions. Read before the Twelfth Collegium Internationale Neuro-Psychopharmacologium Congress, Goteborg, Sweden, 1980.

Index

and eye blinking, 245
foods rich in, 37
functional excess of, 239
and schizophrenia, 55, 240–241
and tardive dyskinesia, 59, 61
Dopamine agonists
growth hormone and, 242–243
prolactin response and, 241–242
See also Amantidine; Apomorphine;
Bromocriptine
Dopamine Beta-Hydroxylase (DBH), 44
Dopamine function
and neuroleptics, 244
and prolactin, 241–242
Dopamine hypothesis of schizophrenia,
240
Dopamine receptors
positron emission tomography and,
247–248
and prolactin, 100
Doxepin, 17, 28, 29
Drug abuse, detection of, 94–95
Drug action, and psychic structures,
228–233
Drug dependence, and benzodiazepines,
10–11
Drug interactions, psychotropic, 191–202
absorption and, 193–194
blocked transport and, 196–198
changes in excretion and, 196
changes in mediator activity with,
198–199
metabolism changes and, 194–196
protein binding and, 194
Drug mediator activity, alteration of,
198–199
Drugs
altered metabolism of, 194–196
cardiac, 212–213
delerium and, 146
effects on psychotherapy of
psychoactive, 228–233
interference with absorption of,
193–194
laboratory assessment of treatment
with, 95–100
placebo effect of psychoactive, 220–221
prescribing combinations of (*see* Polypharmacy, psychotropic)
psychiatric complications of

nonpsychiatric, 207–215
use of multiple psychotropic (*see* Poly-
pharmacy, psychotropic)
See also Antidepressants;
Antihypertensive drugs;
Antipsychotic drugs; *Specific drugs*
DSM-III. *See* Diagnostic and Statistical
Manual of Mental Disorders
DST. *See* Dexamethasone suppression
test

ECT. *See* Electroconvulsive therapy
EEG
and cortical mapping, 254–255
and electroconvulsive therapy, 76,
83–84
sleep studies and, 108–109
See also Average evoked response
Ego, psychic role of, 223, 224
Ego defenses, psychoactive drugs and,
228, 229
Ego libido, scale of, 229–230
Elderly
benzodiazepines and, 11
dexamethasone suppression test and,
102
intellectual deterioration in, 159, 160
and neuroleptic dose, 99
See also Alzheimer's disease
Electroconvulsive therapy (ECT), 71–85
adverse effects of, 75–76
affective disorders and, 72–73
brain damage and, 76–77
chronic pain and, 185–186
effect on central nervous system of,
75–76
electrical stimulus of, 82–83
electrode placement in, 80–81
maintenance, 85
mechanisms of, 74
medication and anesthesia with,
79–80
memory and, 75
morbidity and mortality with, 75
number and spacing of treatments
with, 84–85
possible contraindications to, 78
premedication and, 79–80
schizophrenia and, 73
seizure and, 83–84